M000287250

LIVER TRANSPLANTATION
State of the Art

Other Related Titles from World Scientific

Living Donor Liver Transplantation
2nd Edition
by Sheung Tat Fan, William Ignace Wei, Boon Hun Yong,
Theresa Wan-Chun Hui, Alexander Chiu and Peter Wing-Ho Lee
ISBN: 978-981-4329-75-0

The First Transplant Surgeon: The Flawed Genius of
Nobel Prize Winner, Alexis Carrel
by David Hamilton
ISBN: 978-981-4699-36-5 (hardcover)
ISBN: 978-981-4699-37-2 (softcover)

Contemporary Surgical Management of Liver, Biliary Tract,
and Pancreatic Disease
edited by Dan G Blazer III, Paul C Kuo, Theodore Pappas and
Bryan M Clary
ISBN: 978-981-4293-05-1

Introduction to Organ Transplantation
2nd Edition
edited by Nadey S Hakim
ISBN: 978-1-84816-854-1

Bone Marrow Transplantation Across Major Genetic Barriers
edited by Yair Reisner and Massimo F Martelli
ISBN: 978-981-4271-26-4

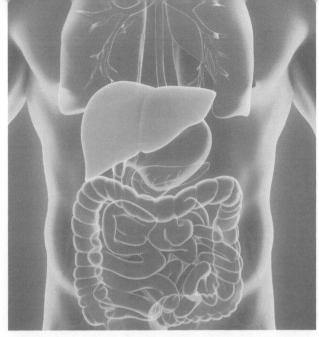

LIVER TRANSPLANTATION
State of the Art

edited by

Abhinav Humar
Amit D. Tevar
Christopher Hughes
University of Pittsburgh, USA

Wϼ **World Scientific**

NEW JERSEY · LONDON · SINGAPORE · BEIJING · SHANGHAI · HONG KONG · TAIPEI · CHENNAI · TOKYO

Published by

World Scientific Publishing Co. Pte. Ltd.

5 Toh Tuck Link, Singapore 596224

USA office: 27 Warren Street, Suite 401-402, Hackensack, NJ 07601

UK office: 57 Shelton Street, Covent Garden, London WC2H 9HE

Library of Congress Cataloging-in-Publication Data
Names: Humar, Abhinav, editor. | Tevar, Amit D., editor. |
    Hughes, Christopher (Christopher B.), editor.
Title: Liver transplantation : state of the art / [edited by] Abhinav Humar,
    Amit Tevar, Christopher Hughes.
Other titles: Liver transplantation (Humar)
Description: New Jersey : World Scientific, [2018] |
    Includes bibliographical references and index.
Identifiers: LCCN 2017048985 | ISBN 9789813234673 (hardcover : alk. paper)
Subjects: | MESH: Liver Transplantation--methods | Tissue Donors
Classification: LCC RD546 | NLM WI 770 | DDC 617.5/5620592--dc23
LC record available at https://lccn.loc.gov/2017048985

British Library Cataloguing-in-Publication Data
A catalogue record for this book is available from the British Library.

Copyright © 2018 by World Scientific Publishing Co. Pte. Ltd.

All rights reserved. This book, or parts thereof, may not be reproduced in any form or by any means, electronic or mechanical, including photocopying, recording or any information storage and retrieval system now known or to be invented, without written permission from the publisher.

For photocopying of material in this volume, please pay a copying fee through the Copyright Clearance Center, Inc., 222 Rosewood Drive, Danvers, MA 01923, USA. In this case permission to photocopy is not required from the publisher.

For any available supplementary material, please visit
http://www.worldscientific.com/worldscibooks/10.1142/10838#t=suppl

Typeset by Stallion Press
Email: enquiries@stallionpress.com

Printed in Singapore

Preface

The field of liver transplantation has undergone remarkable changes in the last 30 years. From a largely experimental field, it has rapidly gone on to become the standard form of therapy to treat patients with liver failure, whether acute or chronic in nature. While areas such as the surgical care of the liver transplant patient or their posttransplant management have become well described in the literature, several new topics are starting to be of interest to individuals who look after liver transplant patients. These include areas such as innovative surgical methods to maximize the donor pool, nonsurgical methods to expand the existing pool of additional donors, the changing face of rejection, and management of infections in the presence of new antivirals to name just a few. This book focuses on these topics along with many others in 16 chapters written by leading experts with experience in the specific area.

Abhinav Humar, Amit Tevar, Chris Hughes
Department of Surgery, University of Pittsburgh

Contents

1. Liver Transplantation for HCC: Moving Beyond Milan

Amit D. Tevar

*Division of Transplantation Surgery, University of Pittsburgh,
Pittsburgh, PA 15213, USA*

1. Introduction

Hepatocellular carcinoma (HCC) remains one of the most common causes of cancer death in the world. The incidence of HCC in regions of the world with endemic hepatitis B and C infection is substantially higher than other areas [1, 2]. Worldwide, the incidence of HCC is the sixth most common diagnosis of cancer and the third cause of cancer death, with the highest incidence rates in Asia and Africa [3]. This is likely a conservative estimate as many HCC diagnosed patients and deaths remain unreported in areas without significant medical infrastructure and reporting mechanisms. There has been a sharp rise in the incidence of HCC in the United States from 1.4/100,000 from 1976 to 1980 to 2.4/100,000 from 1991 to 1995. During this time period, there was also a significant increase in the overall mortality from HCC, with a 41% increase in the mortality rate based on review of the Surveillance, Epidemiology and End Results (SEER) database [4]. More recently in the United States despite a plateau in the overall incidence, there have been further significant increases in the liver cancer mortality from HCC, between 2007 and 2010 (Figure 1). This increase in mortality was found to be localized to African Americans, Hispanics, and white males greater than 50 years of age [5, 6].

Surveillance for HCC has been implemented for cirrhotic and fibrotic patients based on the recommendations of multiple societies. The current

1

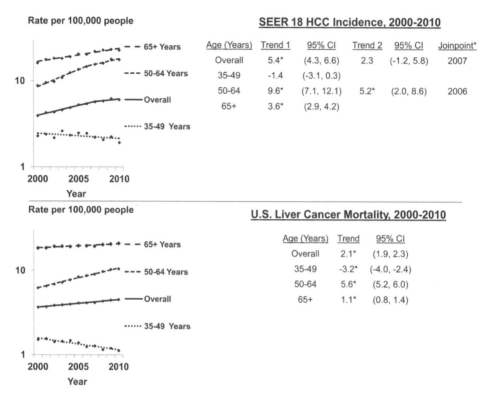

Figure 1. Age-adjusted SEER 18 HCC incidence and United States liver cancer mortality rates by age group and year, 2000–2010. CI: confidence interval; Trend: annual percent change (APC). Joinpoint regression defines when a trend changes. Up to one joinpoint is allowed in the 11-year period. (Reprinted with permission from Ref. [5]. Copyright © 2014 Nature Publishing Group.)

Note: * Slope of trend differs from zero ($p < 0.05$).

guidelines from the American Association of the Study of Liver Diseases (AASLD) suggest that ultrasound examination at an interval of 6 months for screening (Figure 2) [7]. Several studies have demonstrated the utility of a single dynamic imaging modality which demonstrates arterial uptake followed by "washout" in the venous phase to be sensitive for the noninvasive diagnosis of early and late HCC lesions [8, 9].

The staging of HCC remains a problematic and complex problem, as the disease progression and patient survival involves and changes with tumor biology, liver disease, and performance status. As a result, multiple staging algorithms have been proposed and attempted to be validated for prognosis of HCC. The first of these was introduced in 1985 as the OKUDA score and combined liver function and tumor parameters as predictor of survival [10].

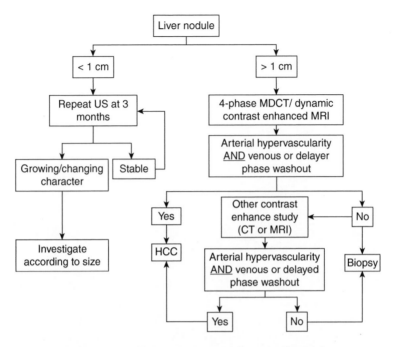

Figure 2.   AASLD Practice Guidelines on HCC [7].

The Italian Cancer of the Liver Italian Program (CLIP) reviewed 435 patients from 16 center and correlated survival based on liver function (Child–Pugh score) and tumor parameters, including portal vein thrombosis and alpha-fetoprotein (AFP) [11]. The Barcelona Clinic Liver Cancer (BCLC) system was introduced in 1999 and linked liver function, tumor parameters, and performance status into four stages: early, intermediate, advanced, and terminal [12]. The system of classification has been subsequently evaluated and validated in large Western and Asian cohorts with an enrollment of 3,892 Asian patients with HCC [13, 14]. Median survival times were noted to be 57.7 months at very early stage and 1.6 months at terminal stage. The BCLC is currently endorsed by European Associations for the Study of the Liver (EASL) and the AASLD and is used in practice throughout Europe and North America (Figure 3).

Several Asian scoring systems have also demonstrated significant survival prediction in the Asian cohort of patients. The Japan Integrated Staging (JIS) was originally released in 2003 and was based on a cohort of nearly 14,000 Japanese patients. Survival prediction is based on Japanese TNM factors (vascular invasion, number and size of lesions) and liver function (CPT Score) [16]. The survival accuracy was further increased in 2006 with

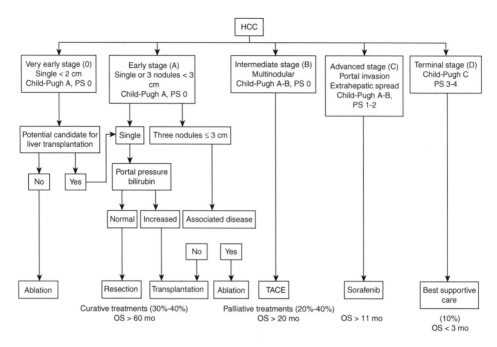

Figure 3. Barcelona Clinic Liver Cancer system. HCC: hepatocellular carcinoma; PS: performance status; TACE: transarterial chemoembolization. (Reprinted with permission from Ref. [15]. Copyright © 2016 The Author(s).)

the use of indocyanine green clearance on a review of 42,269 patients [17] and in 2008 included the addition of three separate HCC tumor markers and is now called the biomarker combined JIS (bm-JIS) [18]. Other Asian classification systems include the Hong Kong Liver Cancer (HKLC) classification system, the Taipei Integrated Scoring (TIS) system, the Advance Liver Cancer Prognostic System (ALCPS), the Chinese University Prognostic Index score, and others [19–22].

2. Liver resection and local regional therapy as curative treatment options

Surgical resection as partial hepatectomy or hemihepatectomy is an effective modality of cure of the HCC in patients with noncirrhotic liver disease without evidence of significant portal hypertension. Approximately 80% of cases of HCC are found in patients with overt cirrhosis worldwide [23]. A very small cohort of patients exist in the East and West with noncirrhotic HCC and can be treated very effectively with primary surgical resection. A meta-analysis of all Eastern and Western studies on noncirrhotic HCC patients and lesions found no demographic patient differences but found that tumors were larger, with more microvascular invasion, in noncirrhotic HCC patients and that noncirrhotic HCC patients had more advanced tumor-node-metastasis (TNM) stage disease compared to cirrhotic patients [24]. In addition, it was noted that there were differences in postoperative morbidity (8.3–55.5%) or mortality (0–6.5%) between both groups. There is an obvious degree of selection bias in the cirrhotic population that undergoes resection as the primary treatment of HCC, but the most important difference that is seen between the two groups is in the disease-free survival (DFS). The largest multicenter report comes from the Liver Cancer Study Group from Japan and their cohort of 6,785 patients treated with resection for HCC [25]. Their cohorts' 1-, 3-, 5-, and 10-year survival rates were noted to be 85, 64, 45 and 21%, respectively. The morbidity and mortality success rate in liver resection (LR) depends on optimizing patient selection and extent of resection to ensure adequate margin and adequate functional liver reserve (FLR) volume after resection. Several studies have demonstrated that adequate FLR be >20% in noncirrhotic livers and >40% in cirrhotics [26–28]. In addition, portal vein embolization is an important tool in the hypertrophy of the remnant liver to ensure adequate volume. A large multicenter study from France, USA, and China reviewing only major (more than segments) LRs for HCC demonstrated 3-, 5-, and 10-year overall survival (OS) of 54, 40, and 27% [29]. Factors predictive of poor long-term survival outcomes included AFP level >1,000 ng/mL, tumor size >5 cm, presence of major vascular invasion, presence of extrahepatic metastases, positive surgical margins, and earlier time period in which the major hepatectomy was performed [29].

Recurrence rates have been demonstrated to be the significant downside to surgical resection as there is an increased risk of *de novo* or recurrent HCC, in comparison to those patients who undergo liver replacement therapy with liver transplant(ation) (LT). Several scoring systems have been developed to predict the recurrence and OS following LR for HCC. These nomograms include the Singapore Liver Cancer Recurrence (SLICER) Score, the Surgery-Specific Cancer of the Liver Italian Program (SSCLIP) scoring system and the Memorial Sloan Kettering Cancer Center scoring system [30–32]. The scores were constructed to predict the 3- and 5-year DFS and all three identified preoperative AFP, vascular invasion and tumor size and independent predictors of successful long-term disease-free outcome. In these cohorts and other single and multi-institutional reviews, the recurrence rate after surgical resection has ranged widely [24, 33–35]. One of the largest series, collected in a prospective fashion, comes from Poon *et al.* and demonstrated 1-, 3-, 5- and 10-year DFS rates were 74, 50, 36, and 22% [33]. Predictors of poor recurrence rates were cirrhosis and number of lesions.

Local regional therapy is an interesting and selective effective modality for treatment of HCC. The experience with this modality comes from the patient in which LT or LR is contraindicated, in which case it has demonstrated prolonged OS. Several indications exist for the use of local regional therapy including as a primary treatment of HCC in those with early disease that are not candidates for LR or LT, a downstaging too for those with tumor size too large for successful transplant, and as a bridge therapy for those that may have a prolonged wait for cadaveric or live donor LT. Commonly used tumor ablative modalities include radiofrequency ablation (RFA), microwave ablation (MWA) or cryoablation. RFA is currently the more commonly used modality for ablative local regional therapy for primary HCC treatment, downstaging, and bridge therapy and works by tissue destruction with frictional heat generation from application of alternating current. The limitations of this modality, as it does require sustained heat generation to ensure tumor tissue necrosis with a margin, includes the "heat sink" effect that does occur from high-flow vasculature found within the liver providing for decreased temperature and therefore ineffective ablation [36]. This limits the use of this modality of lesions in proximity to major vasculature.

The recurrence of lesions and OS are subject to significant selection bias as larger lesions, multifocal disease, and lesions with proximity to vasculature cannot undergo RFA. One of the larger studies of outcomes of early stage HCC treated with RFA as first line therapy demonstrated cumulative local tumor progression rates of 27.0% and 36.9% at 5 and 10 years, respectively and cumulative intrahepatic distant and extrahepatic recurrence rates of 73.1% and 88.5%, and 19.1% and 38.2% at 5 and 10 years, respectively [37]. A similar multicenter Italian group comparing RFA and LR for the initial treatment of early HCC found 4-year OS rates of 74.4% in the resection group vs. 66.2% in the RFA group and 4-year cumulative HCC recurrence rates of 56% in the resection group and 57.1% in the RFA group [38]. Other groups have demonstrated similar results [37–43]. In centers that have extended waiting times for cadaveric LT, RFA has successfully been used as a modality for "bridge therapy" to ablate the main tumor to minimize the risk of tumor progress to a point at which LT is not recommended. This modality has been extensively and successfully used in the United States to avoid waiting-list dropout secondary to tumor progression [36, 44–46].

In addition to RFA, favorable responses to transarterial chemoembolization (TACE), Yttrium-90 radioembolization, and stereotactic body radiation therapy (SBRT) have been obtained and resulted in decreases in waitlist dropout [47–49]. Options for downstaging involve the use of a systematic, multidisciplinary protocol to identify patients that may be able to have tumor reduction to a criteria in which LT would be suitable [50–56]. Multiple groups have demonstrated the benefit of downstaging with various local regional therapy modalities. Several multicenter protocols have been used and the University of California, San Francisco (UCSF) group has demonstrated the use of protocolized TACE, RFA, resection, and alcohol injection used in isolation or conjunction in select patients to successfully reduce tumor burden to LT criteria and decrease waiting-list dropout [57].

3. Liver transplantation

LT remains the ideal modality for the treatment of HCC in the cirrhotic patient. The benefits stem from the oncologic and liver/portal hypertension function. There can be no greater margin for a liver lesion than removal of the entire liver and this allows for removal of not only the known HCC but also the HCC that may not be visible on imaging. Secondly, LT cures not only the liver parenchymal abnormalities of cirrhosis and fibrosis but also the portal hypertension, which plays a considerable role in the perioperative complications seen with LR for HCC in the cirrhotic population. The history of LT for HCC begins with the successful implementation of orthotopic liver transplantation by Thomas E. Starzl, MD. Unresectable HCC in the cirrhotic and noncirrhotic was one of the primary indications for LT in its onset and Iwatsuki and Starzl published in the 1980s several reports of their experience with LT for HCC [58–60]. These results demonstrated then, what is evident now — that advanced stage lesions have a higher recurrence rate and shorter survival and that patients with HCC and cirrhosis did better with LT than resection. As the early experience with LT and HCC was limited to advanced stage lesions that could not undergo LR, the survival and recurrence was expectedly poor with a recurrence rate of 43% and 5-year survival of 39.2% [60]. These dismal outcomes led the Department of Health and Human Services in 1989 to formally list HCC as a contraindication for LT [61].

It became apparent in the early 1990s, as the international experience for LT increased, that patients with cirrhosis and smaller HCC lesions had significantly improved outcomes. Several groups reported single center series with LT for HCC with excellent long-term survival and recurrence outcomes when excluding advanced stage lesions and macrovascular invasion [62–64]. In 1996, Mazzaferro and colleagues reported in the New England Journal of Medicine a sentinel study describing 48 patients undergoing LT with HCC with specific inclusion criteria for eligibility for transplantation of the presence of a tumor 5 cm or less [65] in diameter in patients with single HCC and no more than three tumor nodules, each 3 cm or less in diameter, in patients with multiple tumors [65]. The outcomes from this cohort showed an actuarial 4-year survival of 75%, with a recurrence-free survival (RFS) of 83%. When examining patients within the Milan criteria based on explant liver pathology, the 4-year OS and RFS increased to 85% and 92%, respectively [65]. The findings of successful LT for HCC lesions with the Milan criteria were quickly replicated at multiple other centers and universally adopted as the guideline for the extent of HCC and LT [66–69]. The result of the Milan criteria and predictable excellent RFS allowed LT to be the primary treatment option for this subset of selected patients.

Cadaveric liver organ allocation in the United States during this time period was based on a combination of the Child–Turcotte–Pugh (CTP) score and waiting time on the list. This allowed for patients with early referral and listing for transplant to receive cadaveric transplants very early in their disease progression, disadvantaging those with more advanced liver failure and shorter waiting times, and resulted in significant waiting-list mortality and dropout. No consideration was given at this time for HCC and as a result many patients with early HCC within the Milan criteria did not receive a potentially successful transplant as their tumor size and number enlarged while on the waiting list. In an attempt to increase appropriate allocation of a life-saving scarce, the United Network of Organ Sharing (UNOS) adopted the Model for End-Stage Liver Disease (MELD) allocation system on February 27, 2002, which is currently in use today. The system allows for an objective measure liver function and reserve and accurately predicts 3-month survival on an LT waiting list [70]. The formula is pragmatic and readily available and consists of patient's serum creatinine, bilirubin, and international normalized ratio (INR).

Several groups of end-stage liver disease (ESLD) patients are significantly disadvantaged by the MELD score, as their survival is not reflected by this formula. The HCC patient without significant liver disease progression is disadvantaged and currently patients can receive MELD Exception points.

$$\text{MELD Score} = 0.957 \times \text{Log}_e(\text{creatinine mg/dL}) + 0.378$$
$$\times \text{Log}_e(\text{bilirubin mg/dL}) + 1.120 \times \text{Log}_e(\text{INR}) + 0.643$$

MELD formula, INR: international normalized ratio

Specifically, those patients within the Milan criteria with a T2 lesion may receive extra points to allow for early allocation of cadaveric LT. This has been demonstrated to significantly reduce waiting-list mortality in the HCC population [71–75]. The most current revisions to Organ Procurement and Transplantation Network (OPTN) liver allocation policy were implemented on October 8, 2015.

The inclusion criteria for exception points include the following:

Stage T2 lesions include *any* of the following:

- One lesion greater than or equal to 2 cm and less than or equal to 5 cm in size
- Two or three lesions greater than or equal to 1 cm and less than or equal to 3 cm in size

Prior to applying for an exception, the candidate must undergo a thorough assessment that includes *all* of the following:

1. An evaluation of the number and size of tumors using a dynamic contrast enhanced computed tomography (CT) or magnetic resonance imaging (MRI)
2. A CT or MRI to rule out any extrahepatic spread or macrovascular involvement
3. A CT of the chest to rule out metastatic disease
4. An indication that the candidate is not eligible for resection
5. The candidate's AFP level

Once approved for receipt of exception points based on the above criteria, the center can reapply for additional exception points every 3 months. The patient is kept at their calculated exception for the first two extension cycles (6 months) after which the candidate is assigned a MELD/PELD score equivalent to a 35% risk of 3-month mortality — MELD of 28. For each subsequent extension (every 3m), the candidate will receive additional two points until a cap of 34 is reached [76]. Centers and patients with HCC and cirrhosis outside of Milan criteria can be listed for LT based on each individual center criteria and can receive a cadaveric organ but cannot receive exception points and must be listed on their calculated MELD score. The optimal and often only option for this subset of patients is live donor liver transplant (LDLT). As the outcomes for LT within the Milan criteria have been shown by multiple groups to have good long-term RFS, multiple other centers have proposed and demonstrated excellent survival with expansion of the Milan criteria [77–81]. The expanded criteria included increases in the number and size of tumors to adding degree of differentiation and AFP. The most well known of these comes from is the UCSF Criteria [82]. This study followed the 70 consecutive patients aver 12 years with the following criteria: solitary tumor ≤6.5 cm, or ≤3 nodules with the largest lesion ≤4.5 cm and total tumor diameter ≤8 cm — now known as the UCSF Criteria. LT was demonstrated to have a survival rate of 90% and 75.2%, at 1 and 5 years, respectively, vs. a 50% 1-year survival for patients with tumors exceeding these limits [82]. Other factors found to demonstrate statistically significant poor outcomes included AFP >1,000 ng/mL, total tumor diameter >8 cm, age ≥55 years, or evidence of poorly differentiated tumor on pathology. This study conclusively demonstrated that a carefully selected group of patients with tumor size outside of the Milan criteria could be successfully transplanted with excellent outcomes. Although the UCSF criteria did demonstrate a successful expansion of the Milan criteria, studies have demonstrated that use of the UCSF Criteria based on pretransplant radiographic assessment of HCC has limitations [83, 84]. In a review of 479 HCC patients listed for LT, only a modest number of patients (<45) were suitable for LT and were beyond Milan criteria and within UCSF [85]. In addition, those patients with pre-OLT within UCSF tumor had worse 5-year survival compared to those within Milan.

Another important staging system to predict tumor biology through size comes from the Metroticket project (Figure 4) which used the tumor characteristics of a large retrospective collective cohort of 1,112 LT patients with HCC exceeding the MC from 36 European centers in comparison to 444 patients within the Milan criteria [86]. In the group of patients with HCCs exceeding the criteria, the median size of the largest nodule was 40 mm (range 4–200) and the median number of nodules was four (1–20) and for those transplanted outside the Milan criteria, 5-year OS was 53.6% compared with 73.3% for those that met the criteria [86]. The authors were able to demonstrate increasing hazard ratios with increasing tumor number and size and created a calculator that predicted 5-year survival based on size and number of tumors (http://www.hcc-olt-metroticket.org/#calculator_pre).

Although each of these pre-LT HCC criteria have been shown to effectively predict an acceptable RFS following LT, their limitation lies in that they are using tumor size and number as a surrogate for tumor biology. This is representative surrogate in a majority HCC lesions, but the addition of actual tumor pathology significantly increases the predictive potential. An interesting study from Italy described a single-center experience in which all HCC pre-LT patients underwent lesion pathologic examination prior to listing and

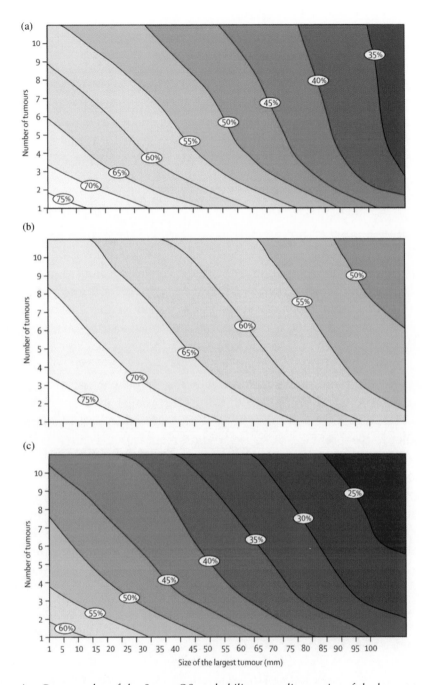

Figure 4. Contour plot of the 5-year OS probability according to size of the largest tumor, number of tumors, and presence or absence of microvascular invasion. (a) Survival estimates according to size and number, not considering microvascular invasion. Survival estimates according to absence (b) or presence (c) of microvascular invasion. Presence of microvascular invasion approximately halves the survival predicted in the absence of the same variable: absent. (Reprinted with permission from Ref. [86]. Copyright © 2009 Elsevier.)

were listed for transplant based on the lesion(s) being moderately or well differentiated and not on tumor size or number. The study showed that despite 38% of patients being outside of the Milan criteria and 42% of patients with HCC pTNM stages III and IV, the 5-year RFS was 92% [80]. The same group showed similar 1- and 3-year recurrence rates in patients outside of Milan, excluded from transplant secondary to macroscopic vascular invasion, metastases, and poorly differentiated disease at percutaneous biopsy [87]. The obvious risk of routine percutaneous biopsy of HCC lesions centers around the complication of tumor track seeding. Although the risk is difficult to quantitate secondary to underreporting, recent meta-analysis reports the median risk of seeding at 2.29% (range = 0–11%) [88, 89]. Several groups have also reported molecular analysis of tumor biopsy as an adjunct to size, number, pathologic grade, and vascular invasion as a predictor of recurrence [90, 91]. A study from the University of Pittsburgh and Mt. Sinai School of Medicine reviewed DNA extracted from tumor samples from paraffin blocks and assigned each tumor a fractional allelic imbalance (FAI) rate index, defined as the number of mutated microsatellite markers divided by the total number of informative markers (out of a possible total of nine markers utilized). Patients transplanted outside of the UCSF criteria had an overall 5-year tumor-free survival of 26.7%, but those patients outside of UCSF criteria with FAI <20% and no macrovascular invasion had a 5-year tumor-free survival rate of 62.5% [91]. In addition to poorly differentiated pathology, the presence of micro and/or macrovascular invasion seen on explanted tissue in both LT and surgical resection of HCC has been clearly demonstrated to be an independent risk factor for poor RFS [66, 92–96].

Biomarkers also serve as important signs of advanced tumor biology, specifically AFP. Pre-LT levels of AFP and progression of AFP levels have been validated to predict poor survival, early recurrence, and poor histologic features of HCC [97–104]. Progression of AFP >15 *ng*/L per month was demonstrated in a European cohort of 153 patients to have significant decrease in OS and RFS vs. those patients without progression (OS 54% vs. 77%; RFS 47% vs. 74%) [97]. This progression of AFP slope of >15 ng/mL/ month was also confirmed in patients who underwent LRT and LT from a six-center European study as an independent predictor of HCC recurrence and patient death in patients within and beyond the Milan criteria [99]. In those patients within the Milan criteria undergoing LT, AFP >1,000 ng/mL was found to be an independent predictor of HCC recurrence. It was also validated to be the best pretransplant variable for prediction of vascular invasion with 1- and 5-year rates of survival without recurrence were 90% and 52.7%, respectively, for patients with an AFP level >1,000 ng/mL and

95% and 80.3%, respectively, for patients with an AFP level ≤1,000 ng/mL [100]. The AFP level >1,000 ng/mL cutoff was found to have excluded 4.7% of patients and resulted in a 20% reduction in HCC recurrence [100]. Several other biomarkers which have shown promise as predictors of HCC recurrence in LT include Lens culinaris agglutinin-reactive alpha-fetoprotein (AFP-L3), and des-gamma-carboxyprothrombin (DCP) [102, 105–107]. A cohort of 313 patients showed that all three biomarkers (AFP, AFP-L3, and DCP) were predictors or HCC recurrence and that combination of AFP >250 ng/mL and DCP >7.5 ng/mL nearly doubles the hazard ratio for recurrence to 5.2 [102].

LDLT continues to be an important tool in the management of the ESLD patient with HCC. It is obviously the only option for ESLD HCC in regions of the world that do not offer deceased donor liver transplant (DDLT). In regions of the world in which a majority of LT is DDLT, it is potentially an underutilized option. The major advantage to LDLT is the elective nature of the LT, which allows HCC patients with a potentially long waiting time to undergo curative LT prior to HCC progression and waiting-list dropout. Recent dropout rates for HCC progression in the United States vary between regions and can be as high as 17% due specifically to HCC progression; and in centers actively listing HCC patients beyond Milan criteria, as high as 28% [47, 108]. A second benefit is the overall impact on the DDLT donor pool as LT seen with LDLT actually does not utilize the DDLT donor pool and therefore decreases waiting time for other ESLD patients on the list that may be listed for other conditions or not have an available or suitable donor. Lastly, the reduced ischemic times and ability to accurately predict size discrepancies allow for LDLT patients to have immediate graft function and excellent graft function in the hands of experienced centers. The downside is the obvious risk or morbidity and mortality to the donor undergoing hepatectomy.

Several multicenter reports have demonstrated interestingly worse recurrence outcomes for LDLT vs. DDLT. The report of nine centers participating in the American Adult-to-Adult Living Donor Liver Transplantation Cohort Study (A2ALL) study found shorter time from listing to transplant (mean 160 vs. 469 days, $p < 0.0001$) and a higher rate of HCC recurrence within 3 years than DDLT recipients (29% vs. 0%, $p = 0.002$) [109]. A Hong Kong experience noted similar rates of recurrence in their LDLT group with a cumulative 5-year recurrence rate of 29% in the LDLT group and 0% in the DDLT group ($p = 0.029$) [110]. There are other conflicting reports about the increased recurrence noted in the LDLT HCC population. A meta-analysis from 2013 found that the combined hazard ratio was 1.59

(95% CI: 1.02–2.49; I(2) = 50.07%) for DFS after LDLT vs. DDLT for HCC [111]. This experience has been shown to be demonstrative of the selection bias for LDLT in more malignant lesions and the benefit of DDLT waiting time in predicting advanced tumor biology with faster progression and dropout of lesions that may have more malignant tumor biology. Regardless, the improved waiting time for carefully selected patients with lesions that will likely grow outside of transplantable size and number does outweigh the risk of recurrence in carefully selected patients.

The field of LT for HCC has evolved considerably from the first series of transplants for unresectable HCC by Dr. Thomas E. Starzl to Mazaferro's description of the excellent outcomes for 48 patients defining the Milan criteria and resulting in the universal acceptance of LT as the preferred treatment option for cirrhotic patients with HCC. Tremendous advances have been made not only in the screening and early detection but also in pretransplant staging and local regional therapy as a form of definitive treatment and as a bridge to successful transplant. The metric for success has been long-term RFS of patients undergoing LT. Tumor biology and the prediction of this remains paramount to the identifying lesions that will have successful long-term outcomes. Although the initial Milan criteria presented in 1996 has withstood the test of time and multiple groups validating this conservative measure of tumor biology over the past 20 years, it has become clear that select patients beyond this criteria can also have excellent RFS.

The pretransplant multidisciplinary patient selection process is the first and most important step in the process, leading to excellent LT outcomes. This process should involve thorough involvement of specific institutional experts that are able to lend their specialized field's insight into the candidacy of these complex patients. This group should include, but not be limited to LT and hepatobiliary surgery, hepatology, oncology, interventional radiology, abdominal imaging radiology, and the transplant team. The candidate and their HCC should not be viewed and labeled in a binary fashion as inside or outside a familiar and unequivocal set of criteria from a singular snapshot of their lesion. Instead, they should be evaluated as patients with two progressive, dynamic disease processes (cirrhosis and HCC) with different rates of progression. A multimodal approach should be used to determine and predict their tumor biology. This should be done not only with classification of patients into a criteria but also with other radiologic, pathologic, and biomarker tools that may aid in the identification of tumors that are beyond the Milan criteria that have favorable biology. Some of these tools include pretransplant biopsy to identify tumor differentiation which may be used in conjunction with FAI and tumor markers AFP, AFP-L3, and DCP to supplement their predictive effectiveness. One of the most important predictors of tumor biology remains it growth in size and/or number or the increase of serum tumor markers over time. This becomes an important diagnostic tool and crucial aspect of waiting-list management as a patient without suitable live donor candidates may have an extended waiting time prior to LT. Locoregional therapy is an important tool not only as a bridge to transplant but also as a downstaging tool for lesions outside of criteria. Closely following response to bridge and downstage interventions will allow for further assessment of tumor biology and for centers to make decisions about allocation of DDLT or LDLT organs. The exact locoregional therapy should be based on the institutional expertise and experience and most commonly involves RFA, selective internal radiation therapy (SIRT), or TACE. Key components to success involve the development and implementation of an institutional protocol for locoregional bridge and downstaging, with specific and clearly stated cutoffs for intervention, surveillance imaging, and biomarker timeframe. Finally, in the pretransplant period, the transplant team must ensure that all treatment options in concordance with the regional allocation regulation and live donor options are thoroughly, systematically, and quickly vetted. This involves the rapid identification and evaluation of potential live donors as the bridge and downstaging algorithm will be potentially avoided. In addition, those patients undergoing LDLT outside of Milan criteria will benefit from further exploration of the lesion's tumor biology, as growth of lesions, response to locoregional therapy, and progression of tumor markers will no longer provide additional information. Posttransplant adherence to a rigorous surveillance system will allow for the early diagnosis and treatment of recurrence. The successful use of LT for the management of this complex disease relies on the careful and thoughtful assessment of each patient's tumor biology, cirrhosis progression, and live donor or cadaveric donor organ options and with this, select patients with favor biology outside of the Milan criteria can undergo LT with excellent long-term RFS.

References

1. Bruix J, Reig M, and Sherman M. Evidence-based diagnosis, staging, and treatment of patients with hepatocellular carcinoma. *Gastroenterology* 2016;150(4):835–53.
2. Perz JF, *et al.* The contributions of hepatitis B virus and hepatitis C virus infections to cirrhosis and primary liver cancer worldwide. *J Hepatol* 2006;45(4):529–38.

3. Jemal A, *et al.* Global patterns of cancer incidence and mortality rates and trends. *Cancer Epidemiol Biomark Prev* 2010;19(8):1893–907.

4. El-Serag HB and Mason AC. Rising incidence of hepatocellular carcinoma in the United States. *N Engl J Med* 1999;340(10)745–50.

5. Altekruse SF, *et al.* Changing hepatocellular carcinoma incidence and liver cancer mortality rates in the United States. *Am J Gastroenterol* 2014;109(4) 542–53. doi: 10.1038/ajg.2014.11.

6. Ha J, *et al.* Race/ethnicity-specific disparities in cancer incidence, burden of disease, and overall survival among patients with hepatocellular carcinoma in the United States. *Cancer* 2016;122(16)2512–23.

7. Bruix J and Sherman M. Management of hepatocellular carcinoma: an update. *Hepatology* 2011;53(3):1020–2.

8. Forner A, *et al.* Diagnosis of hepatic nodules 20 mm or smaller in cirrhosis: prospective validation of the noninvasive diagnostic criteria for hepatocellular carcinoma. *Hepatology* 2008;47(1):97–104.

9. Sangiovanni A, *et al.* The diagnostic and economic impact of contrast imaging techniques in the diagnosis of small hepatocellular carcinoma in cirrhosis. *Gut* 2010;59(5):638–44.

10. Okuda K, *et al.* Natural history of hepatocellular carcinoma and prognosis in relation to treatment. Study of 850 patients. *Cancer* 1985;56(4):918–28.

11. Llovet JM and Bruix J. Prospective validation of the Cancer of the Liver Italian Program (CLIP) score: a new prognostic system for patients with cirrhosis and hepatocellular carcinoma. *Hepatology* 2000;32(3):679–80.

12. Llovet JM, Bru C, and Bruix J. Prognosis of hepatocellular carcinoma: the BCLC staging classification. *Semin Liver Dis* 1999;19(3):329–38.

13. Marrero JA, *et al.* Prognosis of hepatocellular carcinoma: comparison of 7 staging systems in an American cohort. *Hepatology* 2005;41(4):707–16.

14. Wang JH, *et al.* The efficacy of treatment schedules according to Barcelona Clinic Liver Cancer staging for hepatocellular carcinoma—survival analysis of 3892 patients. *Eur J Cancer* 2008;44(7):1000–6.

15. Adhoute X, *et al.* Usefulness of staging systems and prognostic scores for hepatocellular carcinoma treatments. *World J Hepatol* 2016;8(17):703–15. doi: 10.4254/wjh.v8.i17.703.

16. Kudo M, Chung H, and Osaki Y. Prognostic staging system for hepatocellular carcinoma (CLIP score): its value and limitations, and a proposal for a new staging system, the Japan Integrated Staging Score (JIS score). *J Gastroenterol* 2003;38(3):207–15.

17. Ikai I, *et al.* A modified Japan Integrated Stage score for prognostic assessment in patients with hepatocellular carcinoma. *J Gastroenterol* 2006;41(9):884–92.

18. Kitai S, *et al.* A new prognostic staging system for hepatocellular carcinoma: value of the biomarker combined Japan integrated staging score. *Intervirology* 2008;51(Suppl 1):86–94.

19. Hsu CY, *et al.* A new prognostic model for hepatocellular carcinoma based on total tumor volume: the Taipei Integrated Scoring System. *J Hepatol* 2010;53(1):108–17.

20. Yau T, *et al.* Development of Hong Kong Liver Cancer staging system with treatment stratification for patients with hepatocellular carcinoma. *Gastroenterology* 2014;146(7):1691–700.e3.

21. Yau T, *et al.* A new prognostic score system in patients with advanced hepatocellular carcinoma not amendable to locoregional therapy: implication for patient selection in systemic therapy trials. *Cancer* 2008;113(10):2742–51.

22. Leung TW, *et al.* Construction of the Chinese University Prognostic Index for hepatocellular carcinoma and comparison with the TNM staging system, the Okuda staging system, and the Cancer of the Liver Italian Program staging system: a study based on 926 patients. *Cancer* 2002;94(6)1760–9.

23. Fattovich G, *et al.* Hepatocellular carcinoma in cirrhosis: incidence and risk factors. *Gastroenterology* 2004;127(5):S35–50.

24. Zhou YM, *et al.* Outcomes of hepatectomy for noncirrhotic hepatocellular carcinoma: a systematic review. *Surg Oncol* 2014;23(4):236–42.

25. Ikai I, *et al.* Report of the 15th follow-up survey of primary liver cancer. *Hepatol Res* 2004;28(1):21–29.

26. Kubota K, *et al.* Measurement of liver volume and hepatic functional reserve as a guide to decision-making in resectional surgery for hepatic tumors. *Hepatology* 1997;26(5)1176–81.

27. Zorzi D, *et al.* Chemotherapy-associated hepatotoxicity and surgery for colorectal liver metastases. *Br J Surg* 2007;94(3):274–86.

28. Azoulay D, *et al.* Percutaneous portal vein embolization increases the feasibility and safety of major liver resection for hepatocellular carcinoma in injured liver. *Ann Surg* 2000;232(5):665–72.

29. Andreou A, *et al.* Improved long-term survival after major resection for hepatocellular carcinoma: a multicenter analysis based on a new definition of major hepatectomy. *J Gastrointest Surg* 2013;17(1):66–77 (discussion p.77).

30. Cho CS, *et al.* A novel prognostic nomogram is more accurate than conventional staging systems for predicting survival after resection of hepatocellular carcinoma. *J Am Coll Surg* 2008;206(2):281–91.

31. Ang SF, *et al.* The Singapore Liver Cancer Recurrence (SLICER) Score for relapse prediction in patients with surgically resected hepatocellular carcinoma. *PLoS ONE* 2015;10(4):e0118658.

32. Huang S, *et al.* Establishment and validation of SSCLIP Scoring System to estimate survival in hepatocellular carcinoma patients who received curative liver resection. *PLoS ONE* 2015;10(6):e0129000.

33. Poon RT, *et al.* Long-term survival and pattern of recurrence after resection of small hepatocellular carcinoma in patients with preserved liver function: implications for a strategy of salvage transplantation. *Ann Surg* 2002;235(3):373–82.

34. Kanematsu T, *et al.* A 16-year experience in performing hepatic resection in 303 patients with hepatocellular carcinoma: 1985-2000. *Surgery* 2002;131 (1 Suppl):S153–8.

35. Belghiti J, *et al.* Resection of hepatocellular carcinoma: a European experience on 328 cases. *Hepatogastroenterology* 2002;49(43):41–6.

36. Jacobs A. Radiofrequency ablation for liver cancer. *Radiol Technol* 2015;86(6):645–64 (quiz 665–8).

37. Kim YS, *et al.* Ten-year outcomes of percutaneous radiofrequency ablation as first-line therapy of early hepatocellular carcinoma: analysis of prognostic factors. *J Hepatol* 2013;58(1):89–97.

38. Pompili M, *et al.* Long-term effectiveness of resection and radiofrequency ablation for single hepatocellular carcinoma ≤3 cm. Results of a multicenter Italian survey. *J Hepatol* 2013;59(1):89–97.

39. Facciorusso A, *et al.* Conditional survival analysis of hepatocellular carcinoma patients treated with radiofrequency ablation. *Hepatol Res* 2015;45(10): E62–72.

40. Livraghi T, *et al.* Sustained complete response and complications rates after radiofrequency ablation of very early hepatocellular carcinoma in cirrhosis: is resection still the treatment of choice? *Hepatology* 2008;47(1):82–9.

41. Lencioni R, *et al.* Early-stage hepatocellular carcinoma in patients with cirrhosis: long-term results of percutaneous image-guided radiofrequency ablation. *Radiology* 2005;234(3):961–7.

42. Lu DS, *et al.* Percutaneous radiofrequency ablation of hepatocellular carcinoma as a bridge to liver transplantation. *Hepatology* 2005;41(5): 1130–7.

43. Pompili M, *et al.* Percutaneous ablation procedures in cirrhotic patients with hepatocellular carcinoma submitted to liver transplantation: assessment of efficacy at explant analysis and of safety for tumor recurrence. *Liver Transpl* 2005;11(9):1117–26.

44. Vasnani R, *et al.* Radiofrequency and microwave ablation in combination with transarterial chemoembolization induce equivalent histopathologic coagulation necrosis in hepatocellular carcinoma patients bridged to liver transplantation. *Hepatobiliary Surg Nutr* 2016;5(3):225–33.

45. Lee MW, Raman SS, and Asvadi NH. Radiofrequency ablation of hepatocellular carcinoma as bridge therapy to liver transplantation: a 10-year intention-to-treat analysis. *Hepatology* 2017;65(6):1979–90.

46. Bharat A, *et al.* Pre-liver transplantation locoregional adjuvant therapy for hepatocellular carcinoma as a strategy to improve longterm survival. *J Am Coll Surg* 2006;203(4):411–20.

47. Sheth RA, *et al.* Role of locoregional therapy and predictors for dropout in patients with hepatocellular carcinoma listed for liver transplantation. *J Vasc Interv Radiol* 2015;26(12):1761–8 (quiz p. 1768).

48. Hodavance MS, *et al.* Effectiveness of transarterial embolization of hepatocellular carcinoma as a bridge to transplantation. *J Vasc Interv Radiol* 2016;27(1):39–45.
49. Siripongsakun S, *et al.* Loco-regional therapies for patients with hepatocellular carcinoma awaiting liver transplantation: selecting an optimal therapy. *Hepatology* 2016;6(2):306–13.
50. Kulik LM, *et al.* Yttrium-90 microspheres (TheraSphere) treatment of unresectable hepatocellular carcinoma: downstaging to resection, RFA and bridge to transplantation. *J Surg Oncol* 2006;94(7):572–86.
51. Otto G, *et al.* Response to transarterial chemoembolization as a biological selection criterion for liver transplantation in hepatocellular carcinoma. *Liver Transpl* 2006;12(8):1260–7.
52. Vagefi, PA and Hirose R. Downstaging of hepatocellular carcinoma prior to liver transplant: is there a role for adjuvant sorafenib in locoregional therapy? *J Gastrointest Cancer* 2010;41(4):217–20.
53. Gordon-Weeks AN, *et al.* Systematic review of outcome of downstaging hepatocellular cancer before liver transplantation in patients outside the Milan criteria. *Br J Surg* 2011;98(9):1201–8.
54. Green TJ, *et al.* Downstaging disease in patients with hepatocellular carcinoma outside of Milan criteria: strategies using drug-eluting bead chemoembolization. *J Vasc Interv Radiol* 2013;24(11):1613–22.
55. Lei J, Wang W, and Yan L. Downstaging advanced hepatocellular carcinoma to the milan criteria may provide a comparable outcome to conventional Milan criteria. *J Gastrointest Surg* 2013;17(8):1440–6.
56. Lei J, Yan L, and Wang W. Comparison of the outcomes of patients who underwent deceased-donor or living-donor liver transplantation after successful downstaging therapy. *Eur J Gastroenterol Hepatol* 2013;25(11):1340–6.
57. Yao FY, *et al.* A prospective study on downstaging of hepatocellular carcinoma prior to liver transplantation. *Liver Transpl* 2005;11(12):1505–14.
58. Iwatsuki, S, *et al.* Hepatic resection versus transplantation for hepatocellular carcinoma. *Ann Surg* 1991;214(3):221–8 (discussion 228–9).
59. Iwatsuki S and Starzl TE. Role of liver transplantation in the treatment of hepatocellular carcinoma. *Semin Surg Oncol* 1993;9(4):337–40.
60. Iwatsuki S, *et al.* Role of liver transplantation in cancer therapy. *Ann Surg* 1985;202(4):401–7.
61. Fung J and Marsh W. The quandary over liver transplantation for hepatocellular carcinoma: the greater sin? *Liver Transpl* 2002;8(9):775–7.
62. Bismuth H, *et al.* Liver resection versus transplantation for hepatocellular carcinoma in cirrhotic patients. *Ann Surg* 1993;218(2):145–51.
63. Llovet JM, *et al.* Liver transplantation for small hepatocellular carcinoma: the tumor-node-metastasis classification does not have prognostic power. *Hepatology* 1998;27(6):1572–7.

64. Romani F, *et al*. The role of transplantation in small hepatocellular carcinoma complicating cirrhosis of the liver. *J Am Coll Surg* 1994;178(4):379–84.
65. Mazzaferro V, *et al*. Liver transplantation for the treatment of small hepatocellular carcinomas in patients with cirrhosis. *N Engl J Med* 1996;334(11):693–9.
66. Jonas S, *et al*. Vascular invasion and histopathologic grading determine outcome after liver transplantation for hepatocellular carcinoma in cirrhosis. *Hepatology* 2001;33(5):1080–6.
67. De Giorgio M, *et al*. Prediction of progression-free survival in patients presenting with hepatocellular carcinoma within the Milan criteria. *Liver Transpl* 2010;16(4):503–12.
68. Mazzaferro V, *et al*. Milan criteria in liver transplantation for hepatocellular carcinoma: an evidence-based analysis of 15 years of experience. *Liver Transpl* 2011;17(Suppl 2):S44–57.
69. Herrero JI, *et al*. Liver transplantation in patients with hepatocellular carcinoma across Milan criteria. *Liver Transpl* 2008;14(3):272–8.
70. Wiesner RH, *et al*. MELD and PELD: application of survival models to liver allocation. *Liver Transpl* 2001;7(7):567–80.
71. Sharma P, *et al*. Liver transplantation for hepatocellular carcinoma: the MELD impact. *Liver Transpl* 2004;10(1):36–41.
72. Wiesner RH, Freeman RB, and Mulligan DC. Liver transplantation for hepatocellular cancer: the impact of the MELD allocation policy. *Gastroenterology* 2004;127(5 Suppl 1):S261–7.
73. Leung JY, *et al*. Liver transplantation outcomes for early-stage hepatocellular carcinoma: results of a multicenter study. *Liver Transpl* 2004;10(11):1343–54.
74. Zavaglia C, *et al*. Predictors of long-term survival after liver transplantation for hepatocellular carcinoma. *Am J Gastroenterol* 2005;100(12):2708–16.
75. Island ER, *et al*. Twenty-year experience with liver transplantation for hepatocellular carcinoma. *Arch Surg* 2005;140(4):353–8.
76. Policy 9: Allocation of Livers and Liver-Intestines. Organ Procurement and Transplantation Network (OPTN) Policies. Effective September 12, 2017. https://optn.transplant.hrsa.gov/media/1200/optn_policies.pdf#nameddest=Policy_09. Accessed June 29, 2017.
77. Zheng SS, *et al*. Liver transplantation for hepatocellular carcinoma: Hangzhou experiences. *Transplantation* 2008;85(12):1726–32.
78. Onaca N, *et al*. Expanded criteria for liver transplantation in patients with hepatocellular carcinoma: a report from the International Registry of Hepatic Tumors in Liver Transplantation. *Liver Transpl* 2007;13(3):391–9.
79. Ito T, *et al*. Expansion of selection criteria for patients with hepatocellular carcinoma in living donor liver transplantation. *Liver Transpl* 2007;13(12):1637–44.

80. Cillo U, *et al.* Liver transplantation for the treatment of moderately or well-differentiated hepatocellular carcinoma. *Ann Surg* 2004;239(2):150–9.

81. Poon RT, *et al.* Difference in tumor invasiveness in cirrhotic patients with hepatocellular carcinoma fulfilling the Milan criteria treated by resection and transplantation: impact on long-term survival. *Ann Surg* 2007;245(1):51–8.

82. Yao FY, *et al.* Liver transplantation for hepatocellular carcinoma: expansion of the tumor size limits does not adversely impact survival. *Hepatology* 2001;33(6):1394–403.

83. Yao FY, *et al.* Liver transplantation for hepatocellular carcinoma: validation of the UCSF-expanded criteria based on preoperative imaging. *Am J Transplant* 2007;7(11):2587–96.

84. Mazzaferro V, *et al.* Liver transplantation for hepatocellular carcinoma. *Ann Surg Oncol* 2008;15(4):1001–7.

85. Decaens T, *et al.* Impact of UCSF criteria according to pre- and post-OLT tumor features: analysis of 479 patients listed for HCC with a short waiting time. *Liver Transpl* 2006;12(12):1761–9.

86. Mazzaferro V, *et al.* Predicting survival after liver transplantation in patients with hepatocellular carcinoma beyond the Milan criteria: a retrospective, exploratory analysis. *Lancet Oncol* 2009;10(1):35–43.

87. Cillo U, *et al.* Intention-to-treat analysis of liver transplantation in selected, aggressively treated HCC patients exceeding the Milan criteria. *Am J Transplant* 2007;7(4):972–81.

88. Stigliano R, *et al.* Seeding following percutaneous diagnostic and therapeutic approaches for hepatocellular carcinoma. What is the risk and the outcome? Seeding risk for percutaneous approach of HCC. *Cancer Treat Rev* 2007;33(5):437–47.

89. Perkins JD. Seeding risk following percutaneous approach to hepatocellular carcinoma. *Liver Transpl* 2007;13(11):1603.

90. Schmidt C and Marsh JW. Molecular signature for HCC: role in predicting outcomes after liver transplant and selection for potential adjuvant treatment. *Curr Opin Organ Transplant* 2010;15(3):277–82.

91. Dvorchik I, *et al.* Fractional allelic imbalance could allow for the development of an equitable transplant selection policy for patients with hepatocellular carcinoma. *Liver Transpl* 2008;14(4):443–50.

92. Zendejas-Ruiz I, *et al.* Recurrent hepatocellular carcinoma in liver transplant recipients with hepatitis C. *J Gastrointest Cancer* 2012;43(2):229–35.

93. Wai CT, *et al.* Younger age and presence of macrovascular invasion were independent significant factors associated with poor disease-free survival in hepatocellular carcinoma patients undergoing living donor liver transplantation. *Transplant Proc* 2012;44(2):516–9.

94. Hu Z, *et al.* Survival in liver transplant recipients with hepatitis B- or hepatitis C-associated hepatocellular carcinoma: the Chinese experience from 1999 to 2010. *PLoS ONE* 2013;8(4):e61620.

95. Faber W, *et al*. Implication of microscopic and macroscopic vascular invasion for liver resection in patients with hepatocellular carcinoma. *Dig Surg* 2014;31(3):204–9.

96. Barreto SG, *et al*. Cirrhosis and microvascular invasion predict outcomes in hepatocellular carcinoma. *ANZ J Surg* 2013;83(5):331–5.

97. Vibert E, *et al*. Progression of alphafetoprotein before liver transplantation for hepatocellular carcinoma in cirrhotic patients: a critical factor. *Am J Transplant* 2010;10(1):129–37.

98. Sharma P, *et al*. Incidence and risk factors of hepatocellular carcinoma recurrence after liver transplantation in the MELD era. *Dig Dis Sci* 2012; 57(3):806–12.

99. Lai Q, *et al*. Alpha-fetoprotein and modified response evaluation criteria in solid tumors progression after locoregional therapy as predictors of hepatocellular cancer recurrence and death after transplantation. *Liver Transpl* 2013;19(10):1108–18.

100. Hameed B, *et al*. Alpha-fetoprotein level > 1000 ng/mL as an exclusion criterion for liver transplantation in patients with hepatocellular carcinoma meeting the Milan criteria. *Liver Transpl* 2014;20(8):945–51.

101. Jiang L, *et al*. Predictive value of alpha-fetoprotein in the survival of living donor liver transplantation recipients for hepatocellular carcinoma. *Hepatogastroenterology* 2014;61(131):747–51.

102. Chaiteerakij R, *et al*. Combinations of biomarkers and Milan criteria for predicting hepatocellular carcinoma recurrence after liver transplantation. *Liver Transpl* 2015;21(5):599–606.

103. Lai Q, *et al*. Delta-slope of alpha-fetoprotein improves the ability to select liver transplant patients with hepatocellular cancer. *HPB* 2015;17(12): 1085–95.

104. Hong G, *et al*. Alpha-fetoprotein and (18)F-FDG positron emission tomography predict tumor recurrence better than Milan criteria in living donor liver transplantation. *J Hepatol* 2016;64(4):852–9.

105. Inagaki Y, *et al*., Des-gamma-carboxyprothrombin in patients with hepatocellular carcinoma and liver cirrhosis. *J Dig Dis* 2011;12(6):481–8.

106. Ueshima K, *et al*. Des-gamma-carboxyprothrombin may be a promising biomarker to determine the therapeutic efficacy of sorafenib for hepatocellular carcinoma. *Dig Dis* 2011;29(3):321–5.

107. Cheng J, *et al*. Prognostic role of pre-treatment serum AFP-L3% in hepatocellular carcinoma: systematic review and meta-analysis. *PLoS ONE* 2014; 9(1):e87011.

108. Aravinthan AD, *et al*. Liver transplantation is a preferable alternative to palliative therapy for selected patients with advanced hepatocellular carcinoma. *Ann Surg Oncol* 2017;24(7):1843–51.

109. Fisher RA, *et al.* Hepatocellular carcinoma recurrence and death following living and deceased donor liver transplantation. *Am J Transplant* 2007;7(6):1601–8.
110. Lo CM, *et al.* Living donor versus deceased donor liver transplantation for early irresectable hepatocellular carcinoma. *Br J Surg* 2007;94(1):78–86.
111. Grant RC, *et al.* Living vs. deceased donor liver transplantation for hepatocellular carcinoma: a systematic review and meta-analysis. *Clin Transplant*, 2013, 27(1):140–7.

2. Liver Transplantation for Non-HCC Malignancies: Cholangiocarcinoma, Neuroendocrine Tumors, HEHE, and Colorectal Metastases

Daniel Zamora-Valdes* and Julie K. Heimbach*,†

*Division of Transplantation Surgery and the William J.
von Liebig Transplant Center, Mayo Clinic, 200 First Street,
Rochester, MN 55905, USA
†Liver Transplantation Program, Mayo Clinic, 200 First Street,
Rochester, MN 55905, USA

1. Introduction

The surgical management of hepatobiliary tumors is limited by the need to preserve an adequate liver volume, biliary drainage, vascular inflow/outflow, and by underlying parenchymal disease as is present in the vast majority of patients with hepatocellular carcinoma (HCC). Liver transplant(ation) (LT) addresses all of these issues simultaneously but is limited by organ availability. The identification of patients with favorable outcome after transplantation has evolved the field to a point where LT plays an essential role in the multidisciplinary management of HCC and hilar cholangiocarcinoma (CCA). HCC is reviewed extensively in Chapter 1. This chapter focuses on CCA, intrahepatic cholangiocarcinoma (ICC), hepatic epithelioid hemangioendothelioma (HEHE), and secondary hepatic malignancies, including neuroendocrine tumors (NETs) and colorectal carcinoma/cancer (CRC).

As in any other operative oncological therapy, the outcomes of LT for malignant disease are assessed through perioperative morbidity and mortality, disease-free survival (DFS), and overall survival (OS). Perioperative morbidity and mortality among LT recipients with CCA deserves a separate discussion, as neoadjuvant radiation (neo-RT) and surgical staging before LT are associated with increased morbidity. Outcomes are determined by many factors in addition to local and/or regional recurrence as well as distant metastases.

In order to justify the use of a scarce resource, outcomes for patients who undergo LT for hepatic malignancies must be similar to that observed among patients with chronic liver disease without cancer. The use of living donor livers for patients with unresectable hepatobiliary malignancies outside standard criteria is controversial due to the underlying risk to the donor; however, some centers outside the USA do consider LT in these patients with variable results [1–6].

2. Hilar cholangiocarcinoma (CCA)

Early experiences with LT on patients with known or incidental hilar CCA were dismal due to high rates of disease recurrence and poor survival [7, 8]. Results were disappointing even among patients with primary sclerosing cholangitis (PSC) and incidental, early-stage disease; thus, LT alone for patients with hilar CCA is contraindicated [9, 10].

Patients with early-stage hilar CCA often have no or nonspecific symptoms such as weight loss, abdominal pain, night sweats, fatigue, emesis, vomiting, loss of appetite, and pruritus. Jaundice is the hallmark sign that usually prompts cross-sectional imaging and/or cholangiography which leads to the diagnosis. Due to the increased risk of hilar CCA and the availability of effective therapy, many patients with PSC undergo surveillance through cholangiography and brushing [11].

The classic findings of hilar CCA are a malignant-appearing (long, irregular, or asymmetric) stricture on cholangiography and proximal ductal dilation, with or without a mass on cross-sectional imaging. Pathological confirmation of the malignancy is difficult and not always possible. CCA is frequently desmoplastic in nature; endoscopic biopsies and brushings frequently yield paucicellular cytologic specimens difficult to interpret.

Diagnosis is assisted with polysomy detection by fluorescence *in situ* hybridization (FISH) and serum CA 19-9 levels [12]. Both are highly specific but have limited sensitivity [13, 14].

The Mayo Clinic protocol was designed in 1993 with the aim to treat patients with CCA arising in the setting of PSC and early stage unresectable *de novo* CCA. Standard criteria for unresectability include bilateral segmental ductal involvement, encasement of the main portal vein, unilateral segmental ductal involvement with contralateral vascular encasement (not amenable to vascular reconstruction), and an insufficient future liver remnant [15]. These criteria are challenged constantly, as advanced liver resection (LR) techniques with vascular reconstruction show progressively better outcomes [16]. Patients with PSC are typically considered unresectable due to the underlying liver disease as well as the high risk of multifocal CCA. Exclusion criteria include tumor metastases, primary tumor below the cystic duct by cholangiography, *radial* (perpendicular to duct axis) tumor diameter >3 cm, prior attempts of resection with violation of the tumor plane, and diagnostic (malignant cells obtained) transperitoneal fine needle aspiration or biopsy of the primary tumor [17]. Longitudinal extension (regardless of size) of CCA along the duct and vascular encasement is not a contraindication for transplantation.

Early results with neo-RT followed by LT for CCA were promising and has led to adoption of the protocol at multiple centers [18]. Eventually, the United Network for Organ Sharing (UNOS) adopted the Mayo Clinic inclusion/exclusion guidelines and protocol guidelines (requiring neo-RT and operative staging along with protocol review) to enable appropriate prioritization for CCA patients awaiting deceased donor LT. The effectiveness of this combined modality treatment is now generally recognized, and the Center for Medicare and Medicaid Services, as well as other commercial insurance companies now provide coverage for this treatment.

The protocol includes (1) selection of patients with early stage disease (no metastasis and radial tumor diameter <3 cm), (2) high-dose radiotherapy with chemosensitization, (3) operative staging, and (4) LT followed by standard immunosuppression [19].

(1) Careful patient selection: Only patients with early-stage disease without lymph node involvement and/or metastases are included. Clinical staging prior to neoadjuvant therapy includes computerized tomography of the chest and abdomen and a bone scan. Patients usually require biliary drainage to alleviate symptoms, treat cholangitis, and enable the liver to

tolerate neoadjuvant therapy. Endoscopic intervention is preferred over percutaneous cholangiography to reduce the potential risk of tumor dissemination. Although there have been some patients with tube exit-site recurrences, we do not currently exclude patients that have undergone percutaneous cholangiography. Endoscopic ultrasound (EUS) with fine needle aspiration of regional hepatic lymph nodes avoids the morbidity of neoadjuvant therapy for patients destined to fall out of the protocol at operative staging.

(2) High-dose neo-RT has improved the poor results observed with LT alone. The goal of neo-RT prior to staging is to reduce the risk of dissemination of cancer while awaiting transplantation. CCA is a radiosensitive neoplasia; however, hepatotoxicity limits its widespread application in other settings. As with other malignancies, the biological response of the disease to neoadjuvant therapy is useful to assist in the prediction of prognosis [20, 21]. In our experience, around 30% of the patients included in the protocol drop out due to progressive CCA, liver disease decompensation, deconditioning, or positive staging operation.

(3) Operative staging avoids transplantation of patients with regional lymph node and/or peritoneal metastases or locally extensive disease with direct invasion of surrounding structures that was not detected with previous studies. The current rate of positive staging after neo-RT is 18%. Staging is performed after completion of neoadjuvant therapy. Among living donor LT recipients, it is performed the day before the scheduled operation. In deceased donor transplant, staging is typically performed when a patient's Model for End-Stage Liver Disease (MELD) is close to the average score for transplantation in the region. If a patient is too ill to tolerate staging without LT, it may be deferred until an allograft is available, though this requires anticipation of possible reallocation of the liver. Patients with PSC may have adhesions from previous operations for inflammatory bowel disease or colorectal cancer, but the procedure can usually be completed laparoscopically with careful dissection. Some patients have an ostomy that may be a challenge during both staging and transplantation. Any suspicious lesion is biopsied and the perihilar lymph nodes near the hepatic artery and common bile duct are routinely sampled even if they appear normal.

(4) LT achieves a radical resection, avoids future liver problems due to high-dose radiotherapy, and treats underlying liver disease (PSC). Radiotherapy-induced liver damage can be appreciated on liver explants (Figure 1). During LT, the peritoneal cavity is again examined to rule out

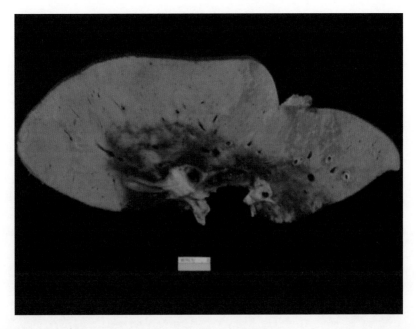

Figure 1. Liver explant from a patient with *de novo* hilar CCA, with a formalin-fixed section showing radiotherapy-induced changes in the liver hilum.

metastatic disease, especially for patients undergoing deceased donor transplantation that may have had a prolonged waiting time between operative staging and transplantation. The liver hilum is not dissected during hepatectomy to avoid tumor dissemination. The hepatic artery, portal vein, and bile duct are transected as close to the duodenum and pancreas as possible. The dissection between the caudate lobe and the inferior vena cava can be challenging and frequently leads to suspicion of tumor invasion; analysis of explanted livers has shown that the loss of the plane between them is due to radiation injury and not cancer. The common bile duct margin is sent for frozen section in patients with PSC and if positive, pancreaticoduodenectomy is performed.

The portal vein in living donor recipients is reconstructed with an ABO-compatible deceased donor iliac vein graft; this allows a tension-free anastomosis and provides length for the placement of a stent if radiation-induced portal vein stenosis occurs later. The hepatic artery is reconstructed with an aortohepatic conduit in deceased donor recipients and to the native hepatic artery in living donor recipients. The bile duct is reconstructed with a Roux-en-Y in all cases.

2.1. *Perioperative morbidity and mortality*

Neoadjuvant therapy is a source of substantial morbidity and an adverse effect on technical difficulty of LT. Patients with hilar CCA are at higher risk of vascular complications due to the radiation therapy. The experience of our center has been recently updated, including 174 cases (1993–2015).

The incidence of hepatic artery complications is high among living donor recipients (thrombosis 5% vs. 15%, $p = 0.043$; stenosis 10% vs. 17%, $p = 0.019$). The incidence of arterial complications in living donor recipients with jump graft reconstruction is higher than among those with native hepatic artery reconstruction. As the injury from radiation therapy is progressive over time, the short interval between the completion of neo-RT and transplantation in living donor recipients typically makes it possible to use the native hepatic artery, while most deceased donor recipients have no other option.

The incidence of portal vein stenosis is high (deceased donor recipients 22.8%, living donor recipients 35%), though management through percutaneous transhepatic dilation and stenting has been highly successful (94% patency rate at 5 years). Screening 4 months and 12 months after transplantation with computed tomography (CT) has reduced the incidence of portal vein thrombosis over time (9% 1993–2006 vs. 2.8% 2007–2015).

2.2. *Disease-free survival (DFS)*

Patients with high-risk features for disease recurrence (residual tumor on explant, perineural invasion and/or positive lymph nodes on explant) undergo immunosuppression with sirolimus and adjuvant chemotherapy in selected cases. Recurrence screening is performed 4 months and 12 months after LT and yearly thereafter. The incidence of recurrence among patients undergoing neo-RT followed by LT is 25% (45 out of 181 patients). Failure from distant metastatic disease is less likely than local or regional disease. Neither resection nor LT have the potential to reduce the risk of distant failure, although effective local control and timely treatment is likely to reduce the risk in either case. The initial recurrence is most often local-regional after LT (~70%; 31 abdominal, 2 drains/ Percutaneous Transhepatic Catheter (PTC) site).

2.3. *Intention-to-treat survival (ITT)*

Neoadjuvant chemoradiotherapy followed by LT for unresectable early-stage *de novo* CCA achieves results comparable to LR for resectable disease [22]. The outcome of patients who fallout of protocol after neoadjuvant

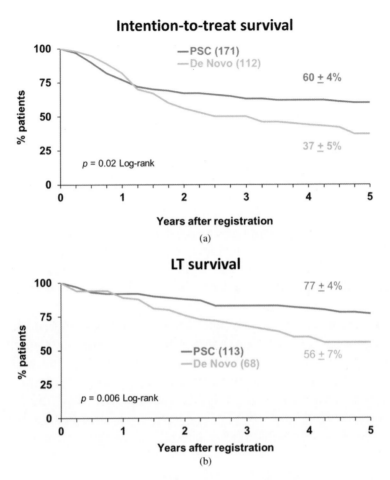

Figure 2. (a) Kaplan–Meier survival intention-to-treat analysis of all patients included in the protocol for CCA at Mayo Clinic as of February 2016. (b) Kaplan–Meier survival analysis of patients undergoing LT after the protocol for CCA at Mayo Clinic as of February 2016.

therapy is similar to those who undergo palliation [23]. Current Mayo Clinic results with over 283 patients enrolled in the neoadjuvant therapy protocol demonstrate intention to treat 5-year survival rates of 60% for patients with underlying PSC and 37% for those with CCA arising *de novo* (Figure 2(a)). Five-year survival rates after transplantation are 77% for patients with underlying PSC and 56% for those with CCA arising *de novo* (Figure 2(b)).

2.4. *Current status and future prospects*

Current outcomes following neoadjuvant therapy and LT for unresectable hilar CCA are very good. Thus questions have been raised about extending the indication to resectable patients. Would an improved survival be observed if neoadjuvant therapy and LT are applied to patients with resectable, presumably earlier stage disease? If so, what would the improvement in survival need to be, compared to that which can be achieved with resection, in order to justify the use of a liver allograft? This question may be addressed in a future randomized trial though it is important to note the crossover between the arms would not be possible, as well as the obvious challenges of organ availability.

3. ICC

ICC has increased significantly during the last four decades (128% from 1973 to 2012), with an annual increase of 4.3% during the last decade (2003–2012). In comparison, hilar CCA incidence has increased by 5% over the same period (annual increase 0.14%) [24]. Although there may be many contributing factors, increased awareness and improvement on molecular diagnosis are likely important. The diagnosis of ICC on cirrhotic patients during screening for HCC could also play a role. Cirrhosis from any cause, alcohol use, diabetes, and obesity are major risk factors for ICC [25]. A meta-analysis showed independent associations of both hepatitis B virus (HBV) and hepatitis C virus (HCV) prevalence with ICC incidence [26]. Furthermore, HBV and HCV genes have been identified in ICCs from patients without cirrhosis [27] Despite the relatively low number of cases (<5% of all *de novo* tumors detected in patients with cirrhosis), ICC is clinically relevant, as it carries a dismal prognosis and has long been considered a contraindication for LT.

ICC tends to originate from the central areas of the liver. Therefore, adequate oncological resection often requires a high volume of nonaffected parenchyma to be resected. Patients with ICC undergo extended hepatectomy (39.3%) more frequently than hemihepatectomy (35%) or minor LRs (less than three segments) (25.7%) [28]. Extended resections are only justified in the setting of potentially R0 resections, as palliative resections do not improve survival [29].

Patients with end-stage liver disease (ESLD) are often not candidates to LR for ICC due to the need for extensive resections in a liver with reduced regenerative capacity. The very limited data to support LT for ICC comes from two recent studies. Through the retrospective analysis of patients who underwent LT and were found to have incidental ICC on the explant, patients with *very early* ICC (single ≤2 cm) were shown to have good survival after LT. A first study identified eight patients from a cohort of 7,876 LT [30, 31], and a second study identified 15 patients from a cohort of 25,016 LT [32]. Of note, none of these 23 patients had a known diagnosis of ICC before LT and none of them underwent transperitoneal biopsy before LT.

Current imaging studies allow patients with *very early* HCC to be diagnosed through noninvasive criteria. ICC, on the contrary, requires histological analysis. Although CA 19-9 could be of assistance in establishing a noninvasive diagnosis, it is not specific and its elevation is associated with a more aggressive biological behavior [33].

3.1. Disease-free survival (DFS)

The 5-year DFS after LT among patients with *very early* ICC (15 patients) is 88%, as opposed to 23% in patients with ICC > 2 cm or multinodularity (33 patients). Factors associated with tumor recurrence were microvascular invasion and poor differentiation of the tumor [32].

3.2. Overall survival (OS)

All studies evaluating patients with ICC who underwent LT are retrospective, with no ITT survival analysis. The OS of patients who have undergone LT even with incidental ICC falls below the expected survival of patients with chronic liver disease without cancer, with the potential exception of patients with single ICC ≤ 2 cm (5-year survival 65–73%).

3.3. Current status and future prospects

LT for ICC is not a standard indication in the USA. Further studies are needed to prove that long-term survival is similar to that observed in patients with chronic liver disease without cancer. At the present time, patients on the waiting list for another indication, found to have an ICC ≤2 cm, may still be candidates for LT in the absence of progression. A promising strategy is the preoperative therapy with intra-arterial Yttrium-90 radioembolization. Rayar *et al.* have shown that this therapy may reduce the size of unresectable ICC, allowing surgical resection in selected cases [34]. Whether or not a similar strategy can be used before LT for ICC will be the subject of future studies [35].

4. Hepatic epithelioid hemangioendothelioma (HEHE)

HEHE is an uncommon low-grade neoplasia, described in 1982 as a tumor of endothelial origin with distinctive histologic features and clinical course [36]. The diagnosis is made usually during the fifth decade of life, with a female-to-male ratio of 3:2. Clinical manifestations are right upper quadrant pain, hepatomegaly and weight loss, though patients may also be asymptomatic. Unlike hepatic infantile hemangioendothelioma, HEHE is not associated with heart failure; most patients (90%) present with bilateral, multifocal liver lesions and 37% have metastasis at the time of diagnosis (lung, peritoneum, lymph nodes, and bone) [37]. Two different patterns of lesions may be present: multiple *peripheral* liver lesions with concentric zones with different signal intensity (Figure 3) and *diffuse* confluent lesions. Macroscopic vascular invasion may cause portal hypertension and/or ascites. A Budd-Chiari-like syndrome secondary to HEHE has been described [38, 39]. Histological diagnosis can be assisted by immunostaining of

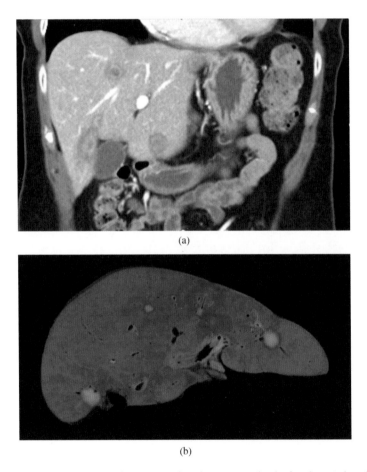

(a)

(b)

Figure 3.   HEHE. (a) Computed tomography showing multiple focal peripherally-located liver lesions with concentric zones of different contrast enhancement (b) Formalin-fixed section of liver explant from the same patient.

endothelial markers (CD31, CD34, factor VIII, and podoplanin) [40]. Biopsy is required, as differentiation from angiosarcoma is of the outmost importance. The prognosis for angiosarcoma is very poor, even after LR (median OS 10 months) [41] or LT (median DFS 5 months, median OS 7 months) [42].

The treatment of HEHE is not standardized. The entity is rare and its biological behavior is difficult to predict. The variable outcome with non-surgical therapies, have led to the suggestion of reserving surgical therapy for those who are resectable/transplantable after an initial period of observation [43]. LR and LT are associated with the highest OS. Due to the extent of the disease at diagnosis, LR is uncommon (9.4% of patients) [37]. LT can provide prolonged survival for HEHE even in the setting of extrahepatic disease, as tumor burden at diagnosis is not a reflection of aggressive tumor biology. HEHE usually presents in patients with normal livers; only a few cases of HEHE arising in the setting of liver disease have been reported [44, 45].

Extrahepatic disease has been usually managed with systemic therapy and/or metastasectomy. The former has not been associated with improved survival and extrahepatic disease may be stable for years after resection of the hepatic disease, making observation a valid alternative [46]. Sequential or combined lung transplantation has been performed in cases with symptomatic thoracic involvement [47].

4.1. *Disease-free survival (DFS)*

The interpretation of DFS in many reports of LT for HEHE is challenging, as many patients have extrahepatic disease at the time of transplantation and thus a more representative outcome may be progression-free survival, which is frequently not reported.

According to the European Liver Transplant Registry (ELTR) among 59 patients transplanted for HEHE), 24% developed recurrent allograft disease after a median time of 49 months (range, 6–98). Long-term survival was achieved through ablation or resection after recurrence in the allograft (five cases, survival 59, 84, 112, 211, and 212 months after LT). DFS at 1, 5, and 10-years are 90%, 82%, and 64%. This report shows no significant influence on DFS by pre-LT treatment, LN status, extrahepatic disease, or vascular invasion [48].

The experience of the Mayo Clinic group has shown that largest tumor size ≥10 cm, number of lesions ≥10, and extent of hepatic involvement greater than or equal to four segments were associated with decreased DFS after LT. Among the surviving patients, after a median follow-up of 41 months, there was no evidence of disease in 68%, stable disease in 26%, and progressive disease in 5% [46].

4.2. *Overall survival (OS)*

The ELTR reported a 5- and 10-year survival after LT of 83% and 72%. Treatment before LT (including LR), lymph node invasion, and extrahepatic disease did not influence OS. Micro and macrovascular invasion significantly reduced OS, although 5-year survival (72%) was still similar to the one observed among patients with chronic liver disease without cancer [48].

4.3. *Current status and future prospects*

HEHE is an accepted indication for LT. However, there are no definitive set of criteria established to provide MELD exception points. Additional MELD points can be granted by the Regional Review Board on a case-by-case basis, but it is not currently a standardized exception [49].

5. Neuroendocrine tumor (NET) liver metastases

NET can originate from a variety of organs and exhibit a highly heterogeneous biological behavior. During the last three decades, a better understanding of its clinical course has allowed distinguishing patients who will progress and die due to the disease, from those who will have an indolent course and benefit from timely therapy. According to a recent analysis of the SEER database, the incidence of NET in the USA has increased over the last 40 years and is now as frequent as testicular cancer, Hodgkin's disease, gliomas, and multiple myeloma [50]. The estimated incidence of all NET primary sites is 5.76 *per* 100,000 *per* year and 3.65 *per* 100,000 *per* year for gastro-entero-pancreatic NET [51]. Symptoms may arise from local compression due to bulky nonfunctional disease (abdominal pain and distention, anorexia, weight loss, nausea) or symptoms secondary to hormone production by functional NETs (serotonin, for small bowel primaries and insulin, gastrin, glucagon, cortisol, vasoactive intestinal peptide, and somatostatin, in order of frequency for pancreatic primaries) [52]. Sixty percent of NET are nonfunctional and at diagnosis, 65% have liver metastases [53]. NET in general are thought be indolent and are associated with favorable outcomes compared to other tumors that metastasize to the liver. LR is performed with

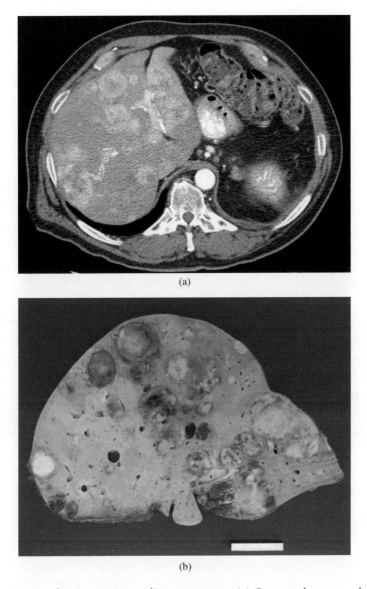

(a)

(b)

Figure 4. Neuroendocrine carcinoma liver metastases. (a) Computed tomography showing multiple focal liver hyperenhancing lesions. (b) Formalin fixed section of liver explant from the same patient.

curative intent (R0) resectable metastases from NET, while TL is an accepted indication for LT for unresectable liver involvement (Figures 4(a) and 4(b)). Although this is a common practice in many centers around the world, there is no robust evidence that R0 resection either through LR or LT is superior to other nonsurgical therapies. However, the collaborative effort of multiple groups has allowed the identification of patients that may benefit from these interventions.

The ELTR has the largest reported series in the literature of LT for NET, with 213 patients between 1982 and 2009 [54]. Before 2000, more aggressive operations such as abdominal exenteration or other major abdominal surgery were performed in addition to LT, adding morbidity and they contributed to worse survival. Other markers of aggressive tumor biology such as poor differentiation, higher tumor burden and hepatomegaly were associated with worse long-term survival. Five-year OS was 52% and DFS was 30%. OS was significantly better in patients with only one unfavorable factor compared to patients with two or three unfavorable factors (79% vs. 38%, $p < 0.0001$).

Mazzaferro *et al.* have recently reported their experience with LT for patients with NET metastases [55]. They included only patients with potentially curative resection of both primary tumor and liver metastases, <60 years of age, no major comorbidities, and no progressive disease during their screening period. The two groups were different in terms of: *first*, larger primary tumors in the non-LT patients (although the extent of liver metastases was similar in two groups); *second*, LT patients were younger (40.5 years vs. 55.5 years); *third*, LT group received more locoregional treatments (40.5% vs. 21.7%) and were less likely to receive continuous treatment with somatostatin analogues (54.8% vs. 89.7%); and *fourth*, LT patients were less likely to have G3 disease (0 vs. 8.7%). Despite these differences and considering the number of variables to take into account, this study allows a comparison between two relatively similar groups who underwent different therapies. The patients in the study underwent LT or other therapies based on the availability of organs through their allocation system, patient compliance and age. The OS was significantly higher in the LT group with 10-year OS 88.8% vs. 22.4%. DFS in the LT patients was 86.9% at 10 years. Eighty-six percent of the patients who received other forms of therapy exhibited progression. The results of this study demonstrated that long-term survival after LT is significantly better than non-LT therapy in patients meeting restrictive criteria.

5.1 *Current status and future prospects*

LT for NET liver metastases is an accepted indication in the USA. Although no definitive set of criteria have been approved to grant MELD exception points, in June 2015, the Liver and Intestinal Organ Transplantation

Committee of the Organ Procurement and Transplantation Network (OPTN)/United Network of Organ Sharing (UNOS) released guidelines for Regional Review Boards (RRBs) evaluating case requests.

(1) Recipient age <60 years.
(2) Only NET primaries with portal venous drainage are considered (lower rectum, esophagus, lung, adrenal gland, and thyroid are not candidates for automatic MELD exception).
(3) Only well to moderately differentiated NETs are considered (mitotic rate <20 per 10 HPF (High Power Field), Ki67 <20%).
(4) Resection of primary NET and extrahepatic disease without evidence of recurrence at least 6 months prior to MELD exception request.
(5) Radiologic characteristics compatible with NET liver metastases.
(6) Unresectable liver metastases.
(7) Tumor metastatic replacement does not exceed 50% of the total liver volume.
(8) Negative metastatic workup (at least one of the three: PET scan, somatostatin receptor scintigraphy and/or Ga^{68}-labeled somatostatin scintigraphy). Exploratory laparoscopy/laparotomy is not required prior to MELD exception request.
(9) Recheck metastatic workup every 3 months. Extrahepatic disease progression should indicate delisting. Patients may be relisted if extrahepatic disease is zeroed and remained so for at least 6 months.

6. Colorectal carcinoma (CRC) liver metastases

CRC is the third most common cancer and the third leading cause of cancer death in men and women in the United States. In 2016 alone, around 134,000 Americans will have CRC, 50% will develop metastases (a large proportion of these in the liver), and 49,000 will die from CRC [56]. Surgery is the only potentially curative therapy. Patients with stage IV disease have a 5-year survival slightly greater than 10%, even after resection of the primary tumor [57]. It is estimated that 20% stage 4 CRC cases are surgical candidates, with an OS of 50–60% [58]. Patients with limited extrahepatic disease (lymph nodes or lung metastases) may still benefit from resection. Perioperative chemotherapy may assist in the selection of patients, as those with controlled systemic disease may benefit from resection.

The surgical management of CRC liver metastases has revolutionized LR. The aggressiveness of surgical therapy has grown as safer resections can be performed after improvements in imaging and surgical techniques, perioperative management and selection and timing of neoadjuvant agents. CRC liver metastases are considered resectable provided that a R0 LR can be tolerated with an adequate remnant, consisting of two contiguous, spared liver segments with sufficient hepatocyte mass, intact vascular inflow, outflow, and biliary drainage. The manipulation of portal inflow and the use of sequential operations have allowed extended resections leaving even only one spared liver segment [59].

Among patients with unresectable CRC liver metastases without extrahepatic involvement, LT has been attempted with variable success. Two cases of CRC liver metastases were among the first LT to ever be performed in 1963 [60]. Early attempts were followed by poor results and the concept was abandoned for a long time [61].

The group of Oslo University Hospital has recently revisited the concept of LT for CRC liver metastases [62]. Some of the reasons that led to this effort are as follows.

First, Norway experienced a very rapid increase in the incidence of CRC with the age-standardized rate for men increasing from 22 to 59 per 100,000/year during the last 50 years [63].

Second, the analysis of LT for CRC liver metastases in the European Liver Transplant Registry (ELTR) showed that graft loss and/or mortality during their early experience were not due to disease recurrence in at least 40% of the cases [64].

Third, the liver allocation system in Norway is part of Scandiatransplant, which also covers Island, Denmark, Sweden, and Finland. Norway was a net exporter of liver allografts in the early 2000s, as more donors were recovered than LT performed in the country. Also, the waiting time for LT was 1 month or less until 2012. These facts allowed the Oslo group to offer liver allografts for patients with CRC liver metastases without compromising the outcome of patients with chronic liver disease. The number of LTs has increased significantly during the last 10 years and thus, the favorable balance of organ supply to demand has since changed [65].

Patients included in the Oslo protocol (1) underwent radical resection of the primary tumor, (2) had a good performance status, and (3) had a minimum of 6 weeks of adequate chemotherapy. Progression during chemotherapy was not a contraindication for LT under the Oslo protocol [66]. Patients with significant weight loss (>10% total body weight in the last 6 months) were excluded. Extrahepatic disease was aggressively ruled out, first through imaging studies and then by staging laparotomy, including frozen section of lymph nodes in the hepatoduodenal ligament. LT is followed by induction with basiliximab and maintenance immunosuppression with steroids, mycophenolate, and sirolimus.

6.1. *Disease free survival (DFS)*

Recurrence screening was performed every 3 months the first year and every 6 months thereafter. Adjuvant chemotherapy was not given after LT. CRC recurred on 90% of the patients, with a median time to recurrence of 6 months; DFS was 35% at 1 year. For comparison, CRC recurs on 62% of the patients undergoing LR after a median time of 13 months [67]. CRC recurrence after LT presents as isolated lung metastasis in 68% of the cases. Unlike the pattern of recurrence observed after LR, isolated liver recurrence after LT is infrequent [68].

6.2. *Overall survival (OS)*

Among patients who underwent LT, OS was 95%, 68%, and 60% at 1, 3, and 5 years, respectively. Three patients were accepted for LT, but were excluded after staging laparotomy showed lymph node involvement; the survival of these three patients was 3–18 months. An ITT survival analysis is not included in the original publication [62]. Patients with progressive disease before LT had a lower 5-year survival (44%) [66].

To allow comparison of a similar group of patients who received palliative chemotherapy, the 21 patients included in the Oslo study were compared with patients with unresectable CRC liver-only metastases treated with palliative chemotherapy (NORDIC VII study, *n* = 47 patients) [69]. There was no difference between the DFS of patients who underwent LT and the progression-free survival of patients who underwent palliative chemotherapy, however, survival after disease recurrence or progression was significantly higher among patients who underwent LT. Five-year OS was significantly higher among patients who underwent LT (NORDIC VII 9% vs. LT 56%).

6.3. *Future prospects*

LT for CRC liver metastases is not an accepted indication in the USA. Further studies are needed to prove that long-term survival is similar to that observed in patients with chronic liver disease without cancer.

The Oslo group has also recently proposed a protocol that allows the use of left-lateral segment (LLS) liver allografts in these cases, either from living donors or split allografts from deceased donors. They have described the technique as "Resection And Partial Liver Segment 2/3 Transplantation With Delayed Total Hepatectomy" (RAPID). Recipient's segments 1–3 are resected, leaving an intentional R2 on the right hemiliver and segment 4. The allograft is implanted through vascular conduits as needed and a hepatico-jejunostomy. The volume of the left-lateral allograft is monitored weekly through CT and the completion total hepatectomy is performed once the volume is deemed adequate [70].

7. Summary

LT and LT following neoadjuvant chemoradiotherapy have become standard therapies for NETs and unresectable hilar CCA, respectively. Similar to LT for HCC, patient selection is essential to ensure acceptable outcomes. HEHE is a rare tumor which is also a suitable indication for LT in selected cases. The role of LT in patients with colorectal metastasis is evolving.

References

1. Soejima Y, Taketomi A, Yoshizumi T *et al*. Extended indication for living donor liver transplantation in patients with hepatocellular carcinoma. *Transplantation* 2007;83:893–9.
2. Lee SG, Hwang S, Moon DB *et al*. Expanded indication criteria of living donor liver transplantation for hepatocellular carcinoma at one large-volume center. *Liver Transpl* 2008;14:935–45.
3. Park YH, Hwang S, Ahn CS *et al*. Long-term outcome of liver transplantation for combined hepatocellular carcinoma and cholangiocarcinoma. *Transpl Proc* 2013;45:3038–40.
4. Moon DB, Lee SG, and Kim KH. Total hepatectomy, pancreatoduodenectomy, and living donor liver transplantation using innovative vascular reconstruction for unresectable cholangiocarcinoma. *Transpl Int* 2015;28:123–6.
5. Itoh S, Ikegami T, Yoshizumi T *et al*. Long-term outcome of living-donor liver transplantation for combined hepatocellular-cholangiocarcinoma. *Anticancer Res* 2015;35:2475–6.
6. Han DH, Joo DJ, Kim MS *et al*. Living donor liver transplantation for advanced hepatocellular carcinoma with portal vein tumor thrombosis after concurrent chemoradiation therapy. *Yonsei Med J* 2016;57:1276–81.
7. Goldstein RM, Stone M, Tillery GW *et al*. Is liver transplantation indicated for cholangiocarcinoma? *Am J Surg* 1993;166:768–71 (discussion 71–2).

8. Meyer CG, Penn I, and James L. Liver transplantation for cholangiocarcinoma: results in 207 patients. *Transplantation* 2000;69:1633–7.
9. Loinaz C, Abradelo M, Gomez R *et al*. Liver transplantation and incidental primary liver tumors. *Transpl Proc* 1998;30:3301–2.
10. Ghali P, Marotta PJ, Yoshida EM, *et al*. Liver transplantation for incidental cholangiocarcinoma: analysis of the Canadian experience. *Liver Transpl* 2005;11:1412–6.
11. Boyd S, Mustonen H, Tenca A, Jokelainen K, Arola J, and Farkkila MA. Surveillance of primary sclerosing cholangitis with ERC and brush cytology: risk factors for cholangiocarcinoma. *Scand J Gastroenterol* 2017;52:242–9.
12. Kipp BR, Stadheim LM, Halling SA, *et al*. A comparison of routine cytology and fluorescence in situ hybridization for the detection of malignant bile duct strictures. *Am J Gastroenterol* 2004;99:1675–81.
13. Navaneethan U, Njei B, Venkatesh PG, Vargo JJ, and Parsi MA. Fluorescence in situ hybridization for diagnosis of cholangiocarcinoma in primary sclerosing cholangitis: a systematic review and meta-analysis. *Gastrointest Endosc* 2014;79:943–50 e3.
14. Liang B, Zhong L, He Q, *et al*. Diagnostic accuracy of serum CA19-9 in patients with cholangiocarcinoma: a systematic review and meta-analysis. *Med Sci* 2015;21:3555–63.
15. Mansour JC, Aloia TA, Crane CH, Heimbach JK, Nagino M, and Vauthey JN. Hilar cholangiocarcinoma: expert consensus statement. *HPB* 2015;17:691–9.
16. Nagino M, Ebata T, Yokoyama Y, *et al*. Evolution of surgical treatment for perihilar cholangiocarcinoma: a single-center 34-year review of 574 consecutive resections. *Ann Surg* 2013;258:129–40.
17. Heimbach JK, Sanchez W, Rosen CB, and Gores GJ. Trans-peritoneal fine needle aspiration biopsy of hilar cholangiocarcinoma is associated with disease dissemination. *HPB* 2011;13:356–60.
18. De Vreede I, Steers JL, Burch PA, *et al*. Prolonged disease-free survival after orthotopic liver transplantation plus adjuvant chemoirradiation for cholangio-carcinoma. *Liver Transpl* 2000;6:309–16.
19. Heimbach JK, Gores GJ, Nagorney DM, and Rosen CB. Liver transplantation for perihilar cholangiocarcinoma after aggressive neoadjuvant therapy: a new paradigm for liver and biliary malignancies? *Surgery* 2006;140:331–4.
20. Darwish Murad S, Kim WR, Therneau T, *et al*. Predictors of pretransplant dropout and posttransplant recurrence in patients with perihilar cholangiocar-cinoma. *Hepatology* 2012;56:972–81.
21. Lehrke HD, Heimbach JK, Wu TT, *et al*. Prognostic significance of the histo-logic response of perihilar cholangiocarcinoma to preoperative neoadjuvant chemoradiation in liver explants. *Am J Surg Pathol* 2016;40:510–8.
22. Croome KP, Rosen CB, Heimbach JK, and Nagorney DM. Is liver transplanta-tion appropriate for patients with potentially resectable de novo hilar cholangiocarcinoma? *J Am Coll Surg* 2015;221:130–9.

23. Sio TT, Martenson JA, Jr., Haddock MG, et al. Outcome of transplant-fallout patients with unresectable cholangiocarcinoma. *Am J Clin Oncol* 2016;39:271–5.
24. Saha SK, Zhu AX, Fuchs CS, and Brooks GA. Forty-year trends in cholangio-carcinoma incidence in the U.S.: intrahepatic disease on the rise. *Oncologist* 2016;21:594–9.
25. Shaib YH, El-Serag HB, Davila JA, Morgan R, and McGlynn KA. Risk factors of intrahepatic cholangiocarcinoma in the United States: a case-control study. *Gastroenterology* 2005;128:620–6.
26. Palmer WC and Patel T. Are common factors involved in the pathogenesis of primary liver cancers? A meta-analysis of risk factors for intrahepatic cholan-giocarcinoma. *J Hepatol* 2012;57:69–76.
27. Perumal V, Wang J, Thuluvath P, Choti M, and Torbenson M. Hepatitis C and hepatitis B nucleic acids are present in intrahepatic cholangiocarcinomas from the United States. *Hum Pathol* 2006;37:1211–6.
28. Hyder O, Marques H, Pulitano C, et al. A nomogram to predict long-term sur-vival after resection for intrahepatic cholangiocarcinoma: an Eastern and Western experience. *JAMA Surg* 2014;149:432–8.
29. Lang H, Sotiropoulos GC, and Fruhauf NR, et al. Extended hepatectomy for intrahepatic cholangiocellular carcinoma (ICC): when is it worthwhile? Single center experience with 27 resections in 50 patients over a 5-year period. *Ann Surg* 2005;241:134–43.
30. Sapisochin G, Rodriguez de Lope C, Gastaca M, et al. "Very early" intrahepatic cholangiocarcinoma in cirrhotic patients: should liver transplantation be recon-sidered in these patients? *Am J Transpl* 2014;14:660–7.
31. Sapisochin G, de Lope CR, Gastaca M, et al. Intrahepatic cholangiocarcinoma or mixed hepatocellular-cholangiocarcinoma in patients undergoing liver trans-plantation: a Spanish matched cohort multicenter study. *Ann Surg* 2014;259:944–52.
32. Sapisochin G, Facciuto M, Rubbia-Brandt L, et al. Liver transplantation for "very early" intrahepatic cholangiocarcinoma: international retrospective study supporting a prospective assessment. *Hepatology* 2016;64:1178–88.
33. Bergquist JR, Ivanics T, Storlie CB, et al. Implications of CA19-9 elevation for survival, staging, and treatment sequencing in intrahepatic cholangiocarcinoma: a national cohort analysis. *J Surg Oncol* 2016;114:475–82.
34. Rayar M, Sulpice L, Edeline J, et al. Intra-arterial yttrium-90 radioembolization combined with systemic chemotherapy is a promising method for downstaging unresectable huge intrahepatic cholangiocarcinoma to surgical treatment. *Ann Surg Oncol* 2015;22:3102–8.
35. Rayar M, Levi Sandri GB, Houssel-Debry P, Camus C, Sulpice L, and Boudjema K. Multimodal therapy including Yttrium-90 radioembolization as a bridging therapy to liver transplantation for a huge and locally advanced intrahepatic cholangiocarcinoma. *J Gastrointest Liver Dis* 2016;25:401–4.

36. Weiss SW and Enzinger FM. Epithelioid hemangioendothelioma: a vascular tumor often mistaken for a carcinoma. *Cancer* 1982;50:970–81.
37. Mehrabi A, Kashfi A, Fonouni H, *et al.* Primary malignant hepatic epithelioid hemangioendothelioma: a comprehensive review of the literature with emphasis on the surgical therapy. *Cancer* 2006;107:2108–21.
38. Walsh MM, Hytiroglou P, Thung SN, *et al.* Epithelioid hemangioendothelioma of the liver mimicking Budd-Chiari syndrome. *Arch Pathol Lab Med* 1998;122:846–8.
39. Hayashi Y, Inagaki K, Hirota S, Yoshikawa T, and Ikawa H. Epithelioid hemangioendothelioma with marked liver deformity and secondary Budd-Chiari syndrome: pathological and radiological correlation. *Pathol Int* 1999;49:547–52.
40. Fujii T, Zen Y, Sato Y, *et al.* Podoplanin is a useful diagnostic marker for epithelioid hemangioendothelioma of the liver. *Mod Pathol* 2008;21:125–30.
41. Zhu YP, Chen YM, Matro E, *et al.* Primary hepatic angiosarcoma: a report of two cases and literature review. *World J Gastroenterol* 2015;21:6088–96.
42. Orlando G, Adam R, Mirza D, *et al.* Hepatic hemangiosarcoma: an absolute contraindication to liver transplantation — the European Liver Transplant Registry experience. *Transplantation* 2013;95:872–7.
43. Thomas RM, Aloia TA, Truty MJ, *et al.* Treatment sequencing strategy for hepatic epithelioid haemangioendothelioma. *HPB* 2014;16:677–85.
44. Ahmad N, Adams DM, Wang J, Prakash R, and Karim NA. Hepatic epithelioid hemangioendothelioma in a patient with hemochromatosis. *J Natl Compr Cancer Netw* 2014;12:1203–7.
45. Baron PW, Amankonah T, Cubas RF, *et al.* Diffuse hepatic epithelioid hemangioendothelioma developed in a patient with hepatitis C cirrhosis. *Case Rep Transpl* 2014;2014:694903.
46. Grotz TE, Nagorney D, Donohue J, *et al.* Hepatic epithelioid haemangioendothelioma: is transplantation the only treatment option? *HPB* 2010;12:546–53.
47. Desie N, Van Raemdonck DE, Ceulemans LJ, *et al.* Combined or serial liver and lung transplantation for epithelioid hemangioendothelioma: a case series. *Am J Transpl* 2015;15:3247–54.
48. Lerut JP, Orlando G, Adam R, *et al.* The place of liver transplantation in the treatment of hepatic epitheloid hemangioendothelioma: report of the European liver transplant registry. *Ann Surg* 2007;246:949–57 (discussion 57).
49. Punch J and Gish RG. Model for end-stage liver disease (MELD) exception for uncommon hepatic tumors. *Liver Transpl* 2006;12:S122–3.
50. Frilling A, Modlin IM, Kidd M, *et al.* Recommendations for management of patients with neuroendocrine liver metastases. *Lancet Oncol* 2014;15:e8–21.
51. Lawrence B, Gustafsson BI, Chan A, Svejda B, Kidd M, and Modlin IM. The epidemiology of gastroenteropancreatic neuroendocrine tumors. *Endocrinol Metab Clin N Am* 2011;40:1–18, vii.

52. Metz DC and Jensen RT. Gastrointestinal neuroendocrine tumors: pancreatic endocrine tumors. *Gastroenterology* 2008;135:1469–92.

53. Panzuto F, Nasoni S, Falconi M, *et al.* Prognostic factors and survival in endocrine tumor patients: comparison between gastrointestinal and pancreatic localization. *Endocr-Relat Cancer* 2005;12:1083–92.

54. Le Treut YP, Gregoire E, Klempnauer J, *et al.* Liver transplantation for neuro-endocrine tumors in Europe — results and trends in patient selection: a 213-case European liver transplant registry study. *Ann Surg* 2013;257:807–15.

55. Mazzaferro V, Sposito C, Coppa J, *et al.* The long-term benefit of liver trans-plantation for hepatic metastases from neuroendocrine tumors. *Am J Transpl,* 2016, 16(10):2892–902.

56. Brenner H, Kloor M, and Pox CP. Colorectal cancer. *Lancet* 2014;383: 1490–502.

57. Stangl R, Altendorf-Hofmann A, Charnley RM, and Scheele J. Factors influenc-ing the natural history of colorectal liver metastases. *Lancet* 1994;343:1405–10.

58. Tzeng CW and Aloia TA. Colorectal liver metastases. *J Gastrointest Surg* 2013;17:195–201 (quiz p. 2).

59. Schadde E, Malago M, Hernandez-Alejandro R, *et al.* Monosegment ALPPS hepatectomy: extending resectability by rapid hypertrophy. *Surgery* 2015;157:676–89.

60. Starzl TE. The saga of liver replacement, with particular reference to the recip-rocal influence of liver and kidney transplantation (1955-1967). *J Am Coll Surg* 2002;195:587–610.

61. Ringe B, Wittekind C, Bechstein WO, Bunzendahl H, and Pichlmayr R. The role of liver transplantation in hepatobiliary malignancy. A retrospective analysis of 95 patients with particular regard to tumor stage and recurrence. *Ann Surg* 1989;209:88–98.

62. Hagness M, Foss A, Line PD, *et al.* Liver transplantation for nonresectable liver metastases from colorectal cancer. *Ann Surg* 2013;257:800–6.

63. Lynge E, Martinsen JI, Larsen IK, and Kjaerheim K. Colon cancer trends in Norway and Denmark by socio-economic group: a cohort study. *Scand J Public Health* 2015;43:890–8.

64. Foss A, Adam R, and Dueland S. Liver transplantation for colorectal liver metastases: revisiting the concept. *Transpl Int* 2010;23:679–85.

65. Fosby B, Melum E, Bjoro K, *et al.* Liver transplantation in the Nordic countries — an intention to treat and post-transplant analysis from The Nordic Liver Transplant Registry 1982–2013. *Scand J Gastroenterol* 2015;50:797–808.

66. Dueland S, Hagness M, Line PD, Guren TK, Tveit KM, and Foss A. Is liver transplantation an option in colorectal cancer patients with nonresectable liver metastases and progression on all lines of standard chemotherapy? *Ann Surg Oncol* 2015;22:2195–200.

67. Butte JM, Gonen M, Allen PJ, *et al.* Recurrence after partial hepatectomy for metastatic colorectal cancer: potentially curative role of salvage repeat resection. *Ann Surg Oncol* 2015;22:2761–71.
68. Hagness M, Foss A, Egge TS, and Dueland S. Patterns of recurrence after liver transplantation for nonresectable liver metastases from colorectal cancer. *Ann Surg Oncol* 2014;21:1323–9.
69. Dueland S, Guren TK, Hagness M, *et al.* Chemotherapy or liver transplantation for nonresectable liver metastases from colorectal cancer? *Ann Surg* 2015;261:956–60.
70. Line PD, Hagness M, Berstad AE, Foss A, and Dueland S. A novel concept for partial liver transplantation in nonresectable colorectal liver metastases: the RAPID concept. *Ann Surg* 2015;262:e5–9.

3. Developments in Donation after Cardiac Death in Liver Transplantation

David P. Foley* and David J. Reich[†]

*Department of Surgery, University of Wisconsin School of
Medicine and Public Health, Madison, WI 53792, USA
[†]Department of Surgery, Drexel University,
College of Medicine, Philadelphia, PA 19129, USA

1. Introduction

Donation after cardiac death (DCD), also referred to as donation after circulatory death and formerly referred to as nonheartbeating donation, has become the fastest growing source of transplant organs in the United States over the past decade [1], bringing full circle the history of organ donation. This chapter reviews the history, ethics, practice guidelines, surgical techniques, clinical outcomes, and challenges of DCD liver transplant(ation) (LT), focusing on the controlled subgroup of DCDs and highlighting recent developments in this field. Profound disparity in supply and demand for transplantable livers causes tragic numbers of end-stage organ failure patients to succumb before receiving a transplant. Based on the 2015 Scientifc Registry for Transplant Recipients (SRTR) Annual Report, although total liver donors and transplants have increased and waiting list time has decreased, waiting-list mortality is approximately 11% and an additional 8% of listed patients were removed from the list due to being too sick to undergo transplant. During 2015, 1,673 patients died without undergoing transplant and another 1,227 were removed due to being too sick [1].

According to Eurotransplant 2015 Annual Report, liver waiting-list mortality was 26% and an additional 6% of wait-listed liver patients were removed as they were sick [2]. In response, one method of increasing the donor pool is to use live donor livers, a high-stake endeavor, and to use expanded criteria organs, including older, hepatitis C virus–positive, hepatitis B core antibody–positive, steatotic, injured, and reduced in size (split) livers. DCD is an additional type of expanded criteria donor, utilized in the United States, Europe, and Asia to boost the number of deceased donors and decrease the dire shortage of transplantable organs. The percentage of deceased donors in the United States that are DCD has grown from 1% in 1996 to 16% in 2015 [1]. Between 2012 and 2015, the number of transplanted DCD livers increased from 263 to 405, a 54% increase. In 2015, 6% of deceased donor LTs performed in the United States and 8% under Eurotransplant were from DCDs [1, 2].

2. Defining donation after cardiac death and the Spanish model

DCD is characterized by irreversible unresponsiveness, apnea, and absence of circulation, in contrast to donation after brain death (DBD), defined by irreversible cessation of all brain functions. Organ ischemia is minimized in DBD because circulatory arrest typically occurs concurrently with perfusion of preservation solution and rapid core cooling. Thus, the procurement procedure does not implicitly involve circulatory dysfunction. Organs recovered from DCD donors are less than ideal because the organs suffer ischemia during the prolonged periods between circulatory dysfunction, circulatory arrest, and subsequent perfusion and cooling. Furthermore, the surgical procedure for DCD organ recovery is demanding, rushed, and with increased potential for vascular injury. It is important to differentiate controlled from uncontrolled DCDs (Figure 1); this chapter will focus on controlled DCD.

2.1. Uncontrolled donation after cardiac death

Uncontrolled DCDs sustain circulatory arrest and either fail to respond to CPR or are declared DOA at the hospital. Uncontrolled DCD is unplanned, so the organs suffer protracted ischemia prior to recovery. Although kidneys tolerate a short period of the resultant warm ischemia, transplant of extrarenal organs from uncontrolled DCDs carries a much greater risk. The Barcelona group has been at the forefront of the use of uncontrolled DCD donors, yielding 1-year liver graft and recipient survival rates of 75% and 90%,

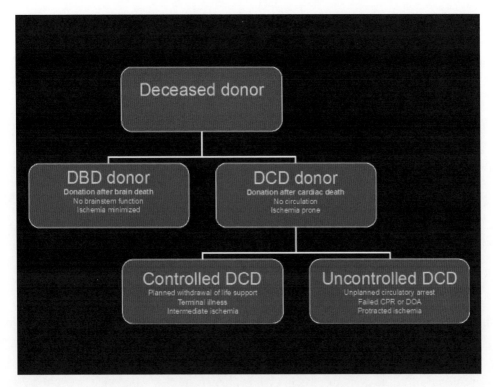

Figure 1. Definitions of various types of deceased donors.

respectively, from 40 uncontrolled DCD LTs performed over an 11-year period [3]. To attain these results they employ various *postmortem* measures, including CPR, femoral vessel cannulation for normothermic extracorporeal membrane oxygenation (ECMO) and normothermic regional perfusion (NRP). These initial measures are performed nonconsensually in Spain, which would be viewed problematically in many other countires, even though organ procurement is aborted in Spain if consent for donation is not ultimately obtained. Without such measures, uncontrolled DCD LT provides prohibitively low graft survival rates; very few are performed in the United States and therefore the remainder of this chapter deals with controlled DCD LT.

2.2. *Controlled donation after cardiac death*

Controlled DCDs provide organs that are exposed to significantly less ischemic damage than those of uncontrolled DCDs and in general offer superior posttransplant function when compared with uncontrolled DCDs.

Controlled DCDs undergo circulatory arrest following planned withdrawal of life support (ventilatory and circulatory support), most often in the operating room, with a donor surgical team readily available. Except in rare circumstances, the potential controlled DCD does not meet brain death criteria but has sustained a catastrophic brain injury or other illness such as end-stage musculoskeletal disease, pulmonary disease, or high spinal cord injury, and has no expectation of meaningful survival as determined by the treating physician(s). The patient's legal decision maker(s) request withdrawal of support, whether or not organ donation is to be pursued. Subsequently, informed consent for organ donation is obtained from them if the patient is otherwise medically suitable for donation. Controlled DCD offers the family and patient with a hopeless prognosis the opportunity to donate when criteria for brain death will not be met prior to cardiac death.

3. Historical perspective

3.1. *The impact of brain death recognition*

During the earliest years of kidney transplant, organ donation amounted to removal of kidneys from patients whose hearts had stopped beating. The first human kidney, liver, and heart transplants, in 1958, 1963, and 1967, respectively, were performed using organs recovered from uncontrolled DCDs. Through the 1960s, determination of death required heartbeat cessation. However, World War II led to the birth of modern critical care, including the use of respirators and CPR. It became possible to re-establish or maintain cardiopulmonary function in severely ill patients, which led neurophysiologists of the 1950s to study irreversible coma. Subsequently, in 1968, the multidisciplinary Ad Hoc Committee of Harvard Medical School to Examine the Definition of Death issued a landmark report that included criteria for the determination of brain death (Harvard Neurologic Definition and Criteria for Death) [4]. In 1980, the Uniform Law Commissioners adopted the Uniform Determination of Death Act (UDODA). According to UDODA, "an individual who has sustained either (1) irreversible cessation of circulatory and respiratory functions, or (2) irreversible cessation of all functions of the entire brain, including the brainstem, is dead" [5]. UDODA has been endorsed by the major American and European medical and legal professional associations and all 50 states have enacted brain death legislation. During the mid-1970s, the practice of recovering organs from DCDs was essentially abandoned. Organs recovered from DBDs are considered more desirable because they are protected from the effects of warm ischemic injury and are less prone to poor graft function. For the following 25 years, virtually all donation was from DBD or live donation.

3.2. Controlled donation after cardiac death liver transplant — early efforts

DCD organ transplant was reintroduced by the University of Pittsburgh transplant program in 1992 [6]. The Pittsburgh program and the program at the University of Wisconsin in Madison, Wisconsin, were pivotal in initiating controlled DCD organ transplant and were the first to describe results of controlled DCD kidney and LT, both in 1995 [7, 8]. The experiences were small and provided survival rates inferior to those after DBD LT, but these pioneering teams' reports were encouraging and provided the impetus to further develop the field of controlled DCD LT. In 2000, Reich *et al.* published the first successful series of controlled DCD LT; at a mean follow-up of 18 months, patient and graft survival rates were 100% and there were no instances of primary nonfunction, hepatic artery thrombosis, or ischemic cholangiopathy [9]. Thereafter, other reports of increasingly larger DCD experiences were published [10–15].

These early experiences with controlled DCD occurred concurrently with the public's increasing reluctance to prolong futile treatment and artificial life support of terminally injured and ill patients and with increasing use of advance directives and health care proxies. In 1997, the Institute of Medicine (IOM) of the National Academy of Science published its first report on DCD [16]. The IOM, commissioned by the Department of Health and Human Services, considered DCD to be an ethical way to address the organ shortage and sought to increase such donations through their follow-up reports of 2000 and 2006 [17, 18]. Starting in 2003, the Department of Health and Human Services organized the Organ Donation and Transplant Breakthrough Collaboratives, mandating increased DCD [19], and leading to a surge in DCD kidney and LT. DCD has also been endorsed by the American Society of Transplant Surgeons (ASTS), the Society of Critical Care Medicine, the United Network for Organ Sharing (UNOS), the Joint Commission on Accreditation of Healthcare Organizations and the Centers for Medicare and Medicaid Services [20–26]. Early estimates were that DCD could increase the deceased donor pool in the United States by over 1,000 donors per year [27]. Indeed, the number of DCD donors steadily increased from only 42 in 1993 to 1,458 in 2015 [1].

4. Controlled donation after cardiac death liver transplant — challenges

4.1. *Ischemic cholangiopathy*

In 2003, the University of Pennsylvania group was the first to report a higher risk of major biliary complications in DCD liver recipients and to caution that DCD biliary epithelium is particularly prone to ischemia-reperfusion injury [14]. Thereafter, enthusiasm for DCD livers has been tempered by widespread experiences of ischemic cholangiopathy, inferior survival, and higher cost after transplant [10, 11, 28–41]. Historically, ischemic cholangiopathy has been reported in 9–50% of DCD recipients [10–15, 33–39]. Ischemic cholangiopathy manifests as biliary strictures and bile cast syndrome, and tends to present within the first few months after transplant (Figure 2).

Ischemic cholangiopathy presents with varying degress of severity. It may resolve with biliary drainage or require repeated long-term endoscopic and/or percutaneous manipulations. One can predict the need for retransplant based on the severity of the bile duct damage. Lee *et al.* studied 44 patients who developed ischemic cholangiopathy after DCD LT [38]. Intrahepatic strictures were defined based on their location and number. Patients with strictures that were described as unilateral focal or at the

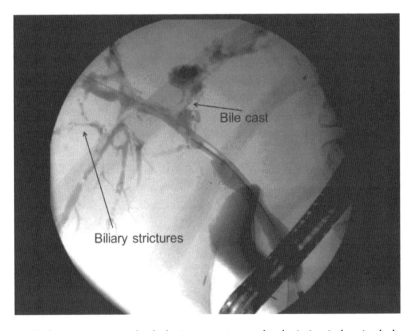

Figure 2. Endoscopic retrograde cholagiopancreatography depicting ischemic cholangiopathy (bile casts and biliary strictures) in a DCD LT recipient.

confluence of the right and left hepatic ducts ($n = 18$) had a good prognosis with percutaneous biliary intervention and none needed retransplantation. In contrast, patients with strictures described as bilateral multifocal ($n = 21$) and diffuse necrosis ($n = 5$) had worse overall outcomes. The authors recommend early retranslpantation in the patients with bilateral multifocal and diffuse biliary necrosis.

In the current Model for End Stage Liver Disease (MELD) score allocation era, retransplantation for DCD LT receipeints with severe ischemic cholangiopathy remains difficult. Ths is due to the fact that despite having severe bile duct damage with occasional bouts of cholangitis; the hepatocellular function in these livers is usually good and thus the physiologic MELD score remains low. UNOS regional review boards are reluctant to grant sufficient MELD exception scores for these patients seeing that their mortality on the wait list is not higher than many others on the transplant list. It is unlikely that the implementation of the new national liver review board will change the current allocation of MELD exception scores for DCD liver recipients with ischemic cholangiopathy. Therefore, patients require prolonged waiting-list time with varying degress of morbidity before being offered another deceased donor liver. This is a major challenge and one that likely contributes to the overall reluctance to transplant DCD livers.

4.2. Inferior results compared with donation after brain death

Numerous single center and pooled registry analyses of controlled DCD LT generally portray outcomes inferior to DBD LT, with patient and graft 1-year survival rates ranging from 74% to 92% and 61% to 87%, respectively [10–15, 28–41]. Review of the SRTR data by Merion *et al.* revealed that, compared with DBD livers, DCD livers carried an adjusted odds ratio for graft failure of 1.85 [30]. A subsequent SRTR review by Merion *et al.* analyzed 1,567 DCD LTs from 2001 through 2009; 3 years post transplant, 64.9% of recipients were alive with functioning grafts, 13.6% required retransplant, and 21.6% died [28]. Since failing DCD livers can survive for an extended period of time, nuanced consideration of intermediate-term graft survival after DCD LT, such as 1-year survival, should account for not only graft losses attributable to death or retransplant but also impending losses in patients with damaged grafts still awaiting retransplant. The 2015 SRTR Annual Report provides updated graft survival outcome curves comparing DCD and DBD liver recipients out to 5 years post transplant (Figure 3) [1]. These analyses demonstrate significantly lower allograft survival for recipients of livers recovered from DCD donors compared to those from DBD donors.

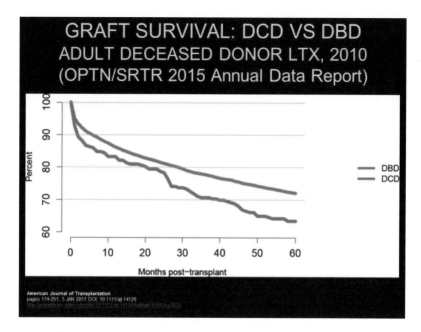

Figure 3.   Graft survival among adult deceased donor LT recipients, 2010, by DCD status. Graft survival estimated using unadjusted Kaplan–Meier methods. DCD, donation after circulatory death; DBD, donation after brain death. (Courtesy of Ref. [42].).

A 2009 report from the Northwestern group revealed that their recipients of DCD livers had a 36% higher incidence of ischemic cholangiopathy compared with their recipients of DBD livers and, primarily for this reason, a 2.1 times greater risk of graft failure and 3.2 times greater risk of retransplant [34]. It is possible that the DCD outcomes of this experienced team are inferior to those reported by other centers because the others were able to use more consistent DCD protocols and stricter selection criteria. For example, the Northwestern group reported variability in the timing of systemic heparinization (before or after withdrawal), location of withdrawal (in or out of the operating room), and source of the donor (local or regional share) for their 32 DCD liver donors. Furthermore, their cohort had a mean age greater than 40 years (43 ± 18) and there was a 9.3% increased odds of ischemic cholangiopathy if the DCD was older than 40 years.

4.3. Costlier liver transplants

The increasing focus on value in healthcare, namely delivery of high-quality and cost-efficient care, has led to several analyses of resource utilization after DCD LT. Both American and European studies bring to bear that DCD, which has the greatest impact on the Donor Risk Index, yields LTs that are costlier than with DBD. Jay *et al.* from the Northwestern group, showed that at their center, higher rates of graft failure and biliary complications translated to increased direct costs for 28 DCD recipients compared with 198 DBD recipients, even after adjustments for recipient MELD score (125.2% of DBD costs, $p = 0.009$) [39]. Singhal *et al.* compared resource use and outcomes of 613 DCD liver allografts with 11,243 DBD liver allografts transplanted from 2007 to 2011, using the University Health System Consortium and SRTR databases [40]. DCD recipients were healthier and had lower MELD scores (17 vs. 19; $p < 0.0001$). Post transplant, there was no difference in length of stay, perioperative mortality, and discharge to home rates. However, DCD allografts were associated with higher direct cost ($110,414 vs. $99,543; $p < 0.0001$), 30-day readmission rate (46.4% vs. 37.1%; $p < 0.0001$), and graft loss.van der Hilst *et al.* prospectively compared cost effectiveness at one year of 89 DCD and 293 DBD LTs at the three Dutch transplant centers between 2004 and 2009 [41]. The cost per life year for DBD was €88,913 compared to €112,376 for DCD, a statistically significant difference, with higher length of stay and complications driving the increased cost of DCD. However, patient and graft survival were similar for DCD and DBD, so the authors advocated for differentiated reimbursement in accordance with the donor source to better accommodate DCD transplantations.

The yield of transplanted livers per donor is markedly lower in the setting of DCD as compared to DBD (Figure 4); in 2015, 27% of DCDs yielded livers that were transplanted as compared to 83% of DBDs in the United States [1]. In the majority of cases of DCD there is no intention to procure the liver for transplant and even when it is procured there is a relatively high discard rate; in 2015 28% of recovered DCD livers were discarded compared to 8% of DBD livers [1]. The significant unease about DCD LT is based upon the resultant cholangiopathy and worse long-term survival; this unease is amplified by centers' and payors' increasing focus on cost of care and by regulatory authorities' oversite of clinical outcomes and rankings [43].

5. Outcomes are improving for donation after cardiac death liver transplantation

Despite lower graft survival seen in DCD LT recipients compared to DBD LTs, recent data suggest that DCD outcomes are improving over time. Of note,

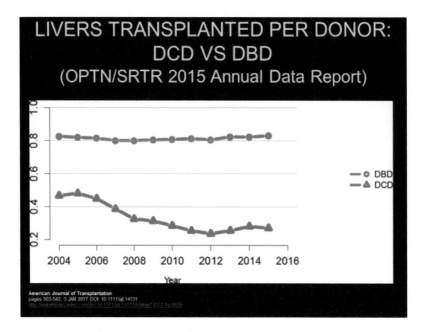

Figure 4. Livers transplanted per donor, by DBD and DCD status. Average number of livers transplanted per donor. Livers divided into segments may account for more than one transplant, the number of livers transplanted may exceed the number recovered. Based on a count of recovered livers that are transplanted, which differs from number of transplant operations. DSA-level means are shown. DSA, donor services area. (Courtesy of the OPTN/SRTR 2015 Annual Data Report: Deceased Organ Donation. Am J Transplant 2017; 17 (Suppl 1): 503–542. doi: 10.1111/ajt.14131. Available at: http://onlinelibrary.wiley.com/doi/10.1111/ajt.14131/full#ajt 14131-fig-0029. Accessed July 1, 2017).

the pooled registry and single center experiences do include cohorts of patients that did well after controlled DCD LT and identify risk factors for worse outcomes. Some single centers that consistently utilize standardized DCD protocols and strict organ selection criteria report excellent results, comparable to DBD LT. DCD LT has not generally resulted in an increased incidence of primary nonfunction (0–12%) or hepatic artery thrombosis (0–9%).

In 2011, the group from Mayo Clinic, Jacksonville, compared 200 DCD LTs to 1,830 DBD transplants [33]. Their patient and graft survivals at 1, 3, and 5 years were not significantly different between DCD and DBD groups. Ischemic cholangiopathy developed in 12% of DCD recipients and half required retransplant. The Mayo group's excellent experience is similar to that reported by Reich *et al.* in their 2006 update; patient and graft survival rates were both 90% at 1 year post transplant and 85% at 2 years; ischemic cholangiopathy developed in 13% of recipients and caused graft failure in 10% [44].

Also in 2011, the King's College group reported their experience with 167 consecutive DCD LTs matched with 333 DBD LTs [45]. No differences in patient and graft survival were found between DBD and DCD recipients at 1, 3, and 5 years. Overall biliary complication rates were similar between the groups (DCD vs. DBD: 19.7% vs. 12.5%; $p = 0.09$). The greatest number of biliary complications that occurred in the DCD group were anastomotic stricture ($n = 16$) and bile leak ($n = 5$). The remainder of biliary complications in the DCD group included nonanastomotic strictures ($n = 2$), ischemic cholangiopathy ($n = 4$) and others ($n = 2$).

In 2016, the Indianapolis group described their experience in significantly reducing their rate of DCD cholangiopathy to zero by optimizing the modifiable risk factors of cold ischemia time, recipient warm ischemia time and the use of thrombolytic flush at the time of procurement [46].

The Oschner Clinic group reported their results of 138 DCD LTs over a 12-year period after modifying multiple steps in their protocol in an attempt to attain better outcomes [47]. They compared a more recent group, 2010–2015 ($n = 100$) to an earlier group, 2003–2010 ($n = 38$). When compared to similar cohort of 435 DBD LT recipients who received a transplant between 2013 and 2016, the early cohort of DCD had lower patient and graft survival compared to DBD recipients. However, the later cohort of DCD recipients had no differences in patient of graft survival compared to the DBD group. In addition, the rate of ischemic type biliary strictures in the recipients was 5% in the early group and 3% in the more recent group.

Croome *et al.* studied the UNOS database to determine if DCD LT outcomes were different over three separate eras between 2003 and 2014 [48]. The eras were divided up into 4-year periods: 2003–2006 (Era 1), 2007–2010 (Era 2), and 2011–2014 (Era 3). Improvements in graft survival were seen between Era 1 and Era 2 and between Era 2 and Era 3. Multivariate analysis that included standard predictors of graft survival revealed Era 2 and Era 3 had a protective effect on graft survival compared to Era 1.

6. Strategies to improve the outcomes of controlled donation after cardiac death liver transplant

6.1. *Young donors, hemodynamically stable donors, short ischemia times, and select recipients yield better results with donation after cardiac death liver transplant*

Two 2006 SRTR analyses of DCD LT focused on risk factors for graft failure. Lee *et al.* showed that a low risk DCD cohort provided similar outcomes to those after DBD; the low risk criteria were donor age less than 45 years, cold ischemia time less than 10 hours and warm ischemia time less than 15 minutes [31]. Mateo *et al.* similarly identified donor risk factors for poor outcome after DCD (warm ischemia time over 30 minutes, cold ischemia time over 10 hours) and also found recipient risk factors, including retransplant, being on life support pre transplant and having a serum creatinine over 2.0 mg/dL. Low-risk DCD grafts transplanted into low-risk recipients provided favorable outcomes, similar to those after DBD [32]. Some advise against using livers from DCDs more than 40–60 years old because they are particularly vulnerable to biliary ischemia and graft loss [11, 14, 35, 49], but others have shown that, selectively, they can provide good outcomes [12, 13, 31, 33, 44, 49].

In their single-center DCD LT anaylsis, the Denver group identified that preoperative donor risk factors for cholangiopathy, included not only age, but also red-cell transfusion, multiple vasopressors use, lower preoperative hemoglobin and lower preoperative oxygen saturation; these were additional to the risk of longer durations of postextubation hypotension, hypoxemia, and time to asystole [49]. Their findings bring to bear that an already ischemic biliary system may be particularly vulnerable subsequent to DCD and transplant.

When deciding on whether to transplant a procured DCD organ, one needs to assess the impact of the various ischemia time intervals (Figure 5). Controlled DCD LT may carry increased risk in the face of true warm ischemia time — the interval between significant (variably defined) hypotension or hypoxemia, and initiation of perfusion — up to and perhaps somewhat beyond 20–30 minutes [12, 13, 44]. Total warm ischemia time — the interval between discontinuation of mechanical ventilation and initiation of perfusion — may extend up to and perhaps somewhat beyond 30–45 minutes [22, 50]. In the Mayo Clinic experience, each minute increase in the asystole-to-cross-clamp duration was associated with a 16.1% increased odds of ischemic cholangiopathy [33]. The risk from DCD livers is lowest when cold ischemia time is kept below 6 hours [28] and is minimized when it is kept below 6–10 hours [22, 50]. In Merion *et al.*'s 2010 SRTR analysis of DCD LT, each hour increase in cold ischemia time was associated with a 6% higher graft failure rate and cold ischemia time between 6 hours and 10 hours was associated with a 64% higher graft failure risk compared to cold ischemia time less than 6 hours [28].

Other factors that may be relevant to the better outcomes with DCD LT at some centers include donor surgeon experience and specifics of the individual DCD protocols such as use and timing of anticoagulant and/or

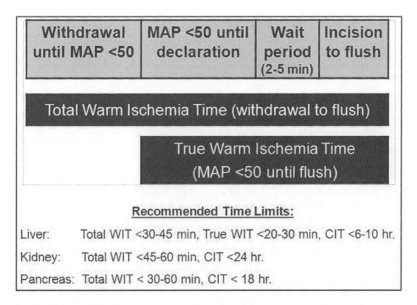

Withdrawal until MAP <50	MAP <50 until declaration	Wait period (2-5 min)	Incision to flush

Total Warm Ischemia Time (withdrawal to flush)

True Warm Ischemia Time (MAP <50 until flush)

Recommended Time Limits:

Liver: Total WIT <30-45 min, True WIT <20-30 min, CIT <6-10 hr.

Kidney: Total WIT <45-60 min, CIT <24 hr.

Pancreas: Total WIT < 30-60 min, CIT < 18 hr.

Figure 5. Recommended ischemia time limits for controlled DCD LT. MAP <50, a drop in mean arterial pressure below 50 mm Hg, is defined by the author as marking the development of significant hypotension and the start of the true warm ischemia time (this point in time is variably defined by others).

vasodilator, withdrawal of support in or out of the operating room, and duration of the wait time between declaration of death and start of surgery [33, 34]. A 2008 SRTR analysis by Selck *et al.* demonstrated higher graft failure within the first 180 days with convergence thereafter; the DCD allografts were more frequently imported from another allocation region [29]. DCD liver biopsies can exclude use of grafts with centrilobular necrosis, steatosis, or other histologic predictors of poor quality.

6.2. *Biliary protection*

The following additional tactics may be considered in an effort to reduce biliary problems after DCD LT: performance of an expeditious *in situ* biliary flush to minimize bile-induced epithelial damage [22, 44], arterial revascularization before or simultaneously with portal revascularization [14, 22], use of a t-tube to facilitate frequent interrogation of the ducts and early intervention to dredge sludge and dilate strictures before casting occurs [22], and liberal use of prophylactic bile acid (ursodeoxycholate) after transplant.

Fung *et al.* first recommended using a thrombolytic in addition to an anticoagulant to decrease periductular microvascular thrombosis and ischemic cholangiopathy after DCD [51, 52]. They attribute their low incidence of ischemic biliary disease after DCD LT to injection of tPA into the donor hepatic artery during the back-table preparation of the allograft. They also use HTK preservation solution rather than the more viscous and particulate University of Wisconsin (UW) solution, to further decrease periductular microvascular thrombosis [51, 52]. However, in a UNOS database analysis by Stewart *et al.*, published in 2009, HTK was associated with an increased risk of graft loss, especially for DCD allografts, when compared to UW preservation [53]. Further analyses need to be performed in order support the notion that increased viscosity of UW solution increases the risk if ischemic cholangiopathy in DCD LT.

Since this previous study advocating for the tPA use in DCD LTs, two additional papers have assessed the effects of using tPA in preventing ischemic cholangiopathy. Seal *et al.* combined data from two institutions, University of Toronto and the Oschner Clinic, to determine the impact of hepatic arterial injection of tPA in DCD LTs. A group of 85 patients who received tPA was compared to 33 DCD liver recipients who did not receive tPA. The doses of tPA and the timing of injection in the recipient were different between the two centers. There was a trend toward lower rates of total biliary strictures in the tPA group compared to control. There were significalty lower rates of diffuse intrahepatic strictures in the tPA group [54].

Subsequently, Bohorquez *et al.* reported the aforementioned Oschner experience; giving DCD liver recipients intraoperative heparin, verapamil, and tPA, and postoperative ASA, was associated with significantly better allograft survival [47]. Because mulitple changes were made in the DCD liver protocol in this study, the true impact of tPA on DCD LT outcomes could not be proven.

The question that remains to be answered is whether DCD livers have an increased risk for microthombi formation compared to DBD livers. A recent study compared biopsies between DCD and DBD livers to answer these questions [55]. Two hundred and eighty-two sections were obtained from 16 discarded DCD livers to assess for the presence of microthrombi. Sections were triple stained with hematoxylin and eosin (H and E), Von Willebrand Factor (VWF), and Fibirn Lendrum (FL) to evaluate the presence of microthrombi. Microthrombi were present in only 1–3% of the VWF stainings without evidence of thrombus formation in paired H and E and FL stainings. An additional analysis of DBD and DCD livers that were transplanted showed no difference in microthrombi formation between the groups and no relationship to the development of ischemic cholangiopathy. Identifying the true etiologic factors that contribute to ischemic cholangiopathy is critical in order to maximize the utilization of these organs. Halldorson *et al.*'s multivariable analysis of a single-center experience with DCD LT showed that recipients induced with antithymocyte globulin as compared with basiliximab had a lower incidence of ischemic cholangiopathy (12.5% vs. 35.2%, $p = 0.011$) and improved 1-year survival (96.1% vs. 75.9%, $p = 0.013$) [56]. They postulated that T cell depletion ameliorates the warm ischemia/inflammation/biliary fibrosis pathway.

6.3. *Recipient selection*

Recipient risk factors for better outcomes after DCD LT have also been identified. Younger, hemodynamically stable, and technically less challenging recipients generally fair better with DCD livers than do other recipients. These may include recipients of primary transplants, those with no previous major upper abdominal surgery, and anticipated uncomplicated transplants that do not require arterial of venous jump grafts for vascular in flow. This is likely related to the importance of keeping cold ischemia time short and placing the liver into a hemodynamically favorable environment to protect against additional ischemia. Severe postreperfusion syndrome has been seen in recipients of DCD LT and thus patients with significant coronary artery disease whose cardiac reserve may be limited are excluded from DCD transplants at some centers. DCD LT is not well suited for patients who would be ill equipped to deal with the burden of biliary complications (increased hospital visits and interventions, percutaneous tubes), such as patients who live far from the transplant center and/or have poor social support.

The risk–benefit ratio of DCD LT is improved if donor and recipient risk factors are not compounded. The current MELD allocation and distribution system creates regional disparities in the utilization of DCD livers in that transplant centers in less competitive organ procurement organizations (OPOs) can select ideal recipients for DCD livers whereas centers in more competitive OPOs must typically accept DCD liver offers for candidates high on the match runs or lose access to the offers. Additional understanding of the various risk factors and risk interactions is needed.

Some groups advise caution when considering whether to use a DCD liver for a PSC patient. A UNOS database analysis showed DCD transplant incrementally reduced graft survival time in PSC patients, compared to non-PSC patients [57]. Another multicenter group identified a significantly higher risk of intrahepatic biliary strictures in DCD recipients who underwent a Roux-en-Y hepaticojejunostomy for the bile duct anastomosis; they hypothesized that increased exposure of the DCD ischemic bile ducts to the gut microbiome and toxins in the setting of a Roux-en-Y hepaticojejunostomy may aggravate the biliary damage [58].

After the implementation of Share 35 policy, more patients with HCC have been receiving livers from ECD and DCD donors and waiting-list mortality for LT candidates with HCC has increased [59]. Some previous studies have suggested that transplanting DCD livers into patients with HCC may have a deleterious effect on long-term outcome due to increased HCC recurrence [60]. However, more recent analyses suggest that DCD LT in itself does not increase the risk of HCC recurrence compared to DBD LT [61] or impact cancer-related survival [62]. With low physiologic MELD scores and HCC exception scores, DCD LT appears to be a good option for patients with HCC provided that the risk of cholangiopathy remains low.

7. Donation after cardiac death practice guidelines

DCD protocols and techniques vary among OPOs and transplant centers. Best practice guidelines for DCD organ procurement and transplant are available and cover many aspects of the endeavor, including donor criteria, consent, withdrawal of support, operative technique, ischemia times, recipient considerations, and biliary issues. In 2009, Reich and colleagues published evidence-based recommendations on controlled DCD on behalf of the ASTS [22]. The ASTS recommendations attempt to address the unique challenges posed by DCD organ procurement and transplant and to facilitate improvement in outcomes. They complement guidelines published earlier by UNOS [23–25], the IOM [16–18], the Society of Critical Care Medicine [26], and in a multiorganization national conference report [49].

8. Ethicolegal issues and professionalism

8.1. *Basic principles*

DCD organ procurement honors the donor's wishes, brings some comfort to the family, and benefits the recipients. However, as DCD develops, relevant ethical and logistical issues have stimulated scrutiny, discussion and debate among lay and medical communities. The IOM's original study of

DCD was organized partly in response to a well-publicized, controversial 1997 60 minutes CBS television report that negatively portrayed DCD initiatives and led to public skepticism about organ donation in general [16]. Some ethicolegal principles pertinent to DCD include the following: individuals may not be killed for their organs or killed as a result of the removal of their organs (the "dead donor" rule), patients must not be jeopardized in order to facilitate organ procurement, euthanasia is prohibited, informed consent and respect for family wishes must not be violated, and the autonomous right of patients to refuse treatment must be upheld [6, 16, 22, 26, 63–66]. It is imperative to ensure that there is no conflict of interest between the duty to provide optimal patient care and the desire to recover organs for transplant [22, 64–66]. Specifically, the rationale for withdrawal of life support and the determination of death must be extricable from the decision to recover organs. Therefore, the patient care and organ donor teams need to be completely separate.

Even though DCD procurement is often hectic, the donor surgical team should behave courteously and respectfully at the donor facility. The risks and benefits of DCD organ transplant, including the possibility and implications of biliary complications, should be discussed with transplant candidates during the transplant evaluation process [22].

8.2. Donation after cardiac death from executed prisoners is a violation of human rights

There are numerous reports of violations of human rights and international ethics standards in the organ procurement practices in China [67, 68]. Over 90% of the organs transplanted in China before 2010 were procured from prisoners. International condemnation led Chinese officials in December 2014 to announce that the country would completely cease using organs harvested from prisoners. However, there are reports that organs from executed prisoners are still being used for transplant in China. A major loophole exits in that prisoner donation with written consent, notwithstanding the coercive context, is classified by the Chinese government as voluntary citizen donation rather than prisoner donation. The international community has called for additional reforms of organ donation in China, including Chinese laws that specifically outlaw use of prisoner organs even if consent is obtained, and these reforms prohibit procurement of organs from incompletely executed, still-living prisoners — reportedly still performed at some Chinese hospitals.

8.3. *Controversial ethics topics*

Several issues related to the ethics and laws of DCD organ procurement remain sources of debate. Interventions that improve the chance of successful donation rather than directly benefiting the donor are permitted, as long as they are consensual, do not hasten death or harm the donor, and are not prohibited by the local procurement protocol. That said, there are differing views regarding use of anticoagulants, vasodilators, and intravascular cannulae placed *premortem* [18, 22, 24–26, 50, 65]. Medications routinely provided for patient comfort are permitted even if they might hasten death; these are given at the discretion of the patient's treating care team and procurement team members shall not participate in decisions regarding the use of such agents [22, 26, 50]. A highly publicized lawsuit involved the professional behavior of a surgeon who became involved in administration of narcotic and anxiolytic during an attempted DCD [69].

Another issue that is debated is whether determination of death for a DCD requires loss of cardiac electrical activity or if absence of heart sounds, pulse, and blood pressure are sufficient criteria, just as it is for patients who are not organ donors [6, 17]. Ultimately, the donor hospital and care team have the responsibility for defining and declaring patient death. Another important ethical question that impacts upon the warm ischemic time endured by DCD organs relates to the duration of the waiting period used to assure irreversible death. Autoresuscitation after 1 minute of pulselessness has not been reported in the literature [64]. However, different waiting times from circulatory arrest to initiation of organ procurement surgery have been prescribed by various groups, ranging from 2 minutes to 10 minutes [16–18, 22, 26, 50, 63–65]. The ASTS recommends 2 minutes [22], the Society of Critical Care Medicine recommends 2–5 minutes [26] and the IOM recommends 5 minutes [16–18].

9. Identifying appropriate candidates for potential donation after cardiac death

9.1. *Donation after brain death is preferable to donation after cardiac death*

Enthusiasm about the option of DCD ought to be tempered by the realization that both the yield of transplantable organs from DCDs and the outcomes of DCD organ transplants are not generally as favorable as with DBDs. Therefore, when it seems that DBD will be possible, DCD should not be viewed as an equally acceptable alternative. A potential organ donor's family and healthcare providers should be encouraged to wait for completion of a brain death protocol when brain death seems present or imminent. This approach is important even if brain death protocols might be viewed as cumbersome at a time when hospitals are increasingly pressed to empty critical care beds and transplant professionals strive to expedite organ donation.

9.2. *Organ procurement organization efforts*

Potential DCDs are identified by mandatory referral of dying patients to the OPO, pursuant to local state laws [27]. DCD can provide genuine expansion of the donor pool if DBD is not feasible. Such situations include a request for withdrawal of life support when there is catastrophic injury and either brain death is not imminent or a brain death protocol is precluded because of hemodynamic instability or a family's absolute refusal to wait. Strong OPO initiatives are crucial for increasing DCD and certain OPOs have developed highly successful DCD programs [27, 70]; in 2016, 16% of the deceased donors that yielded transplants from the Gift of Life Donor Program OPO of the Delaware Valley donor service area involved DCD (77/473) [71]. There have been attempts to develop a system that predicts the time to cardiac death after withdrawal of support from a particular potential DCD, to help identify when it is worth pursuing organ donation, but no model has performed reliably [72].

10. Preoperative maneuvers and operative strategy for donation after cardiac death organ procurement

10.1. *Preparation*

The DCD protocol used by the author and those at other programs in our OPO is summarized in Table 36–1. The donor surgery should be performed by a surgeon who is familiar with the ethics and laws of DCD, knows the OPO DCD protocol and is experienced in rapid procurement techniques. Communication between the DCD surgeon and the donor coordinator(s) and operating room personnel about conduct of the operation, prior to withdrawal of support, facilitates cooperation and speediness of the recovery. Upon withdrawal of support, a flow sheet should be filled out by a coordinator in the operating room, documenting hemodynamic measurements every minute and the times of discontinuation of mechanical ventilation, cessation of cardiorespiratory function, waiting period, declaration of death, incision, and perfusion of each organ (Figure 6). After procurement, this information is critical for assessing ischemic injury [22, 25, 50].

GIFT OF LIFE DONOR PROGRAM

TITLE: Operating Room Donation After Cardiac Death Flow Sheet

Patient Name________________ UNOS#________________

INTRAOPERATIVE MANAGEMENT

Blood Drawn	Date___/___/___	Time___:___	(EST)
Heparin Administered	Date___/___/___	Time___:___	(EST)
Entered OR	Date___/___/___	Time___:___	(EST)
Withdrawal of Support	Date___/___/___	Time___:___	(EST)
Pronouncement	Date___/___/___	Time___:___	(EST)
Incision	Date___/___/___	Time___:___	(EST)
Cross-Clamp	Date___/___/___	Time___:___	(EST)

Time From Withdrawal to Pronouncement ________minutes

Time From Pronouncement to Cross-Clamp ________minutes

Total Warm Ischemic Time (withdrawal to cross-clamp) ________minutes

Flush Solution ______ 1st Liter in @____:____ Total Flush ________cc

Family Present for Withdrawal ☐ Yes ☐ No Location of Withdrawal ☐ OR ☐ ICU ☐ PACU ☐ Other__________

Care and Comfort Administered ☐ Yes ☐ No Was Patient Extubated ☐ Yes ☐ No

START TIME____:____ **HEMODYNAMIC MEASUREMENTS**

	@ Start	Min 1	Min 2	Min 3	Min 4	Min 5	Min 6	Min 7	Min 8	Min 9	Min 10	Min 11	Min 12	Min 13	Min 14	Min 15	Min 16	Min 17	Min 18	Min 19
HR																				
BP																				
RR																				
SPO2																				
	Min 20	Min 21	Min 22	Min 23	Min 24	Min 25	Min 26	Min 27	Min 28	Min 29	Min 30	Min 31	Min 32	Min 33	Min 34	Min 35	Min 36	Min 37	Min 38	Min 39
HR																				
BP																				
RR																				
SPO2																				
	Min 40	Min 41	Min 42	Min 43	Min 44	Min 45	Min 46	Min 47	Min 48	Min 49	Min 50	Min 51	Min 52	Min 53	Min 54	Min 55	Min 56	Min 57	Min 58	Min 59
HR																				
BP																				
RR																				
SPO2																				

Figure 6. Gift of Life Donor program DCD operating room flow sheet. (Courtesy of Ref. [71].)

10.2. *Super-rapid surgical technique*

Most surgeons who procure DCD organs use some modification of the super-rapid technique described by the Pittsburgh group [7, 9, 22, 73, 74]. Ideally, patients undergo withdrawal of support in the operating room. Otherwise, transporting the DCD to the operating room after declaration of death may exclude subsequent LT because of excessive hepatic ischemia. To minimize operating and ischemic times, the potential donor should be prepared and draped prior to withdrawal of support. Instruments for rapid entry and aortic cannulation should be chosen, as depicted (Figure 7). The cannula and tubing should be flushed and placed on the field, maintaining the containers of preservation solution in an ice bucket to prevent warming. During this prepping and draping it is critical to recognize that the potential DCD donor is a patient who is still alive. Comfort care is provided at the discretion of the patient's care team, without any involvement of the donor team.

According to most OPO DCD protocols, heparin and a vasodilator are administered. Following the above preparatory maneuvers the surgical team

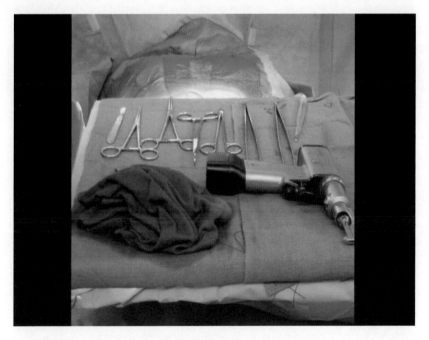

Figure 7. Example of instruments for rapid entry and aortic cannulation; to minimize operating time, the potential donor should be prepared and draped prior to withdrawal of support (instruments include a scalpel, a pair of kocher clamps, a moist towel, metzenbaum scissors, a right-angle clamp, a moist umbilical tape, two kelly clamps, a sternal saw, abdominal and sternal retractors, and a flushed cannula and tubing connected to preservation solution in an ice bucket).

should exit the operating room and wait until potential procurement, to avoid conflict of interest during withdrawal of support and declaration of death. The family can be given the opportunity to be present after the surgical team leaves, until cessation of cardiorespiratory function. If the patient is not declared dead within the time frame stipulated by the local procurement protocol, then donation is aborted and the patient is returned to the ward for comfort care [16, 22, 24, 25]; in the rare instances that this occurred in our OPO, the patient always expired within the next few hours.

Postmortem, a midline laparotomy is performed. Upward traction on two Kocher clamps placed on each side of the umbilicus expedites rapid entry without injury to the viscera. A large scalpel is used to incise all layers of the abdominal wall. A moist towel is used to retract the small intestine to the right while the sigmoid colon is retracted to the left. Although not pulsatile, the aorta is easily palpated just above its bifurcation on the left side of the vertebral column. Metzenbaum scissors are used to clear the retroperitoneum over a small segment of distal aorta in preparation for cannulation. There is no need to dissect out the inferior mesenteric artery. A right-angle clamp is used to pass a moist umbilical tape around the distal aorta, which will be used to secure the cannula. Distally, the aorta is clamped with a Kelly clamp. Next, the cannula is passed cephalad through an aortotomy and secured with the umbilical tape. The flush should be started immediately at this point, without waiting to cross-clamp the proximal aorta or vent the vena cava Using this approach, flush is typically initiated within 2–3 minutes of incision.

The surgeon should not be disturbed to see a dark, purple, and somewhat engorged liver at initial inspection, as this is the typical appearance of a DCD liver. Assessment of liver quality is best left until after perfusion, at which point the liver should appear normal. Next, the round and falciform ligaments are divided sharply. The knife is used to open from the suprasternal notch to the abdomen. Median sternotomy is performed with a pneumatic saw and a Finochietto sternal retractor is placed. It is this author's preference to clamp the thoracic rather than supraceliac aorta during superrapid procurement. The descending thoracic aorta can be easily accessed through the left thoracic cavity just above the diaphragm. The vena cava is vented above the diaphragm. A Balfour retractor is placed across the upper abdomen. Ice slush should be placed on the abdominal organs simultaneously with the sternotomy. Approximately 5 L of cold UW solution, containing dexamethasone 16 mg/L and insulin 40 U/L, is infused through the adult DCD aorta. In order to provide a clear effluent, 1 L is used before sternotomy, cross-clamping, and venting, and then 4 L afterward. Approximately twice this volume is necessary when using histidine–tryptophan–ketoglutarate (HTK) solution.

Since all the visceral dissection is performed in the cold, without blood flow and without having had opportunity to assess pulses, particular care must be taken not to damage vital structures. The hepatoduodenal ligament is divided from right to left as close to the duodenum as possible, taking care to preserve the hepatic artery. First, the common bile duct is divided and the biliary tree flushed with chilled preservation solution through an opening in the gallbladder and through the common duct directly. Expeditious performance of this maneuver may reduce bile-induced epithelial damage and ischemic cholangiopathy following DCD LT. The portal vein is divided at the confluence of the superior mesenteric and splenic veins. The gastroduodenal and right gastric arteries need not be clearly delineated.

The left-lateral segment of the liver is elevated by dividing the left triangular ligament. It is safest to assume that there is a replaced or accessory left hepatic artery arising from the left gastric artery. Therefore, the lesser omentum and left gastric artery should be separated from the lesser curvature at the level of the stomach. The splenic artery is divided to the left of the midline, far from the celiac axis, and then dissected toward the aorta, so that it can be rotated to the right for exposure of the superior mesenteric artery, which lies deep to it.

Unless the plan is to procure the DCD pancreas, discussed below, the head of the pancreas should be taken with the liver to avoid transecting an aberrant right hepatic artery and to expedite organ extraction time. After a Kocher's maneuver, the duodenum and pancreatic head are elevated and retracted caudally to expose the superior mesenteric artery which is then dissected down to the aorta. Care is taken not to transect an accessory or replaced right hepatic artery by avoiding dissection on the right side of the superior mesenteric artery. Rather than taking extra time to search for a right branch, it is safest to assume that one exists and to take a common patch of superior mesenteric and celiac arteries with the liver. An aortotomy is performed between the superior mesenteric and right renal arteries and extended to provide the arterial patch.

The left diaphragm is then divided down toward the Carrel patch. The suprahepatic inferior vena cava is divided. The right diaphragm is then divided down to the upper pole of the right kidney. The infrahepatic inferior vena cava is then transected just above the renal veins. The liver is extricated and immediate back-table portal flush with 1 L of chilled UW solution is performed; some cannulate and flush the portal system *in situ* via the inferior mesenteric vein. It is particularly important to perform back-table inspection and trimming of the DCD liver well in advance of the recipient surgery, to ensure that it is safe to transplant the organ.

Adding whole-organ pancreatectomy to hepatectomy during a superrapid recovery carries risk for transecting an aberrant right hepatic artery because there is no opportunity to palpate arterial pulsations in the DCD. Meticulous *in situ* dissection in search of a right branch can significantly increase extraction time. Therefore, the DCD liver is typically removed with the pancreatic head to avoid injuring an aberrant right hepatic artery. We do not routinely procure DCD whole pancreata when procuring DCD livers, unless there is favorable donor body habitus, short warm ischemia time and other aspects of the individual case are optimal [75]. Alternatively, the liver and pancreas may be removed *en bloc*.

Bilateral nephrectomies may be performed after hepatectomy. The kidneys can be kept *en bloc* for machine perfusion, or separated and sent directly to the recipient centers. Even though DCD organ procurement is a rushed procedure, it is still crucial to perform careful donor exploration in an effort to discern the possibility of unrecognized malignancy or infection.

10.3. *Premortem cannulation technique, with or without extracorporeal membrane oxygenation*

The *premortem* cannulation technique, described by Groth and colleagues in Stockholm, Sweden [76] decreases the rush inherent with the super rapid recovery technique and may decrease warm ischemia time, particularly if withdrawal of support is performed outside the operating room. The technique requires consensual, pre-extubation (*premortem*) femoral vessel cannulation [16–18, 22, 24, 25, 50]. Femoral artery and femoral vein cannulae are inserted under local anesthesia. After declaration of death, cold preservation solution is immediately infused via the femoral artery cannula and the femoral vein cannula is opened to gravity to decompress the venous system. Thereafter, median sternotomy and midline abdominal incisions are made and the intra-abdominal organs are topically ice cooled and then removed *en bloc* or separately. One modification of this technique is to perform the femoral vessel dissection under local anesthesia without *premortem* cannulation. If the patient expires in the required time frame, then rapid *postmortem* cannulation of the femoral vessels is performed. This approach, which is currently used by the Universtiy of Wisconsin group, avoids femoral vessel intervention in cases where the donor does not progress to death in the required time frame.

The University of Michigan group and others use *premortem* cannulation in conjunction with *postmortem*, normothermic ECMO to restore the flow of warm oxygenated blood to the intra-abdominal organs during the interval between death and organ procurement [77]. This technique is also known as extracorporeal support and as normothermic regional perfusion (NRP). Not only does it facilitate unhurried procurement, it may also improve graft function. To prevent resumption of circulation to the heart and brain, an occlusion balloon catheter is introduced in the contralateral femoral artery and inflated in the descending aorta. Their most recently published report demonstrates successful use of ECMO in 37 controlled DCD recoveries. Thirteen livers were successfully transplanted. One- and two-year graft survival rates were 85.7% and 71.4%, respectively. Biliary strictures and primary nonfunction (PNF) were reported in one patient each (14.7%) [78].

This use of NRP in the donor after the declaration of death has been reported in other European centers more recently. In a recent report from the United Kingdom, NRP was used in 21 controlled DCD donors [79]. Eleven livers were transplanted and only one pateient sustained primary nonfunction. The first week median peak ALT was 389 IU/L. In Italy, DeCarlis *et al.* started the first Italian series of DCD LT using NRP in six uncontrolled and one controlled DCD donor [80]. *Ex vivo* hypothermic machine perfusion was also used in select cases to decrease the effects of static cold storage. Patient and graft survival were 100% after a mean follow up of 6.1 months and there were no cases of ischemic cholangiopathy in the group. The first Spanish series of using NRP in controlled DCD was reported recently. Minambres *et al.* performed abdominal NRP to resotre blood flow before organ recovery in 27 controlled DCD donors [81]. Eleven DCD livers were recovered and transplanted. The 1-year graft survival was 91% with no cases of ischemic cholangiopathy. The authors concluded that regional NRP in DCD donors is feasible and may lead to better outcomes after DCD LT. More studies are necessary to truly ascertain the benefit of NRP in DCD LT.

11. Donation after cardiac death liver transplant research and the potential of *ex vivo* machine perfusion

A major focus of DCD LT research involves preservation methods to decrease the ischemic insult of DCD. In renal transplant, pulsatile *ex vivo*

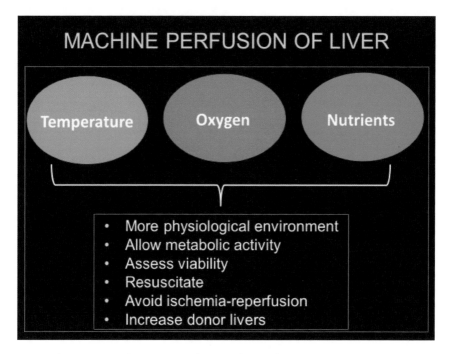

Figure 8.   The promise of *ex vivo* machine perfusion for donor liver preservation, assessment, and resuscitation.

machine perfusion of kidneys is used to reduce delayed graft function DGF and improve outcomes. In LT, the current paradigm of static hypothermic preservation may eventually change to dynamic, *ex vivo* machine perfusion. This approach reduces hypothermic injury; permits oxygenation, recharging of adenosine triphosphate (ATP) cellular energy stores and further reconditioning of donor livers; enables other treatments to potentially resuscitate the liver; and allows for testing to predict which livers are likely to perform well (Figure 8). Such benefits are particularly appealing to apply to DCD livers, given the thought that the DCD warm ischemic insult depletes ATP and makes the liver, particularly the biliary tree, prone to damage from the second ischmic injury of reperfusion. Multicenter trials and smaller efforts are attempting to assess machine perfusion for DCD and other extended criteria livers, and whether hypothermic or normothermic preservation is better for reducing the ischemia-reperfusion injury and cholangiopathy. Chapter 4 is fully dedicated to the topic of machine perfusion of the liver. Other areas of research relate to the use of thrombolytic for DCD LT, the risks, benefits, utility, and costs of DCD LT, and organ allocation policy for retransplant of recipients with failed DCD livers.

12. Conclusions

DCD has been embraced by various professional societies and federal governmental agencies in many countries as an effective way to deal with the shortage of transplantable organs. Ideally, patients who are brain dead, or will likely soon become so, should donate organs according to brain death protocols because the yield of transplantable organs from DCDs and outcomes of DCD LT are generally not as favorable as with heartbeating donors. The increased risk of ischemic cholangiopathy after DCD LT can be mitigated by adherence to recommended best practice DCD protocols, careful selection of DCD organs and recipients, and rapid procurement by surgeons familiar with DCD operative techniques. The current agenda of those working to advance the field of DCD LT involves further identification of risk factors for graft failure after transplant and research into organ preservation methods to decrease the ischemic insult of DCD.

References

1. Organ Procurement and Transplantation Network (OPTN) and Scientific Registry of Transplant Recipients (SRTR). OPTN/SRTR 2015 Annual Data Report. Rockville, MD: Department of Health and Human Services, Health Resources and Services Administration; 2016. Available at: https://srtr.transplant.hrsa.gov/annual_reports/Default.aspx. Accessed July 1, 2017.
2. Annual report. Eurotransplant International Foundation, 2015. Available at: http://www.eurotransplant.org/cms/mediaobject.php?file=AR_ET_20153.pdf. Accessed July 1, 2017.
3. Blasi A, Hessheimer AJ, Beltrán J, *et al*. Liver transplant from unexpected donation after circulatory determination of death donors: a challenge in perioperative management. *Am J Transplant* 2016;16:1901–08.
4. A definition of irreversible coma: report of the Ad Hoc Committee of the Harvard Medical School to Examine the Definition of Brain Death. *JAMA* 1968;205:337–40.
5. UDODA — Guidelines for the determination of death: report of the medical consultants on the diagnosis of death to the President's Commission for the Study of Ethical Problems in Medical and Biomedical and Behavioral Research. *JAMA* 1981;246:2184–86.
6. DeVita MA, Vukmir R, Snyder JV, *et al*. Procuring organs from a non-heartbeating cadaver: a case report. *Kennedy Inst Ethics J* 1993;3:371–85.
7. Casavilla A, Ramirez C, Shapiro R, *et al*. Experience with liver and kidney allografts from non-heartbeating donors. *Transplantation* 1995;59:197–203.
8. D'Alessandro AM, Hoffmann RM, Knechtle SJ, *et al*. Successful extrarenal transplantation from non-heartbeating donors. *Transplantation* 1995;59:977–82.

9. Reich DJ, Munoz SJ, Rothstein KD, *et al.* Controlled non-heart-beating donor liver transplantation: a successful single center experience, with topic update. *Transplantation* 2000;70:1159–66.

10. Abt PL, Desai NM, Crawford MD, *et al.* Survival following liver transplantation from non-heart-beating donors. *Ann Surg* 2004;239:87–92.

11. Foley DP, Fernandez LA, Leverson G, *et al.* Donation after cardiac death: the University of Wisconsin experience with liver transplantation. *Ann Surg* 2005;242:724–31.

12. Muiesan P, Girlanda R, Jassem W, *et al.* Single-center experience with liver transplantation from controlled non-heartbeating donors: a viable source of grafts. *Ann Surg* 2005;242:732–38.

13. Fukumori T, Kato T, Levi D, *et al.* Use of older controlled non-heart-beating donors for liver transplantation. *Transplantation* 2003;75:1171–74.

14. Abt P, Crawford M, Desai N, *et al.* Liver transplantation from controlled non-heart-beating donors: an increased incidence of biliary complications. *Transplantation* 2003;75:1659–63.

15. Manzarbeitia CY, Ortiz JA, Jeon H, *et al.* Long-term outcome of controlled non-heartbeating donor liver transplantation. *Transplantation* 2004;78:211–15.

16. Institute of Medicine, National Academy of Sciences. *Non-Heart-Beating Organ Transplantation: Medical and Ethical Issues in Procurement.* Washington, DC: National Academies Press, 1997.

17. Institute of Medicine, National Academy of Sciences. *Non-Heart-Beating Organ Transplantation: Practice and Protocols.* Washington, DC: National Academies Press, 2000.

18. Institute of Medicine, National Academy of Sciences. *Organ Donation: Opportunities for Action.* Washington, DC: National Academies Press, 2006.

19. Health Resources and Services Administration, Department of Health and Human Services. The donation and transplantation community of practice. January 28, 2010. Available at: http://www.healthcarecommunities.org/SearchResult.aspx?searchtext=DCD%20transplant. Accessed June 13, 2013.

20. Joint Commission on Accreditation of Healthcare Organizations. Health care at the crossroads: Strategies for narrowing the organ donation gap and protecting patients. June 2004. Available at: http://www.jointcommission.org/assets/1/18/organ_donation_white_paper.pdf. Accessed June 13, 2013.

21. Centers for Medicare and Medicaid Services (CMS), Department of Health and Human Services. Medicare and Medicaid Programs: conditions for coverage for organ procurement organizations (OPOs). Final rule. *Fed Regist* 2006;71:30981–1054.

22. Reich DJ, Mulligan DC, Abt PL, *et al.* ASTS recommended practice guidelines for controlled donation after cardiac death organ procurement and transplantation. *Am J Transplant* 2009;9:2004–11.

23. United Network of Organ Sharing. *Donation after Cardiac Death: A Reference Guide.* Richmond, VA: UNOS, 2004.

24. Attachment III to Appendix B of the OPTN [Organ Procurement and Transplantation Network] Bylaws. Model Elements for Controlled DCD Recovery Protocols. [Updated March 23, 2007] Available at: http://optn.transplant. hrsa.gov/policiesandBylaws2/bylaws/OPTNByLaws/pdfs/bylaw_167.pdf. Accessed June 13, 2013.

25. United Network for Organ Sharing. Critical Pathway for Donation after Cardiac Death. Available at: http://www.unos.org/docs/Critical_Pathway_ DCD_Donor.pdf. Accessed June 13, 2013.

26. Recommendations for nonheartbeating organ donation. A position paper by the Ethics Committee, American College of Critical Care Medicine, Society of Critical Care Medicine. *Crit Care Med* 2002;29:1826–31.

27. Edwards JM, Hasz RD, Robertson VM. Non-heart-beating organ donation: process and review. *AACN Clin Issues* 1999;10:293–300.

28. Mathura AK, Heimbach J, Steffick DE, *et al.* Donation after cardiac death liver transplantation: predictors of outcome. *Am J Transplant* 2010;10:2512–19.

29. Selck FW, Grossman EB, Ratner LE, *et al.* Utilization, outcomes, and retransplantation of liver allografts from donation after cardiac death: implications for further expansion of the deceased-donor pool. *Ann Surg* 2008;248:599–607.

30. Merion RM, Pelletier SJ, Goodrich N, *et al.* Donation after cardiac death as a strategy to increase deceased donor liver availability. *Ann Surg* 2006;244:555–62.

31. Lee KW, Simpkins CE, Montgomery RA, *et al.* Factors affecting graft survival after liver transplantation from donation after cardiac death donors. *Transplantation* 2006;82:1683–88.

32. Mateo R, Cho Y, Singh G, *et al.* Risk factors for graft survival after liver transplantation from donation after cardiac death donors: an analysis of OPTN/ UNOS data. *Am J Transplant* 2006;6:791–96.

33. Taner CB, Bulatao IG, Willingham DL, *et al.* Events in procurement as risk factors for ischemic cholangiopathy in liver transplantation using donation after cardiac death donors. *Liver Transpl* 2012;18:100–11.

34. Skaro AI, Jay CL, Baker TB, *et al.* The impact of ischemic cholangiopathy in liver transplantation using donors after cardiac death: the untold story. *Surgery* 2009;146:543–52.

35. de Vera ME, Lopez-Solis R, Dvorchik I, *et al.* Liver transplantation using donation after cardiac death donors: long-term follow-up from a single center. *Am J Transplant* 2009;9:773–81.

36. Fujita S, Mizuno S, Fujikawa T, *et al.* Liver transplantation from donation after cardiac death: a single center experience. *Transplantation* 2007;84:46–9.

37. Maheshwari A, Maley W, Li Z, *et al.* Biliary complications and outcomes of liver transplantation from donors after cardiac death. *Liver Transpl* 2007;13:1645–53.

38. Lee, H. W., Suh, K.-S., Shin, W. Y.: *et al.* Classification and prognosis of intrahepatic biliary stricture after liver transplantation. *Liver Transpl* 2007;13:1736–42.

39. Jay CL, Lyuksemburg V, Kang R, *et al.* The increased costs of donation after cardiac death liver transplantation: caveat emptor. *Ann Surg* 2010;251:743–8.

40. Singhal A, Wima K, Hoehn RS, *et al.* Hospital resource use with donation after cardiac death allografts in liver transplantation: a matched controlled analysis from 2007 to 2011. *J Am Coll Surg* 2015;220:951–8.

41. van der Hilst C.S, IJtsma AJC, Bottema JT, *et al.* The price of donation after cardiac death in liver transplantation: a prospective cost-effectiveness study. *Transpl Int* 2013;26:411–8.

42. Israni AK, *et al.* OPTN/SRTR 2015 annual data report: deceased organ donation. Am J Transpl, 2017, 17(Suppl 1):503–42. doi: 10.1111/ajt.14131. Available at: http://onlinelibrary.wiley.com/doi/10.1111/ajt.14131/full#ajt14131-fig-0029. Accessed July 1, 2017.

43. Reich DJ. Quality assessment and performance improvement in transplantation — Hype or hope? *Curr Opin Organ Transplant* 2013;18:216–21.

44. Reich DJ. Donation after cardiac death. In: Busuttil RW, Klintmalm GB, Eds. *Transplantation of the Liver*, 3rd ed. Philadelphia, PA: WB Saunders, 2015, pp. 557–69.

45. Oliveira ML, Jassem W, Valente R, *et al.* Biliary complications after liver transplantation using grafts from donors after cardiac death. Results from a matched control study in a single large volume center. *Ann Surg* 2011;254:716–22.

46. Kubal C, Mangus R, Fridell J, *et al.* Optimization of perioperative conditions to prevent ischemic cholangiopathy in donation after circulatory death donor liver transplantation. *Transplantation* 2016;100:1699–704.

47. Bohorquez H, Seal JB, Cohen AJ, *et al.* Safety and outcomes in 100 consecutive donation after circulatory death liver transplants using a protocol that includes thrombolytic therapy. *Am J Transplant* 2017;17:2155–64.

48. Croome KP, Lee DD, Keaveny AP, *et al.* Improving national results in liver transplantation using grafts from donation after cardiac death donors. *Transplantation*, 2016;100:2640–7.

49. Chirichella TJ, Dunham CM, Zimmerman MA, *et al.* Donor preoperative oxygen delivery and post-extubation hypoxia impact donation after circulatory death hypoxic cholangiopathy. *World J Gastroenterol* 2016;22:3392–403.

50. Bernat JL, D'Alessandro AM, Port FK, *et al.* Report of a national conference on donation after cardiac death. *Am J Transplant* 2006;6:281–91.

51. Fung JJ, Eghtesad B, and Patel-Tom K. Using livers from donation after cardiac death donors — a proposal to protect the true Achilles heel. *Liver Transpl* 2007;13:1633–6.

52. Hashimoto K, Eghtesad B, Gunasekaran G, *et al.* Use of tissue plasminogen activator in liver transplantation from donation after cardiac death donors. *Am J Transplant* 2010;10:2665–72.

53. Stewart ZA, Cameron AM, Singer AL, *et al.* Histidine–tryptophan–ketoglutarate (HTK) is associated with reduced graft survival in deceased donor livers, especially those donated after cardiac death. *Am J Transplant* 2009;9:286–93.

54. Seal JB, Bohorquez H, Reichman T, *et al.* Thrombolytic protocol minimizes ischemic-type biliary complications in liver transplantation from donation after circulatory death donors. *Liver Transpl* 2015;21:321–8.

55. Verhoeven CJ, Simon TC, de Jonge J, *et al.* Liver grafts procured from donors after circulatory death have no increased risk of microthrombi formation. *Liver Transpl* 2016;22:1676–87.

56. Halldorson JB, Bakthavatsalam R, Montenovo M, *et al.* Differential rates of ischemic cholangiopathy and graft survival associated with induction therapy in DCD liver transplantation. *Am J Transplant* 2015;15:251–8.

57. Sundaram V, Choi G, Jeon CY, *et al.* Donation after cardiac death liver transplantation in primary sclerosing cholangitis: proceed with caution. *Transplantation* 2015;99:973–8.

58. Goldberg DS, Karp SJ, McCauley ME, *et al.* Interpreting outcomes in DCDD liver transplantation: first report of the multicenter IDOL Consortium. *Transplantation* 2017;101:1067–73.

59. Croome KP, Lee DD, Harnois D, *et al.* Effects of the share 35 rule on waitlist and liver transplantation outcomes for patients with hepatocellular carcinoma. *PLoS ONE* 2017;12:1–9.

60. Croome KP, Wall W, Chandok N, *et al.* Inferior survival in liver transplant recipients with hepatocellular carcinoma receiving donation after cardiac death liver allografts. *Liver Transpl* 2013;19:1214–23.

61. Croome KP, Lee DD, Burns JM, *et al.* The use of donation after cardiac death allografts does not increase recurrence of hepatocellular carcinoma. *Am J Transplant* 2015;15:2704–11.

62. Khorsandi SE, Yip VS, Cortes M, *et al.* Does donation after cardiac death utilization adversely affect hepatocellular cancer survival? *Transplantation* 2016;100:1916–24.

63. Kootstra G: The asystolic, or non-heartbeating, donor. *Transplantation* 1997; 63:917–21.

64. Whetstine L, Bowman K, and Hawryluck L: Pro/con ethics debate: is nonheart-beating organ donation ethically acceptable? Crit Care 2000;6:192–5.

65. Bell MDD. Non-heart beating organ donation: old procurement strategy — new ethical problems. *J Med Ethics* 2003;29:176–81.

66. Arnold RM and Younger SJ. Time is of the essence: the pressing need for comprehensive non-heart-beating cadaveric donation policies. *Transplant Proc* 1995;27:2913–21.

67. Allison KC, Caplan A, Shapiro ME, *et al.* Historical development and current status of organ procurement from death-row prisoners in China. *BMC Med Ethics* 2015;16:1–7.

68. Paul NW, Caplan A, Shapiro ME, *et al.* Human rights violations in organ procurement practice in China. *BMC Med Ethics* 2017;18:1–9.

69. Rubenstein S. California surgeon cleared of hastening organ donor's death. Health Blog. Goldstein J, lead writer. *The Wall Street J*, December 19, 2008.

http://blogs.wsj.com/health/2008/12/19/california-surgeon-cleared-of-hastening-organ-donorsdeath. Accessed June 13, 2013.

70. Reiner M, Cornell D, and Howard RJ. Development of a successful non-heart-beating organ donation program. *Prog Transplant* 2003;13:225–31.

71. Nathan HM and Hasz RD. Gift of Life Donor Program: 2016 Annual Report. Philadelphia: Gift of Life Donor Program, Inc., 2016.

72. Suntharalingam C, Sharples L, Dudley C, *et al*. Time to cardiac death after withdrawal of life-sustaining treatment in potential organ donors. *Am J Transplant* 2009;9:2157–65.

73. Olson L, Davi R, Barnhart J, *et al*. Non-heart-beating cadaver donor hepatectomy "the operative procedure". *Clin Transplant* 1999;13:98–103.

74. Reich DJ. Donation after cardiac death organ procurement and transplantation. In: Humar A, Sturdevant ML. Eds. *Atlas of Organ Transplantation*, 2nd ed. London: Springer, 2015, pp. 25–36.

75. Jeon H, Ortiz JA, Manzarbeitia CY, *et al*. Combined liver and pancreas procurement from a controlled non-heart-beating donor with aberrant hepatic arterial anatomy. *Transplantation* 2002;74:1636–9.

76. Yamamoto S, Wilczek HE, Duraj FF, *et al*. Liver transplantation with grafts from controlled donors after cardiac death: a 20-year follow-up at a single center. *Am J Transplant* 2010;10:602–11.

77. Magliocca JF, Magee JC, Rowe SA, *et al*. Extracorporeal support for organ donation after cardiac death effectively expands the donor pool. *J Trauma* 2005;58:1095–102.

78. Rojas-Peña A, Sall LE, Gravel MT, *et al*. Donation after circulatory determination of death: the University of Michigan experience with extracorporeal support. *Transplantation* 2014;98:328–34.

79. Oniscu GC, Siddique A, Dark J, *et al*. Dual temperature multi-organ recovery from a Maastricht category III donor after circulatory death. *Am J Transplant* 2014;14:2181–6.

80. De Carlis R, Di Sandro S, Lauterio A, *et al*. Successful donation after cardiac death liver transplants with prolonged warm ischemia time using normothermic regional perfusion. *Liver Transpl* 2017;23:166–73.

81. Miñambres E, Suberviola B, Dominguez-Gil B, *et al*. Improving the outcomes of organs obtained from controlled donation after circulatory death donors using abdominal normothermic regional perfusion. *Am J Transplant* 2017;17:2165–72.

4. Machine Preservation of Livers for Transplantation

Paulo Fontes, Arjan van der Plaats, Roberto Lopez,
Kyle Soltys, Wallis Marsh, Ruy Cruz, Banan Babak,
William R Light, and Christopher Hughes

*Department of Surgery, University of Pittsburgh, Pittsburgh,
PA 15213, USA*

1. Background

Organ perfusion was initially attempted in mid-19th century by Loebel, who reported his preliminary perfusion studies of isolated organs in 1849. Langendorf developed a simple and nonpulsatile organ perfusion apparatus that consisted of a perfusate reservoir and a siphon tube attached to the organ in1895 (Figure 1). The organ was perfused by gravity in an open system without recirculation of the perfusate [1]. In 1903, Kuliabko published intriguing studies on heart revival after death. He used a similar Langendorf's apparatus while perfusing an infant heart 30 hours after the death of the child. He described faint right atrial movements seen 20 minutes after *in vitro* perfusion, which were apparently followed by right ventricle motion and subsequent left ventricle contractions [2]. Knowlton and Starling introduced the first heart–lung preparation in 1912, by combining active perfusion with blood oxygenation [3]. His heart–lung preparation was rather innovative since oxygenators and perfusion pumps were not available yet. Bainbridge and Evans reported the first successful kidney perfusion experiments in 1914. They used two dogs for each experiment (one for heart–lung preparations and one for kidneys) and perfused the kidneys both *in* and *ex situ*. They achieved sustainable blood flow *ex vivo* while

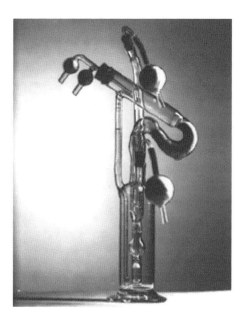

Figure 1.   Langendorf organ perfusion apparatus, 1895.

keeping the temperature and vasculature pressures within physiological ranges. This normothermic kidney perfusion yielded normal arterial blood gases values while allowing the kidney to produce urine [4]. Carrel joined Rosenberg in 1930 to develop a new automated perfusion system composed by a combined metal and glass pump. Despite creating a highly efficient system based of well-crafted mechanical components, their outcomes were rather disappointing regarding organ function. Organ perfusion experiments became rather routine during the second and third decades of 20th century. However, none of the perfusion circuits could be used for long-term extracorporeal maintenance of the organs since the devices were open and unable to be properly sterilized. Charles Lindbergh devised a new all-glass apparatus at the Rockefeller institute in 1935, being the first one capable to provide flow under pulsatile pressures and within sterile conditions [5]. From 1935 to 1939, near 900 experiments were carried out using the flawless Lindbergh–Rockefeller perfusion system, revealing the great technical and operational features of this new device [6]. In the former Soviet Union, innovative perfusion research was conducted in dog models, where kidneys and limbs were successfully transplanted after machine preservation by Lapchinsky. He conducted additional experiments focused on extended *ex vivo* preservation with perfusion devices. He preserved dog limbs for 28 hours under hypothermic conditions (2–4°C) using cooled blood for the first hours and switching to warm perfusion for 1 hour prior to transplantation. He achieved 42% early postoperative survival after transplantation for the limb model. Later on, 50% of the surviving dogs rejected their limbs, 25% died from additional complications and 25% achieved long-term survival [7]. Further experiments with the same dog model showed reasonable recipient survival using autografts. In the mid 1960s the Naval Medical Research Institute, MD, USA became interested in *ex vivo* organ perfusion. In spite duplicating the Lindbergh organ perfusion apparatus, the results were much below expectations. Lindbergh was further invited to assist the research institute, where he successfully reproduced and validated his previous experiments [8]. Kidney transplantation was clinically attempted in the early 1960s in spite the lack of progress in organ preservation. The first human kidneys were successfully transplanted in identical twin cases despite the absence of proper preservation techniques leading to an extended warm ischemia time (WIT). It became clear to the field that clinical transplantation would not evolve without major new developments in organ preservation. Early attempts to induce total body hypothermia in living kidney donors [9] were performed with the technology initially developed for open heart procedures [10]. Hypothermia was further utilized by Lillehei [11] as a way to extend organ preservation by immersing small bowel loops in iced saline before doing autotransplants. A similar approach was taken by Shumway while developing early experimental models for heart and heart–lung transplantation [12]. Hypothermia was readily accepted as beneficial for organ preservation in the 1960s, despite the lack of technological developments in solutions and machine perfusion (MP) devices. Subsequent preclinical experiments in dogs showed the beneficial effect of hypothermia by infusing cold solutions through the portal vein in liver allografts prior to transplantation. These animals were the first survivors from orthotopic liver transplantation [13]. The same principle was applied in clinical kidney transplantation, where cold lactated Ringer's or low-molecular-weight dextran solutions were infused through the renal artery in kidney allografts immediately after the initial procurement [14]. Continuous hypothermic perfusion of cadaveric livers and kidneys allografts became routine long before brain death was accepted as a clinical condition for organ donation. The first human liver transplant was conducted after the cadaveric allograft was perfused *ex vivo* by a machine perfusion developed by Starzl and his Denver group (Figure 2).

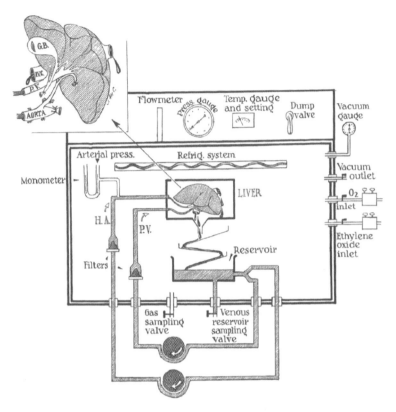

Figure 2.   Starzl's machine perfusion device for liver preservation.

This MP technique was successfully utilized for the first 11 liver transplantations performed in humans [15]. A similar MP device was further introduced by Kestens in 1969, creating a new *in situ* liver preservation technique that led to favorable outcomes in the first human transplantations in Belgium [16]. Despite these successes, MP technology was temporary abandoned with the introduction of new hypothermic solutions for cold storage (CS). Ackerman and Barnard [17] reintroduced the Carrel/Lindberg MP system by perfusing kidney allografts with continuous low flow using a perfusate primed with blood and oxygenated within a hyperbaric chamber. *Ex vivo* oxygenation appeared to be a feasible technique and it was further utilized for the preservation of hepatic allografts [18]. Unfortunately, the complex technical and operational features involved in effective *ex vivo* oxygenation precluded further dissemination of this technique while creating a positive environment for new developments in organ and tissue preservation solutions that would

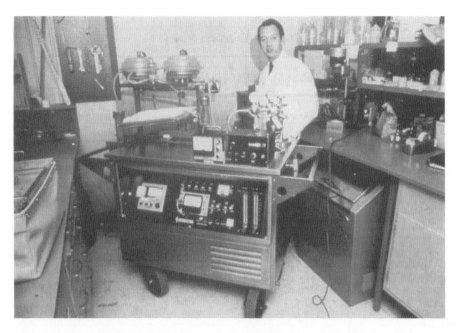

Figure 3.   Belzer's initial device for kidney perfusion.

sustain prolonged hypothermia. Belzer discarded the use of hyperbaric chamber in combination with blood products and developed a new preservation solution for CS, showing remarkable results in a 72-hour kidney preservation model [19]. Their new solution was further optimized as the first blood-free perfusate for MP. Belzer's team introduced hypothermic machine perfusion (HMP) (Figure 3), using cryoprecipitated plasma as the perfusate in a protocol involving 17-hour preservation prior to kidney transplantation [20]. They extended their studies with HMP and developed a hyperconcotic heterostarch-based solution, the University of Wisconsin machine perfusion solution (MPS), which became the gold standard MPS for several decades [21]. The MPS was unsuccessful in liver preservation and MP technology was further abandoned after the successful introduction of CS solutions, which became the new standard for organ preservation. New attempts to resurrect MP were again tried in 1990. Pienaar achieved a remarkable 87.5% survival in a liver transplant dog model where they utilized HMP for 72 hours, using pulsatile perfusion through the portal vein with high pressures (16–18 mmHg) and switching the Na+/K+ ratio of their original MPS solution [22]. This model couldn't be further reproduced and MP became again an elusive technology. Subsequent developments in MP were further promoted by Dutkowski, who introduced the concept of end-ischemic hypothermic oxygenated perfusion (HOPE) for liver preservation [23] where they reintroduced MP for a short period prior to organ implantation. Their extensive studies in rodents and pre-clinical large animal models showed their ability to reduce endothelial shear stress while minimizing the release of reactive oxygen species (ROS) by providing a short period (1–3 hours) of oxygenation under hypothermic conditions and without the use of a professional oxygen carrier (OC) molecule within the perfusate. They developed a pressure-sealed chamber capable to deliver intermittent positive/negative pressure with an amplitude of 8 mbar, producing physiological flow profiles between 32–36 mL/minute. This fluctuating and oscillating pressure-controlled perfusion through the portal vein, was thought to progressively restore mitochondrial function and promote effective ATP reconstitution during a short but effective perfusion time [24–27]. Normothermic (37°C) MP was also reintroduced by Neuhaus [28] in 1993 and further optimized by Friend [29] in 2009. HMP (4°C) was reintroduced again by Guarrerra in 2005. He described their basic operational features on a swine model, where livers were successfully perfused hypothermically through the portal vein (continuous flow) with a new preservation solution Vasosol (Holdings East, Glenmoore, USA) developed by his group. They conducted 12 hours HMP of pig livers using dual perfusion (PV: 3–5 mmHg, HA: 12–18 mmHg) without additional oxygenation with 100% survival after transplantation [30]. They modified the University of Wisconsin-MPS by adding antioxidants, metabolic substrates and vasodilators. Guarrera [31] pioneered the clinical applications in MP in the USA by conducting a successful feasibility trial with 20 patients in 2009. Their liver allografts were perfused from 4–7 and the CIT time remained below 12 hours. Despite the lack of active oxygenation during HMP, sustainable pO_2 levels were achieved (mean of 137.2 mmHg) with room air interchange at the organ chamber. Furthermore, the proinflammatory expression was less pronounced in HMP when compared to their CS control group [32]. In addition, HMP liver recipients had significantly shorter hospital stay and lower biochemical hepatic injury markers. This study showed the safety and efficacy of HMP when compared to CS. A subsequent clinical trial was conducted by Friend in Oxford, UK, where a new NMP device utilizing human red blood cells (RBCs) as the OC solution [33].

2. Rationale for the use of MP devices

MP devices have evolved around the idea of providing sustained flow (continuous and/or pulsatile) through the liver allografts to enhance/extend organ preservation while minimizing ischemia reperfusion injuries. The main issues involved in MP are the following:

1. Provision of continuous circulation and better flow through the macro and microcirculation,
2. Provision of effective oxygenation to fulfil/repair the organ's metabolic demands,
3. Removal of metabolic waste products and toxins,
4. Create an opportunity to assess organ function and viability,
5. Enhance clinical outcomes by promoting organ rescue/amelioration *ex vivo* prior to implantation, allowing the use of expanded criteria donors (ECDs),
6. Extend preservation time without imposing further ischemia-reperfusion injuries (IRIs),
7. Promote the *ex vivo* administration of cytoprotective and immunomodulatory substances,
8. Improve transplant outcomes by decreasing the incidence of early graft dysfunction and PNF, which would impact directly on the length of hospital stay, subsequent posttransplant admissions and improved graft and patient survival rates.

3. Advantages of MP

3.1. *Assessment of liver function and viability*

One of the main disadvantages of CS is its inability to assess organ function and viability before transplantation. Given that ECD livers are associated with higher risks of posttransplant complications, assessment of their functionality and viability before graft implantation remains very critical. MP systems provide a unique opportunity for *ex vivo* manipulations before organ transplantation (Table 1). During MP, the liver is metabolically active, and the key elements of hepatocyte metabolism can be measured in real time. Several "viability markers" have been suggested by different research groups (lactate, INR, ATP etc.) [34]. Ongoing MP clinical trials have focused on the sensitivity and the specificity of these markers in predicting liver's function post transplantation. Reliable predictive markers are seminal for the decision process involved in allocation and utilization of ECDs. Effective *ex vivo* management during MP has the potential to increase organ utilization by decreasing the current and unacceptable discard rate (50% for DCDs). Volumetric measurement of bile production has been proposed as a reliable marker for graft viability during MP [35]. Perfusate samples can be

Table 1.   Risks & benefits of MP.

Advantages	Disadvantages
Lower incidence of delayed graft function	Higher cost in the short term
Continuous monitoring of parameters	Logistic issues during procurement
Decrease vasospasm	Endothelial injury is possible
Ability to provide metabolic support	Logistic issues during preservation
Potential for pharmacologic manipulation	Possible equipment failure
Immunomodulation	Infection
Control of inflammation (DAMPs)	
Biomarkers to predict organ function	

serially obtained for acute real-time assessment of graft function during MP. Besides liver enzymes, cytokines/chemokines and the production of coagulation factors have been additionally considered as potential markers for graft injury and synthetic function. In MP systems providing full oxygenation, the need for additional oximetry assays in both the perfusate and the tissues are important variables that require continuous measurement [59]. Due to the differences in perfusion protocols involving flow, temperature, and oxygenation rates, the liver allografts can display variable functional features when perfused under hypothermic, subnormothermic (sNM), and normothermic (NM) conditions. Accurate and reliable measurements for graft function and viability before transplantation remain crucial for the extended use of ECDs. Therefore, with further developments in MP technology, the determination of specific biomarkers related to graft viability and subsequent postreperfusion outcomes remains critical for the field. In this regard, further assessment of bile composition and conjugation should be another important measurement of liver function during MP. Furthermore, the subsequent development of better diagnostic tools (*e.g.* confocal microscopy and biomarkers) to monitor MP protocols will greatly extend the impact of this technology.

3.2. *Prolonged preservation*

CS allows a rather limited cold ischemia time (CIT) for liver preservation (usually <14 hours) before transplantation. This technical limitation continues to hold liver transplantation as a semiemergency procedure. MP protocols, however, enable prolonged preservation time and allow a wider window for organ allocation, recipient selection and preparation and further operational delays within the transplant center (e.g., completion of ongoing elective surgical procedures competing for additional resources). Also, this approach would theoretically enable remote organ sharing between transplant centers.

3.3. *Allograft reconditioning*

MP systems provide an ideal platform to treat, repair, optimize and recover ECD livers. Expression of genes and biosynthesis of proteins are hampered under hypothermic conditions, making further pharmacological reconditioning of the allografts unfeasible during CS. Also, the unique *ex vivo* access to the liver allograft before transplantation provided by MP should prevent recipient's systemic exposure to the agents that could be used for reconditioning. In this scenario, the MP system is supplemented with the agent of interest and the liver is continuously assessed overtime. ECD livers showing early signs of anticipated changes/improvements could be subsequently accepted by the primary center and utilized for transplantation. Pharmacological reconditioning during MP also aims the minimization of potential ischemia-reperfusion injuries (IRI) acquired prior and during the initial procurement. In a recently published study from the Toronto group, an anti-inflammatory cocktail was made by mixing sevoflurane, alprostadil, *n*-acetylcysteine, and carbon monoxide. The cocktail was then injected into perfusion solution of MP device [36]. This study showed that inflammatory signaling pathways could be manipulated during preservation period and this approach has the potential to improve transplant outcomes. In another study, Banan *et al.* showed that supplementing the EMP device with defatting agents (exdenin-4 and L-carnitine) reduces IRI and has the potential to reduce the fat content of discarded steatotic livers before transplantation [37].

4. MP modalities

Regarding the temperatures utilized during MP protocols, the field has been divided among hypothermic (HMP), subnormothermic (sNM MP) and normothermic (NM MP) systems [47]. Most modern MP devices are now capable to deliver dual pressures, meaning that pulsatile can be simultaneously provided at the arterial system while continuous pressures are delivered at the venous bed. These devices also utilize centrifugal pump units,

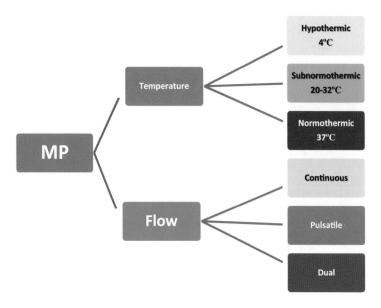

Figure 4.   Modalities of machine perfusion based on flow and temperature.

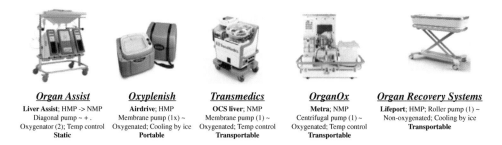

Figure 5.   Current medical devices for liver machine perfusion.

that are pressure driven. This implicates in a tight flow control within a given pressure range (Figure 4).

5. MP devices

MP devices (Figure 5) require CE approval in Europe. In the USA, these devices require FDA approval as class II medical devices, which are required to receive and initial Investigational Device Exemption (IDE) before starting feasibility clinical trials. The FDA requires a mandatory pairing between the medical device and a given perfusate and the final approval restricts the exclusive use of the device with the original perfusate. Pivotal multicenter clinical trials (100 patients with a 1-year follow-up) are required for the final FDA approval.

6. Basic principles for MP

6.1. *Perfusion*

Restoration of active circulation through the explanted organ is a key function of MP systems. The principal objective of this recirculation is to support active cellular metabolism by providing continuous supply of nutrients and oxygen, while continuously removing metabolic waste products and preserving vascular and endothelial structures through fluid dynamic stability. The characteristics of perfusion strongly depend on the required application and/or therapy, thus temperature, and the type of organ are keys to determine perfusion ranges (e.g., flows and pressures). Design criteria for perfusion pumps include low energy consumption, light-weight, small-size, operable in both hypothermic as normothermic conditions and affordable and ease of use. Basically, there are two main blood pump types: positive displacement pumps and rotary pumps (Figure 6). Displacement pumps include roller pumps, membrane pumps and piston pumps, and are based on the principle of forcing fluid forwards [38]. A roller pump uses two or more rollers that generate a peristaltic movement by squeezing a fluid-containing tube alternately. Depending on the number of rollers, the resulting flow is pulsatile or near-continuous. Membrane pumps consist of a flexible membrane that separates the fluid from a driving medium, in most cases compressed air. The driving volume alternately moves the membrane up and down, and subsequently the fluid is forced in and out the membrane pump. The membrane pump is a purely a pulsatile pump. Unidirectional flow can be obtained using in and out flow valves.

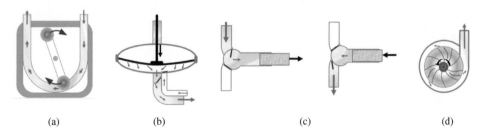

(a) (b) (c) (d)

Figure 6. Different types of pumps utilized in machine perfusion devices. (a) roller pump, (b) membrane pump, (c) piston pump, (d) rotary pump.

6.2. Oxygenation

To sustain effective aerobic metabolism, oxygen must be provided, transported and effectively delivered to all oxygen demanding cells in the organ being perfused, meaning that oxygen delivery (DO_2) needs to exceed oxygen consumption (VO_2). VO_2 is the volume of oxygen consumed by tissues per minute [39]. Large differences are seen in VO_2 between different tissues [40, 41]. The major oxygen demanding organs are liver (20.4%), brain (18.4%), heart (11.6%) and kidney (7.2%) regarding total body oxygen consumption when baseline physiological values at measured at rest. VO_2 rates change per the organs and tissues' metabolic rates. More importantly, oxygen demand and consumption require active dynamic regulation during MP. There are two important factors to be considered regarding oxygen demand during MP. The first one is the temperature. Lower temperatures decrease the metabolic rate while lowering oxygen demand according van 't Hoff's principle [38] (Figure 7).

Oxygen demand needs to be matched by oxygen delivery, which brings an important issue regarding the presence of professional oxygen carrier (OC) in the perfusate. Hemoglobin remains the most potent OC available, having the capacity to promote a 70-fold increase in the oxygen content of blood and perfusates when compared to only dissolved oxygen [42]. By providing a 3, 6 kPa oxygen tension, the oxygen content can be increased significantly if the OC has a standard (24 or higher) p50. In other words, when an OC is present in a perfusion solution, it is not necessary to provide excessive oxygenation since a small amount of oxygen will result in sufficient oxygen content to be properly delivered to the tissues. Paradoxically, when red blood cells (RBCs) or OC are present in the perfusate, 100% or carbogen (95% O_2/5% CO_2) is used to actively oxygenate the organ. Furthermore, the higher the temperature of the MP intervention, the higher are the oxygen

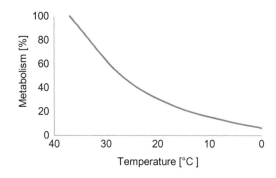

Figure 7.   Correlation between organ temperature and metabolic rate.

requirements to support aerobic metabolism. This implicates in the upmost need of effective OC in this MP systems. However, OC are only seen in the mid- and normothermic MP applications. Active oxygenation is intended to promote higher oxygen concentrations, which can also generate undesirable levels of reactive oxygen species (ROS) if the mitochondrial function is not preserved. Excessive ROS can lead to impaired tissue integrity due to uncontrolled oxidative stress [43]. This detrimental environment can be found in some of the hypothermic applications of MP. OC should be very useful in prolonged HMP, by avoiding high levels of ROS as a byproduct of hyperoxygenation in temperature ranges (4–17°C) where some of the mitochondrial enzymes (e.g., translocases) are still not fully functional.

6.3. *Methods for ex vivo oxygenation*

There are two possible ways to deliver oxygen to an organ *ex vivo* with MP devices [44]:

1. Persufflation (PSF, gaseous oxygen perfusion) is an older method in which oxygen is provided directly intravascular. The principal barrier is the risk for *in vivo* embolization post transplant. PSF may increase the risk of endothelial vascular damage. Depending on gaseous oxygen concentration, PSF may also induce further hyperoxic damage. Desiccation is another potential risk if the gas mixture is not properly humidified during long-term preservation. PSF resembles iatrogenic gas embolization and it doesn't allow the delivery of nutrients like liquid perfusion. PSF appears to be less efficient at removing waste products.
2. Membrane oxygenation (MO): Membrane oxygenators are based on the utilization of microporous, silicon or polypropylene membranes. MO van be divided in three different types:
    2.1. Plaque oxygenators: These devices promote blood and gas flowing in opposite sides of the membrane. These are built with microporous membranes of expanded polypropylene, folded in a Z-shape, resembling an accordion.
    2.2. Spiral Oxygenators: The membrane oxygenator is rolled around a central axis resembling a spiraled ball of yarn. These are a derivative of the old model of the Kobolov's oxygenator that utilized silicon membranes.
    2.3. Hollow fiber oxygenators: This is the most common type of oxygenator currently used. They are manufactured with microporous

polypropylene membranes, constituted by capillary fibers positioned in parallel bunches or as skeins, forming hollow, capillary fibers or capillary membranes. These oxygenators are divided into two subgroups, per the type of blood circulation.

A.   Inside the capillary blood flow: In this model, the blood/perfusate circulates inside the capillary fiber bunches and the gas circulates outside, in opposite directions. There is a pressure gradient produced by the resistance of fibers on the passage of the blood/perfsuate. Micro thrombosis is a potential risk, which would compromise the oxygenator function.

B.   Inside the capillary gas flow: In this model, gas passes through the capillary fiber bunches which are immersed in blood/perfusate. This configuration reduces the gradient between blood/perfusate and gas, reducing considerably the mechanical trauma produced by the passage of blood inside the capillaries. This method also allows a reduction in the membrane's area, optimizing the utilization of the apparatus.

Nowadays, the most common used oxygenators are the hollow fiber microporous polypropylene membrane oxygenators, having outstanding surface-area-to-volume ratios. The blood/perfusate can flow inside the polypropylene fibers (intraluminal flow), or around the fiber bundles (extraluminal). The extraluminal design has advantages over the intraluminal design because of enhancement of gas exchange by passive mixing of the blood/perfusate, thereby allowing reduction of the gas exchange surface area [45].

6.4. *Temperature*

Temperature control is one of the most critical performances in MP devices. Most thermocouple sensors are based on the Seebeck effect. Resistance temperature detectors (RTD) are progressively replacing the thermocouple because of their greater accuracy, stability and repeatability [46]. The resistance of RTD's changes depending on the temperature. An electrical current causing self-heating of the detector needs to flow through a RTD to allow resistance measurements of the RTD. This self-heating effect can influence temperature measurements depending on the cooling capacity of the medium of interest. Besides, the temperature sensor can heat up the perfusate when measuring very small volumes. This shouldn't be an issue for MP devices since in organ perfusion the volume of fluid is relatively high. Accurate temperature measurements require further verification of the sensor's is suitability for the

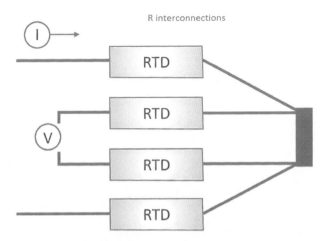

R interconnections

Figure 8.   Graphic representation of a modern heating monitoring system composed on four resistance temperature detectors.

medium to be measured. Temperature control is an important safety issue for MP devices and accurate measurement by a four-wire RTD should be preferred (Figure 8).

6.5. *Pressure*

MP devices can provide continuous (through the portal vein) and pulsatile (through the hepatic artery) flow to the liver during the preservation protocols. In most medical sensors, the pressure is measured relatively to ambient pressures. These measurements are taken by the difference between the pressure in the perfusion loop and the atmospheric pressure, characterizing them as Gauge pressor sensors (Figure 9). A deflecting membrane with a piezoresistive elements is a common base for pressure sensors. Since the change in resistance of these elements is small, the interconnection of these elements on the membrane is done in a special way.

One side of the membrane is connected to the medium with the pressure of interest, while the other side is venting to the ambient air. The venting port should not be blocked. Blocking the vent port will result in a pressure change on the ambient side of the membrane due to the expansion of the blocked medium by temperature. This change in pressure reading will not be immediate but will develop over time when temperature changes. MP devices have safety requirements to provide arterial and venous pressures within a given range. Most MP protocols are conducted with pressures lower then physiological ranges for the arterial bed (20–40 mmHg). The portal

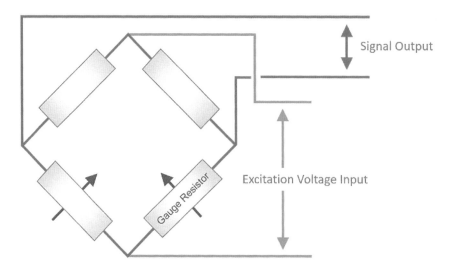

Figure 9. A Wheatstone bridge, the interconnection of four piezoresistive elements, that can accurately measure small changes in resistance.

pressures are kept at physiologic ranges (4–6 mmHg). Higher pressures and flows over extended periods of time can cause early endothelial cell damage within the allografts. When measuring pressure in MP devices, attention should be paid to the vent port, since blocked pressure readings are largely influenced by temperature. The static pressure should always be measured perpendicular to the flow, otherwise the flow will influence the pressure reading. This also applies for the additional pressure lines, which should also be perpendicular to the flow. Finally, resistance of the perfusion tubing and height differences (most commonly between the monitor and the organ chamber) should be considered since it can generate a pressure deviation depending on length, radius, flow rate and height.

6.6. *Flow*

Flow is the amount of solution that flows through the organ per time interval and is a very important parameter in MP protocols. Although flow measurement in principle is a simple procedure by using a stopwatch and a balance (volume per time), in MP this would have further implications. Electromagnetic flow sensors are instantaneous flow sensors that are made to measure pulsatile flow. They operate with any electrical conductive liquid. The measurement of perfusate flow with electromagnetic flow probes uses the principle described by Faraday (1832) in his law of electromagnetic induction. Ultrasonic flow meters use an ultrasound signal that is emitted from a transducer, deflected

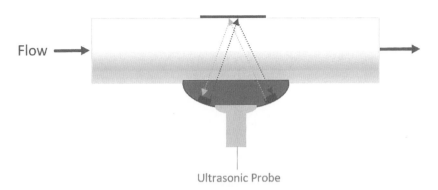

Figure 10. Schematic representation of an ultrasonic probe utilized to measure flow in a machine perfusion device.

and then captured by an ultrasonic transducer to determine flow. This type of flow probe consists of a probe body containing two ultrasonic transducers as well as an acoustic reflector (Figure 10). Upon excitation, the transducer emits a wave of ultrasound that traverses the vessel and rebounds on the acoustic reflector and is detected by the second transducer. When the ultrasonic wave travels upstream the transit time is increased dependent on the flow. A very short time later, receiver becomes transmitter and transmitter becomes receiver, causing the ultrasonic wave to travel downstream and the transit time is decreased dependent on the flow. The difference in time between the upstream measurement and the downstream measurement is related to flow, increasing flow will increase the time difference. Both sensor types can measure pulsatile flow and are both used in MP systems. However, when MP systems are based on using a cellular aqueous perfusion solutions, electric conductivity must be considered when using electromagnetic flow sensors. Ultrasonic sensors can be applied with all solutions. The two measurement techniques are in some extend sensitive to turbulent flow. In the electromagnetic technique, the distance between the electrodes must be known. However, in the ultrasonic technique the inner diameter of the tubing is the main parameter to be determined. Additional safety measures call for proper isolation of the electrodes within the electromagnetic flow probe from potential hazardous voltages.

7. Clinical experience

7.1. *Liver-HMP: hypothermic oxygenated perfusion (HOPE)*

Dutkowski conducted a pilot study with the Organ Assist device (Liver Assist®) in which oxygenated portal perfusion was used for DCD livers

(n = 8) and was compared with standard cold stored DBD livers (n = 8) [48]. This protocol involved only a pressure-controlled portal vein perfusion for a short period (1–2 hours). UW gluconate solution was recirculated at a temperature of 10°C with an oxygen tension between 40 kPa and 60 kPa. The perfusion pressure was adjusted below 3 mmHg to prevent endothelial shear stress. HOPE conditions were maintained for about 1–2 hours until the recipient hepatectomy was completed. DCD liver allografts preserved with MP/HOPE displayed excellent early function with low enzymatic profile (AST/ALT) when compared to matched donors after brain death (DBD) liver allografts preserved under CS. The intensive care unit (ICU) was shorter for the MP/HOPE livers (not significant) and the length of hospital stay was comparable. However, the total costs during hospital stay were significantly lower in the DCD liver recipients. This was the first clinical trial showing that cadaveric liver allografts treated by HOPE with the Liver Assist® device can be safely and effectively preserved before transplantation. More importantly, the initial follow up revealed low reperfusion injury and no incidence of ischemic cholangiopathy on this high-risk DCD population. The same group completed an additional multicenter study with end-ischemic oxygenated HMP, focusing primarily on the performance of the treatment [49]. An additional set of HOPE-treated DCD livers (n = 25) were matched and compared with CS DCD liver grafts (n = 50) from two well-established European programs. Criteria for matching included duration of warm ischemia and key confounders summarized in the balance of risk score. On a second cohort of patients, perfused and unperfused DCD livers were compared with liver allografts from standard DBD (n = 50), also matched to the balance of risk score, serving as baseline controls. DCD livers preserved with MP/HOPE had a significant decrease in graft injury when compared with matched cold-stored DCD livers regarding peak ALT (1239 vs. 2065 U/L, p = 0.02), intrahepatic cholangiopathy (0% vs 22%, p = 0.015), biliary complications (20% vs. 46%, p = 0.042), and 1-year graft survival (90% vs. 69%, p = 0.035) (Figure 11). The authors reported no graft failure due to intrahepatic cholangiopathy and no incidence of primary nonfunction (PNF) in the MP/HOPE-treated livers, whereas 18% of unper-fused DCD livers had graft failure requiring retransplantation. In addition, MP/HOPE DCD livers achieved similar results as control donation after DBD in all investigated endpoints. Porter and his Groningen, Netherlands group did a similar study with human DCD livers in an early clinical pilot study (Figure 12).

Their preliminary results showed increased portal and arterial perfusion during the MP/HOPE protocol. ATP reconstitution significantly increased during perfusion and subsequently after reperfusion. Unfortunately, no

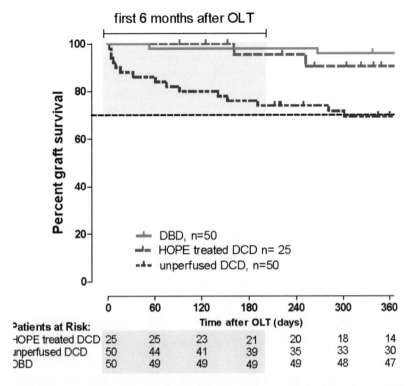

Figure 11. Graft survival curve comparing grafts obtained from DCD liver allografts and treated with cold storage (unperfused) and HOPE (machine perfusion). The baseline comparison (top curve) represents the graft survival from donors after brain death (DBD).

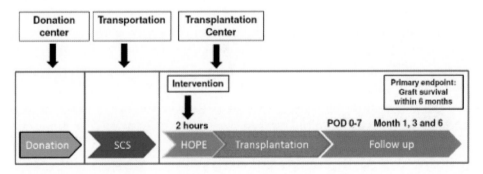

Figure 12. Methodology for Porter's study in MP and HOPE after initial preservation with cold storage (SCS).

control data is available yet. These initial experiments with MP/HOPE in DCD human livers showed optimistic results but further randomized (multicenter) trials might be needed to prospectively analyze the effects of MP/HOPE in comparison to CS [50]. An upcoming multicenter randomized clinical trial using the Liver Assist® device is being organized with centers in France, The Netherlands, Spain, Sweden, Switzerland and the United Kingdom. The focus will be on end-ischemic hypothermic oxygenated liver perfusion in both DCD and DBD livers. The primary end point will be the incidence of ischemic cholangiopathy at the 6th month follow-up. Secondary end points will include patient survival, PNF, initial poor function (IPF), biochemical analysis (AST/ALT), and the duration of ICU and hospital stay.

7.2. *Liver-sNMP: clinical data*

The Pittsburgh group had promising results (100% survival) in their proof-of-concept preclinical studies (swine model) using a new OC solution at 21°C with the Liver Assist® device over a 9-hour period of preservation [59]. The first clinical trial with sNMP utilized a controlled oxygenated rewarming (COR) protocol was successfully conducted by the Bonn/Essen group in January 2016 [51]. In their first clinical series where six patients were enrolled, cadaveric livers initially preserved with CS and allocated by the rescue offer mechanism by Eurotransplant, were subjected to MP (Liver Assist® device) under slow controlled oxygenated rewarming (COR) for 90 minutes before organ implantation. All organs were procured at distant hospitals and cold flushed with UW or HTK (Custodiol) solution. The COR protocol was carried out only if the planned application time of 90 minutes would not prolong the overall CIT. After conventional back table preparation, the grafts were prepared for cannulation of the hepatic artery and the portal vein. Pulsatile perfusion pressure was used for the hepatic artery, while continuous perfusion pressure was used for the portal vein. In this series, perfusion pressures were set to 25 mmHg (60 bpm) at the hepatic artery and 2–4 mmHg at the portal vein. Custodiol-N (Dr. Köhler Chemie, Bensheim, Germany) was used as perfusion solution. During the MP priming protocol, 2 L of Custodiol-N were recirculated through the system at 10°C. The solution was oxygenated with an $FiO_2 = 100\%$. Initial oxygen partial pressures in the perfusate were around 500 mmHg during the 90-minute period. After initial hypothermic perfusion at 10°C, the temperature was gradually increased to 12°C, 16°C, and 20°C after 30, 45, and 60 minutes, respectively. At the completion of the COR protocol, MP was carried out for 90 minutes and the perfusate's temperature was elevated to 20°C. The COR data was compared to a historical cohort of 106 patients. This multicenter patient population had comparable graft (all rescue offer organs) and recipient factors. The recipients of liver allografts treated by MP/COR had a significant reduction (50%) in peak

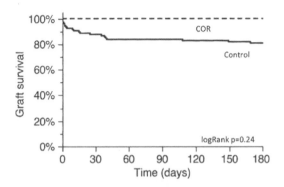

Figure 13. Graft survival curve comparing liver allografts treated with controlled oxygenated rewarming (COR) and liver allografts preserved under cold storage (Control).

serum transaminases after transplantation compared to untreated controls (AST 563.5 vs 1204 U/L, p = 0.023). After a 6-month follow-up period, graft survival was 100% in the COR group and 80.9% in the controls (p = 0.24). Respective patient survival was 100% and 84.7% (p = 0.28) (Figure 13). Real-time assessment of glucose concentration in the perfusion solution correlated well with postoperative synthetic graft function ($r2$ = 0.78; p < 0.02). All treated recipients had normal liver function after a 6-month follow-up and are well and alive. This first clinical application of sNM MP with COR showed that controlled graft rewarming after cold storage is a feasible and safe method, in standard clinical practices where the livers are procured and transported under CS, and improves early transplantation outcome in this small series. Clinical trials using continuous and prolonged sNM MP are in preparation by Tim Berendsen from the Boston group.

7.3. Liver-NMP: clinical data

The world's first discarded human liver was transplanted in Birmingham, UK in 2014 after 7 hours of NMP with the Liver Assist® device. MP parameters showed that the portal (blue) and arterial (red) flow rates increased within the first 2 hours, and were sustained within physiological ranges for the next 5 hours. Glucose decreased and pH was corrected to near physiological levels. The lactate levels decreased from 14 to normal levels in the first 2 hours (Figure 14). Bile production reached 22 grams in 7 hours, which was considered a high bile output when compared to previous studies. The liver had normal function after reperfusion and the patient was discharged home on the 11th postoperative day.

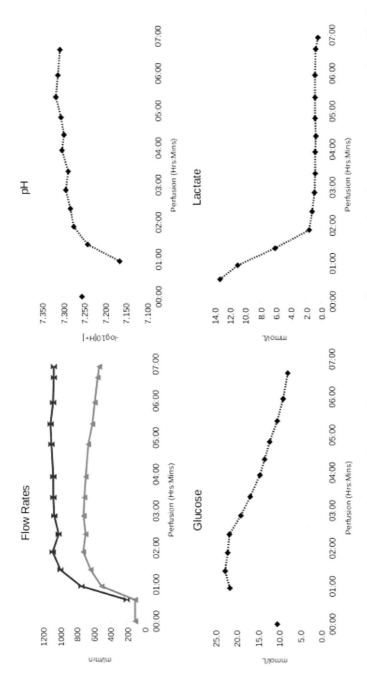

Figure 14. Graphic representation of the machine perfusion parameters (Flow rates) and perfusate's measurements for pH, Glucose and Lactate over a 7-hour period.

NMP was also successfully implemented in an early clinical trial in Oxford, UK, completed in 2015, where 20 patients were treated. The Oxford group utilized the OrganOx® device, after extensive preclinical experimentation [53]. This device utilizes RBCs as their OC at 37°C. The authors reported a median preservation time of 9.3 hours (3.5–18.5) for the NMP group and 8.9 hours (4.2–11.4) for the CS control group. Both groups had similar 30-day graft survival (100% NMP and 97.5% CS). As seen on previous experiments, the peak AST levels were significantly lower ($p = 0.03$) in the NMP group.

A third MP device was successfully transitioned into clinical applications in 2016, when Markmann conducted NMP experiments with the OCS™ Liver System (TransMedics, Cambridge, MA). This device utilizes RBCs as the perfusate and brings a new level of technical sophistication to the field by providing precise monitoring of the perfusion parameters over time through a resourceful digital panel.

8. Future developments

8.1. *Novel oxygen carriers*

Guidelines to assure effective *ex vivo* oxygenation in MP systems continue to evolve. Due to the substantial reduction of the metabolic rate under sub-normothermia, it has been conjectured that adequate oxygenation of the graft could be properly achieved without the use of professional oxygen carriers [52]. Washed RBCs are currently seen as the primary and most accessible vehicle to assure oxygenation and CO_2 removal in MP settings. The use of RBCs in MP systems (both with centrifugal and rotational pumps) has been clearly associated with progressive hemolysis due to the unavoidable mechanical injuries imposed on the RBC membranes in prolonged perfusion sessions [54, 55]. Hence, the necessity of cell-free OC in the MP devices has been one of the most important challenges of the field of *ex vivo* perfusion. Several OC have been investigated (e.g., PFC nanoparticles), but so far the HBOC molecules have shown the most promising results [56–58]. Our group has pioneered the utilization of a bovine-derived HBOC solution in sNMP system, providing sustainable oxygenation through the sinusoids, the arterial microcirculation and the peribiliary plexus of the extrahepatic bile duct system [59]. This system combines a low hemoglobin concentration (Hb = 3.5 g/dl) with a stable HES-based colloid, which is further enhanced by additional buffers, impermeant, hepatic growth factors (e.g., insulin), and reactive oxygen species scavengers. This

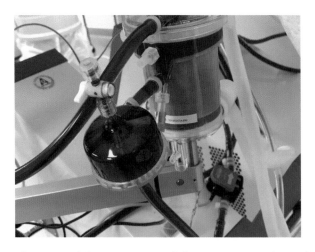

Figure 15. Image from one of the oxygenators of the Liver Assist® device showing the color change in the human-derived HBOC solution observed in the perfusate after effective oxygenation.

ex vivo HBOC solution showed no signs of deleterious oxidation of the hemoglobin component, which was significantly lower than the previous methemoglobin levels previously reported from *in vivo* applications with a higher hemoglobin concentration (13 g/dL). The *ex vivo* utilization of the HBOC/HES-based colloid solution has additional advantages over RBCs. It eliminates the risk of hemolytic reactions while sustaining low viscosity. Additional benefits of cell-free OC products would be greater availability, long storage life, universal compatibility, and minimal likelihood of transmitting blood-borne infections [57]. Our group has recently conducted a series of experiments to validate a new human-derived HBOC (VIR-XV1) developed by VirTech Bio Inc, Natick, MA. These experiments aimed to test the efficacy of this new OC solution, developed exclusively for *ex vivo* utilization in organ and tissue preservation (Figure 15).

9. Conclusions

(1) The HBOC molecule showed great stability over a 12-hour period; (2) the HBOC molecule show great efficacy in providing prolonged hepatic oxygenation while completely removing CO_2 to values below detectable levels; (3) the MP/HBOC system was able to sustain normal hepatic function (e.g., lactate clearance, normal liver enzymes and sustained pH) over a 12-hour period; (4) in spite of low Hb (3 g/dL) levels, the pO2 was sustained between 400 and 500 mmHg; (5) histological analysis showed

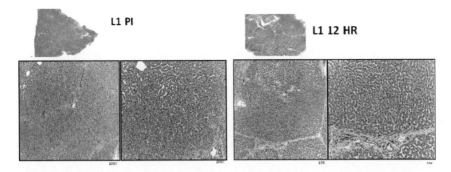

Figure 16. Liver biopsies taken at baseline before the initial procurement (PI) and after 12 hours of preservation (12 HR). The tissues were stained by H&E and analyzed with different magnitudes (10X and 20X). A blind analysis performed by the pathologist couldn't differentiate between the two samples, meaning that the hepatic tissue sustained complete integrity under MP/HBOC preservation over a 12-hour period.

normal anatomical hepatic features after 12 hours of *ex vivo* preservation with the new HBOC; (6) the new HBOC didn't cause sinusoidal debris and SEC detachment after 12 hours of MP as previously seen with a bovine-derived HBOC [59] (Figure 16); (7) mitochondrial function was sustained within normal range during the 12-hour *ex vivo* period; (8) the magnitude of NO oxidation (nitrite and nitrate levels) was 10–100X lower than previous published data with a bovine-derived HBOC; (8) hepatocytes sustained full cell integrity (EM analysis) over the 12-hour period, which includes normal anatomical features for the mitochondria. Taken together, these parameters indicate the HBOC stayed intact and fully functional during the 12-hour study.

References

1. Bing R. The perfusion of whole organs in the Lindbergh apparatus with fluids containing hemocyanin as respiratory pigment. *Science* 1938;87:554–5.
2. Kuliabko. Weltere Studein fiber die Wiederbebung des Herzens. *Pflug Arch* 1903;xvcii:539.
3. Knowlton FP and Starling EH. The influence of variations in temperature and blood-pressure on the performance of the isolated mammalian heart. *J Physiol* 1912;44:206–19.
4. Bainbridge FA and Evans CL. The heart, lung, kidney preparation. *J Physiol* 1914;48(4):278–86.
5. Carrel A and Lindbergh CA. The culture of whole organs. *Science* 1935;81:2112.

6. Lindbergh CA. An apparatus for the culture of whole organs. *J Exp Med* 1935;75:415.

7. Lapchinsky AG. Recent results of experimental transplantation of preserved limbs and kidneys and possible use of technique in clinical practice. *Ann NY Acad Sci* 1960;87:539–71.

8. Lindbergh CA. *Autobiography of Values*. New York: Hartcourt Brace Jovanovich, 1978.

9. Starzl TE, Brittain RS, Stonington OG, Coppinger RW, and Waddell WR. Renal transplantation in identical twins. *Arch Surg* 1963;86:600.

10. Owens TC, Prevedel AE, and Swan H. Prolonged experimental occlusion of thoracic aorta during hypothermia. *Arch Surg* 1955;70:95.

11. Lillehei RC, Goott B, and Miller FB. The physiologic response of the small bowel of the dog to ischemia including prolonged in vitro preservation of the bowel with successful replacement and survival. *Ann Surg* 1959;150:543.

12. Lower RR and Shumway NE. Studies on orthotopic homotransplantations of the canine heart. *Surg Forum* 1960;11:18.

13. Starzl TE, Kaupp HA Jr, Brock DR, Lazarus RE, and Johnson RV. Reconstructive problems in canine liver homotransplantations with special reference to the postoperative role of hepatic venous. *Surg Gynecol Obstet* 1960;111:733.

14. Starzl TE. *Experience in Renal Transplantation*. Philadelphia: Saunders, 1964, pp. 68–71.

15. Marchioro TL, Huntlev RT, Waddell WR, and Starzl TE. Extracorporeal perfusion for obtaining postmortem homografts. *Surgery* 1963;54:900.

16. Kestens PJ, Otte JB, Alexandre GP, et al. Human orthotopic liver graft. *Acta Chir Belg* 1970;69:285–303.

17. Ackerman JR, and Barnard CN. A report on the successful storage of kidneys. *Br J Surg* 1966;53:525.

18. Brettschneider L, Daloze PM, Huguet C, Porter KA, Groth DG, Kashiwagi N, Hutchison DE, and Starzl TE. The use of combined preservation techniques for extended storage of orthotopic liver homografts. *Surg Gynecol Obstet* 1968;126:203.

19. Belzer FO, Ashby BS, Dunphy JE. 24-Hour and 72 hour preservation of canine kidneys. *Lancet* 1967;2:530.

20. Belzer FO, Ashby BS, Huang JS, et al. Etiology of rising perfusion pressure in isolated organ perfusion. *Ann Surg* 1968;168:382–9.

21. Belzer FO, Southard JIH. Principles of solid-organ preservation by cold storage. *Transplantation* 1988;45:673.

22. Pienaar BH, Lindell SL, Van Gulik T, et al. Seventy-two-hour preservation of the canine liver by machine perfusion. *Transplantation* 1990;49:258–60.

23. Dutkowski P, Schonfeld S, Odermatt B, et al. Rat liver preservation by hypothermic oscillating liver perfusion compared to simple cold storage. *Cryobiology* 1998;36:61–70.

24. Dutkowski P, Graf R, and Clavien PA. Rescue of the cold preserved rat liver by hypothermic oxygenated machine perfusion. *Am J Transplant* 2006;6:903–12.

25. Dutkowski P, de Rougemont O, and Clavien PA. Machine perfusion for 'marginal' liver grafts. *Am J Transplant* 2008;8:917–24.

26. Schlegel A, Graf R, Clavien PA, *et al*. Hypothermic oxygenated perfusion(HOPE) protects from biliary injury in a rodent model of DCD liver transplantation. *J Hepatol* 2013;59:984–91.

27. Dutkowski P, Schlegel A, de Oliveira M, *et al*. HOPE for human liver grafts obtained from donors after cardiac death. *J Hepatol* 2014;60:765–72.

28. Neuhaus P and Blumhardt G. Extracorporeal liver perfusion: applications of an improved model for experimental studies of the liver. *Int J Artif Organs* 1993;16:729–39.

29. Brockmann J, Reddy S, Coussios C, *et al*. Normothermic perfusion: a new paradigm for organ preservation. *Ann Surg* 2009;250:1–6.

30. Guarrera JV, Estevez J, Boykin J, *et al*. Hypothermic machine perfusion of liver grafts for transplantation: technical development in human discard and miniature swine models. *Transplant Proc* 2005;37:323–25.

31. Guarrera JV, Henry SD, Samstein B, *et al*. Hypothermic machine preservation in human liver transplantation: the first clinical series. *Am J Transplant* 2010;10:372–81.

32. Guarrera JV, Henry SD, Samstein B, *et al*. Hypothermic machine preservation facilitates successful transplantation of "orphan" extended criteria donor livers. *Am J Transplant* 2015;15:161–9.

33. Vogel T, Brockman JG, Quaglia A, *et al*. The 24-hour normothermic machine perfusion of discarded human liver grafts. *Liver Transpl* 2017;23:207–20.

34. Bruinsma BG, Sridharan GV, Weeder P, *et al*. Metabolic profiling during ex-vivo machine perfusion. *Sci Rep* 2015;6:1–13.

35. Op den Dries S, Sutton M, Lisman T, and Porte R. Protection of bile ducts in liver transplantation: looking beyond ischemia. *Transplantation* 2011;92:373–9.

36. Selzner M, Goldaracena N, Echeverri J, Kaths JM, Linares I, Selzner N, *et al*. Normothermic ex vivo liver perfusion using Steen solution as perfusate for human liver transplantation: first North American results. *Liver Transpl* 2016;22:1501–8.

37. Banan B, Xiao Z, Watson R, Xu M, Jia J, Upadhya GA, *et al*. Novel strategy to decrease reperfusion injuries and improve function of cold-preserved livers using normothermic ex vivo liver perfusion machine. *Liver Transpl* 2016;22:333–43.

38. van der Plaats A, 'T Hart NA, Verkerke GJ, Leuvenink HG, Ploeg RJ, Rakhorst G. Hypothermic machine preservation in liver transplantation revisited: concepts and criteria in the new millennium. *Ann Biomed Eng* 2004;31(4):623–31.

39. McLellan SA and Walsh TS. Oxygen delivery and haemoglobin. *Crit Care Pain* 2004;4(4):123–6.

40. Klabunde RE. *Cardiovascular Physiology Concepts*, 2nd ed. Baltimore, MD: Lippincott Williams & Wilkins, 2011.
41. Boushel R, Langberg H, Olesen J, *et al*. Monitoring tissue oxygen availability with near infrared spectroscopy (NIRS) in health and disease. *Scand J Med Sci Sports* 2001;11:213–222.
42. Bhagavan NV. *Medical Biochemistry*, 2nd ed. Boston: Jones and Bartlett Publishers, 1978.
43. 'T Hart NA, van der Plaats A, Faber A, Leuvenink HG, Olinga P, Wiersma-Buist J, *et al*. Oxygenation during hypothermic rat liver preservation: an in vitro slice study to demonstrate beneficial or toxic oxygenation effects. *Liver Transpl* 2005;11:1403–11.
44. Drummond M, Braile D, Lima-Oliveira AP, *et al*. Technological evolution of membrane oxygenators. *Braz J Cardiovasc Surg* 2005;20:432–7.
45. Gaylor JDS. Membrane oxygenators: influence of design on performance. *Perfusion* 1994;9:173–80.
46. Jones DP. *Biomedical Sensors*. Sensors Technology Series. New York: Momentum Press, 2010.
47. Karangwa SA, Dutkowski P, Fontes P, *et al*. Machine perfusion of donor livers for transplantation: a proposal for standardized nomenclature and reporting guidelines. *Am J Transplant* 2016;16:2932–42.
48. Dutkowski P, Schlegel A, de Oliveira M, *et al*. HOPE for human liver grafts obtained from donors after cardiac death. *J Hepatol* 2014;60(4):765–72.
49. Dutkowski P, Polak WG, Muiesan P, Schlegel A, Verhoeven CJ, Scalera I, DeOliveira ML, Kron P, and Clavien PA. First comparison of hypothermic oxygenated perfusion versus static cold storage of human donation after cardiac death liver transplants. An International-matched case analysis. *Ann Surg* 2015;262:764–71.
50. Op den Dries S, Sutton ME, Karimian N, *et al*. Hypothermic oxygenated machine perfusion prevents arteriolonecrosis of the peribiliary plexus in pig livers donated after circulatory death. PLos ONE 2014;9(2):e88521.
51. Hoyer DP, Mathé Z, Gallinat A, Canbay AC, Treckmann JW, Rauen U, Paul A, and Minor T. Controlled oxygenated rewarming of cold stored livers prior to transplantation: first clinical application of a new concept. *Transplantation* 2016;100(1):147–52.
52. Minor T and Paul A. Hypothermic reconditioning in organ transplantation. *Curr Opin Organ Transplant* 2013;18:161–7.
53. Liu Q, Nassar A, Farias K, *et al*. Sanguineous normothermic machine perfusion improves hemodynamics and biliary epithelial regeneration in donation after cardiac death porcine livers. *Liver Transpl* 2014;20:987–99.
54. Benedetti M, De Caterina R, Bionda A, *et al*. Blood — artificial surface interactions during cardiopulmonary bypass. A comparative study of four oxygenators. *Int J Artif Organs* 1990;13:488–97.

55. Kameneva M, Undar A, Antaki JF, *et al*. Decrease in red blood cell deformability caused by hypothermia, hemodilution and mechanical stress: factors related to cardiopulmonary bypass. *ASAIO* 1999;45:307–10.

56. Jahr JS, Mackenzie C, Pearce LB, Pitman A, Greenburg AG. HBOC-201 as an alternative to blood transfusion: efficacy and safety evaluation in a multicenter phase III trial in elective orthopedic surgery. *J Trauma* 2008;64:1484–97.

57. Jahr JS, Walker V, and Manoochehri K. Blood substitutes as pharmacotherapies in clinical practice. *Curr Opin Anesthesiol* 2007;20:325–30.

58. McNeil JD, Propper B, Walker J, Holguin L, Evans L, Lee K, *et al*. A bovine hemoglobin-based oxygen carrier as a pump prime for cardiopulmonary bypass; reduced system lactic acidosis and improved cerebral oxygen metabolism during low flow in a porcine model. *J Thorac Cardiovasc Surg* 2011;142:411–7.

59. Fontes P, Lopez R, van der Plaats A, *et al*. Liver preservation with machine perfusion and a newly developed cell free oxygen carrier solution under subnormothermic conditions. *Am J Transplant* 2015;15:381–94.

5. Living-Donor Hepatectomy: Laparoscopic and Robotic Techniques

Salvatore Gruttadauria*, Giovanni B. Vizzini*, Duilio Pagano*,
Bruno G. Gridelli*, and Angelo Luca†

*Department for the Treatment and Study of Abdominal Diseases
and Abdominal Transplantation, IRCCS–ISMETT
(Istituto Mediterraneo per i Trapianti e Terapie ad alta specializzazione)/
UPMC, Via E. Tricomi 5, 90127, Palermo, Italy
†Department of Diagnostic and Therapeutic Services, IRCCS–ISMETT
(Istituto Mediterraneo per i Trapianti e Terapie ad alta specializzazione)/
UPMC, Via E. Tricomi 5, 90127, Palermo, Italy

1. Introduction

Laparoscopic liver surgery has been a major advancement in surgery over
the last three decades reducing postoperative pain, blood loss, and morbidity
when compared with open liver surgery [1]. This has led to the development
of new instrumentation and technologies, including robotic platforms,
which are expanding the limits of minimally invasive liver surgery.

Living-donor liver transplantation (LDLT) for both children and adults
has become a well-established therapeutic option for patients in need of liver
replacement, particularly in countries with no or limited access to cadaver
organ donation. The major concern of LDLT is donor safety, and initiatives
of the international transplantation community aim at improving safety,
reducing complications and expanding access to this life saving procedure [2].

Laparoscopic live-donor hepatectomy (LLDH) was initially developed
for pediatric LT and, subsequently, for adult patients. Whereas LLDH for

pediatric recipients today is performed regularly by several centers, the diffusion of LLDH for adults, because of its higher complexity, is still quite limited [3].

Three LLDH techniques have been developed by some of the most experienced liver transplant(ation) (LT) centers: the pure or totally laparoscopic hepatectomy (PLH) [4], the hand-assisted method, and the laparoscopic-assisted or hybrid technique (LADH) [5–8].

Most of the LLDHs reported in literature are laparoscopic left-lateral sectionectomies (LLLSs) for adult-to-pediatric LDLT, and laparoscopic right hepatectomies (LRHs) for adult-to-adult LDLT [9,10]. LLLS was first introduced in pediatric LT by Cherqui and colleagues in 2002 [11]. LLLS is now fully established as a standard procedure for liver procurement in pediatric referral centers. Laparoscopic liver procurement for adult transplantation is more challenging because of the greater liver parenchyma mass required by the adult metabolism.

The use of robotic techniques has been explored as a way to render the procedure easier and safer, but still has a very limited diffusion [12].

The aim of this chapter is to provide a summary of the most relevant LLDH techniques for both pediatric and adult living-donor transplantation. The robotic approach to liver graft procurement for LDLT, and our Center's experience with some LLDH surgical techniques will also be described.

2. Adult-to-pediatric living-donor liver transplantation (LDLT)

2.1. *Laparoscopic left-lateral sectionectomies (LLLS)*

The number of clinical studies reporting the outcome of LLLS cases has increased over the last few years, validating the safety and effectiveness of LLLS for resection of benign and malignant liver lesions. This surgical procedure is also being increasingly applied in adult-to-pediatric LDLT (Table 1).

In 2002, Cherqui and colleagues described the first LLLS for living-related LT in a pediatric recipient in *The Lancet* where they reported two LLLSs performed in two adult donors using five ports and a small suprapubic incision to retrieve the grafts. There were no complications and the transplanted allografts rapidly recovered their function, suggesting the feasibility of LLLS for adult-to-child LDLT [11].

Following this first report, Soubrane *et al.* presented a larger series in 2006, comparing 16 LLLS with 14 open procedures. Two hepatic artery thromboses were reported among the recipients of laparoscopic group, and

Table 1. LLLS: published series

Authors	Number of donors	Operative time (minutes)	Blood loss (cc)	Length of stay (days)	Warm ischemia time (minutes)	Donor complication(s)	Recipient complication(s)
Cherqui (2002)	2	360–420	150–450	5–7	4–10	0	1 (hepatic artery thrombosis)
Troisi (2009)	1	—	—	7	6	0	NO
ISMETT (2012)	11	458	—	5.9	5	2 (1 pleural effusion, 1 incision hematoma)	4 (2 portal vein thrombosis, 1 biliary stenosis, 1 cava stenting)
Yu (2012)	15	331	410	7.1	5.8	0	2 (1 portal vein stenosis, 1 biliary stricture)
Troisi (2014)	1	—	—	2	4	0	NO
Scatton (2015)	67	275	82	—	9	6 (2 bile leak, 1 biliary stricture, 1 incision hematoma, 1 bladder injury, 1 ulcer)	18 (5 hepatic artery thrombosis, 3 portal vein thrombosis, 10 biliary complications)
Soubrane (2006)	16	320	18.7	11	10	3 (1 bile leak, 2 incision hematoma)	6 (2 hepatic artery thrombosis, 1 retransplantation due to portal vein thrombosis, 3 biliary strictures)
Kim (2011)	11	330	396	6.9	6	0	2 (1 portal vein stenosis, 1 biliary stricture)
Samstein (2015)	17	478	177	4.3	—	2 (1 hernia, 1 bile leak)	2 (1 hepatic artery thrombosis, 1 portal vein thrombosis)

one in the open group. This data was mistakenly used by some authors to conclude that LLLS carries an increased risk of recipient vascular complications compared to the open approach [8].

Other series were also reported by Kim *et al.* in 2011 (11 LLLS), and by Yu and Kim in 2012 with a larger donor group (15 LLLS) confirming the safety, feasibility, and reproducibility of the procedure. This consists in the resection of Coinaud segments 2 and 3, including the left hepatic artery, the left portal vein, the left hepatic vein, and the left bile duct. Parenchymal dissection is performed along the falciform ligament, up to the origin of the left hepatic vein. A 7–8 cm suprapubic incision is usually performed to extract the graft [13,14].

These three studies showed that the laparoscopic approach had advantages in terms of less postoperative pain and morbidity, cosmetic benefits, and reduced blood loss. There were no surgical, vascular, or infectious complications in the LLLS group, while worse recipient outcomes were reported in the two open approach groups, including two patients with portal vein stenosis, one with acute rejection, and one death. The costs of the laparoscopic procedures were higher than those of open surgery [15].

In 2015, Scatton presented the largest case series, with 67 living donors — 62 LLLS and five laparoscopic left hepatectomies (LLHs), while Samstein compared 17 LLLSs with 20 open procedures. In both series, there was a shorter period of hospitalization and an earlier return to work. In the Samstein series, there were only minor complications in the donors, and no primary graft failure in the recipients. The 1-year graft and patient survival was 91% in the LLLS group and 85% in the open group [16,17].

3. Adult-to-adult living-donor liver transplantation (LDLT)

3.1. *Laparoscopic right hepatectomies (LRH)*

Particularly in Western countries, a sufficient partial liver graft for an adult LDLT recipient usually requires a right lobe in order to provide an adequate hepatic parenchymal volume. The widespread diffusion of LRH is limited by crucial technical issues, such as the detachment of the right liver from the retrohepatic vena cava, and the specific skeletonization and division of the vascular and biliary pedicles to allow a safe deep parenchymal transection [10,18,19].

Three different surgical minimally invasive options have been developed in living-donor liver donation surgery: the totally laparoscopic method, the laparoscopic-assisted method, and the hand-assisted method (Table 2) [20].

Table 2. Laparoscopic full-left hepatectomy: published series.

Authors	Number of donors	Operative time (minutes)	Blood loss (cc)	Length of stay (days)	Laparoscopic assisted method (yes/no)	Donor complication(s)	Recipient complication(s)
Oya (2011)	4	529–645	100–1,100	9–22	Yes	0	N/A
Soyama (2012)	9	456	520	—	Yes	1 (portal vein thrombosis with relaparotomy)	N/A
Takahara (2015)	13	380	200	8	Yes	3 (3 biliary complications)	N/A
Kurosaki (2006)	10	363	302	11	Yes	0	3 early graft losses
Marubashi (2013)	14	435	353	10.3	Yes	2 (2 delayed gastric emptying)	N/A
Soyama (2015)	41	398	475	—	Yes	3 (1 duodenal ulcer, 1 portal vein thrombosis, 1 ileus)	N/A
Troisi (2013)	4	487.5	50	5	No	1 (right posterior duct leak treated with Roux-en-Y)	2 (1 cholestasis, 1 redo laparotomy for hepatic artery dissection + intrahepatic abscesses)
Samstein (2013)	2	368	125	4	No	0	1 (bile leak)
Samstein (2015)	5	478	173.3	4.27	No	2 (1 hernia, 1 bile leak)	N/A
Takahara (2015)	3	482	69	8.5	No	1 (biliary fistula)	N/A

In 2006, Koffron, in Chicago, reported a successful case of hand-assisted LRH that used two laparoscopic ports and a subxiphoid midline incision for hand assistance during liver mobilization and direct vision during dissection. Kurosaki, in Japan, reported three laparoscopic-assisted LRHs with right liver mobilization under laparoscopic view, using three to five operative trocars, and completing the dissection under direct vision through a 12-cm laparotomy. Donor postoperative courses were uneventful in both series [21,22].

Laparoscopic-assisted LRH was later reported in a number of comparative and case-matched series. The largest studies, by Baker in 2009 (33 cases), Ha in 2013 (20 cases), Zhang in 2014 (25 cases), and Makki in 2014 (26 cases) reported shorter operative times, comparable blood losses, significantly shorter hospital stays, less analgesic use, and comparable donor complication rates and recipient outcomes [23–26].

In 2012, Choi reported 40 donors who underwent single-port laparoscopic-assisted LDH, for which graft mobilization was performed under laparoscopic vision using a right subcostal single port. Parenchymal transsection was completed in an open fashion extending the single port incision. Intraoperative complications consisted in a right hepatic vein injury, an adrenal gland bleeding requiring conversion, a diaphragmatic injury, and a capsular hematoma. Recently, other groups have reported successful pure LRH: Soubrane in 2012 (one case), Rotellar in 2013 (one case), Han (two cases), Takahara (three cases), and Kim (three cases) in 2015, describing uneventful postoperative courses in all donors. These studies reported no surgical or infectious complications resulting from laparoscopic organ procurement. Pure LRH resulted in less wound-related morbidity, as well as more rapid recovery, with better cosmetic results compared to open liver surgery for living-related liver donation (Table 3) [4,5,27–29].

3.2. Laparoscopic left hepatectomies (LLH)

While right lobe procurement provides more liver parenchyma for the recipient, exposing the donor to higher risks related to the small remnant donor liver, the use of the left lobe, leaving more hepatic parenchyma to the donor, increases the recipient's risk of small-for-size syndrome (SFSS).

For these reasons, the right lobe is usually the transplanted graft in adult-to-adult LDLT, especially in Western countries. Only recently has the left graft received renewed interest because of the morbidity and mortality related to right lobe procurement, and of the development of new techniques for the prevention and treatment of SFSS [22].

Table 3. Pure laparoscopic living donor right hepatectomy: published series

Authors	Number of donors	Operative time (minutes)	Blood loss (cc)	Length of stay (days)	Warm ischemia time (minutes)	Robotic surgery (yes/no)	Donor complication(s)	Recipient complication(s)
Soubrane (2013)	1	480	100	7	12	No	0	N/A
Rotellar (2013)	1	480	100	4	3	No	0	N/A
Han (2015)	2	N/A	N/A	9	N/A	No	0	N/A
Takahara (2015)	3	482	69.5	8.5	N/A	No	1 (biliary fistula)	N/A
Kim (2015)	3	458	240	7.8	4.8	No	0	N/A
Giulianotti (2012)	1	480	350	5	35	Yes	1 (portal vein stenosis)	0
ISMETT (2012)	1	720	460	7	5	Yes	0	1 (hepatic artery thrombosis)

It was recently reported that for every 5% reduction of the minimum requirement for graft weight (GW)/standard liver volume (SLV) ratio, the rate of adult LDLT using left liver graft could be doubled. Also, if the minimum GW/SLV ratio for successful LDLT was reduced to 25%, a left liver graft could be used in two-thirds of all adult LDLTs [30].

Reports of LLH for LDLT have been relatively limited, particular the totally laparoscopic ones: there are 91 reported cases of laparoscopic-assisted left hepatectomies (LALHs) and only 14 cases of pure LLH (Table 4). LLH procurement allows retrieving the second, third, and fourth Coinaud segments, with or without the first segment, including the left branch of the portal vein, the left hepatic artery, and the left and middle hepatic veins. Graft extraction is usually performed through a 10–12 cm incision. Three comparative studies, by Kurosaki in 2006 (10 LALH including the caudate lobe vs. 13 open ones), by Marubashi in 2013 (14 LALH vs. 79 open procedures), and by Soyamain in 2015 (41 LALH vs. 137 open resections), showed longer operative times (435 min. vs. 383 min.), comparable blood losses (300–475 mL), but less postoperative pain with reduced use of analgesics (3.2 vs. 3.7 days of analgesic use; 1.2 times vs. 3.8 per day), and shorter hospital stays (10 days vs. 18 days). Complications were minor and there was no donor mortality [22,31,32].

In 2013, Troisi published the first case series of four donors who underwent total LLH (lobes 2–4, with or without the caudate lobe), followed by Samstein with two case reports, and later in 2015 with five more LLH, and by Takahara with three LLH.

These papers showed LLH is feasible and, although operative times were longer, the advantages were a lower blood loss, and a shorter hospital length of stay [5,17]. Reported donor complications were one bile leak treated with hepaticojejunostomy, a biliary fistula that required external biliary drainage, and an incisional hernia. Recipient outcomes were not described, with the exception of Samstein who reported one relaparotomy for bile leak, with no hepato-specific complications related to SFSS [33].

With more experience and a better understanding of the mechanisms of graft injury in SFSS, there is evidence that minimum graft size safety limit can be lowered, and a higher proportion of LDLTs using left liver graft can be performed. Successfully extending the selection criteria for LLH will expand the donor pool by removing inadequate size of the graft or liver remnant as a reason for rejecting a donor, and improve the safety of the donor operation [34].

Table 4. Laparoscopy-assisted right hepatectomy: published series

Authors	Number of donors	Operative time (minutes)	Blood loss (cc)	Length of stay (days)	Incision length (cm)	Hand assistance (yes/no)	Incision type	Donor complication(s)
Kurosaki (2006)	3	363	302	11	12	Yes	Midline	0
Koffron (2006)	4	235	150	3	5	Yes	Midline	0
Koffron (2007)	20	—	—	—	—	Yes	—	—
Suh (2009)	7	489	—	10	9	Yes	Transverse	1 (fluid collection. required percutaneous drainage)
Baker (2009)	33	265	417	4.3	5	Yes	Midline	2 (1 small bowel injury, 1 biloma)
Soyama (2012)	6	456	520	—	12	Yes	Midline	1 (portal vein thrombosis)
Nagai (2012)	4	389	350	6.3	10	Yes	Midline	—
Ha (2013)	20	335	290	10.7	10–12	Yes	Subcostal	0
Choi (2014)	11	483	307.8	9	9	Yes	Transverse	—
Zhang (2014)	25	385	378	7	12	Yes	Midline	1 (bleeding)
Makki (2014)	26	702	336	—	9	Yes	Midline	1 (pleural effusion)
Suh (2015)	14	334	298	10.2	9	Yes	Transverse	0
Takahara (2015)	25	—	—	—	—	Yes	—	2 (2 biliary complications)
Soyama (2015)	25	411	600	—	12	Yes	Midline	3 (1 duodenal ulcer, 1 portal vein thrombosis, 1 ileus)
Choi (2012)	20	383	870	12.1	15	No	Subcostal	4 (1 diaphragmatic hernia, 2 pleural effusions, 1 biliary stricture)

4. Robotic donor hepatectomy

Robot-assisted surgery was developed to address the limitations of conventional laparoscopy, allowing better tissue dissection and precise intracorporeal suturing. It was accomplished recreating the human hand's degrees of freedom, providing dexterity and precise movements, with complex algorithms able to minimize physiologic tremor. The three-dimensional view and magnification of the operative field increase visual perception [12].

Robot-assisted liver surgery has been progressively utilized for oncologic diseases in centers with extensive and skilled performance, reporting encouraging complication rates and similar perioperative outcomes between open, laparoscopic, and robotic approaches [35].

However, although existing data are promising and deserve further investigation, given the higher cost, the cost-effectiveness ratio of robotic procedures is not favorable [36].

Giulianotti and colleagues reviewed the literature on robotic liver resection and its application to liver donation, and described the first robot-assisted right living-donor hepatectomy (RLDH) carried out with the Da Vinci-S® robotic surgical system (Intuitive Surgical, Inc., Sunnyvale, CA, USA) [37].

The procurement was performed inserting four robotic trocars and one laparoscopic access, and completed with a 7-cm subumbilical midline minilaparotomy access for hand-assistance graft retrieval maneuvers. The donor developed portal vein stenosis 6 months after the procedure, successfully treated with balloon dilatation. The postoperative course of the recipient was uneventful.

In 2012, our group at ISMETT, in Palermo, in collaboration with a team from the University of Pisa, performed the second robotic RLDH leveraging our extensive LT experience and Pisa's experience in major robotic hepatic resections. The donor was a 46-year-old male who volunteered to donate his right liver to his 50-year-old brother affected with HCV-related cirrhosis (Figure 1). The fully robotic procedure was performed with four robotic ports and one accessory laparoscopic port (Figure 2). The right lobe was extracted from a 10-cm suprapubic incision, with a graft warm ischemia time of 5 minutes. The procedure lasted 12 hours, and blood loss was 460 mL. The donor's postoperative course was uneventful, and he was discharged on postoperative day 7. He is back to normal life, with normal liver function. The recipient developed acute early postoperative hepatic artery thrombosis, successfully treated with thrombolysis. On postoperative day 47, the recipient was discharged and is currently in good clinical conditions, with normal hepatic function [38].

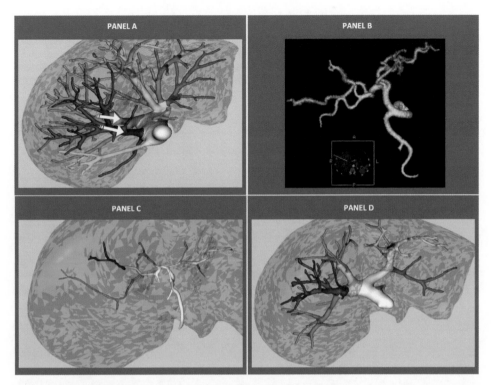

Figure 1. Preoperative imaging study of the donor using the MEVIS Hepavision® system in order to obtain a more detailed analysis of the outflow venous drainage. Panel A: two large accessory hepatic veins (white narrows) draining the right lobe along with the right hepatic vein. Panel B: conventional hepatic artery anatomy. Panel C: normal biliary tree anatomy. Panel D: presence of the short right portal vein.

5. The ISMETT experience

Our group performs a mid-high volume of hepatobiliopancreatic procedures, and includes surgeons with a strong laparoscopic background. This has allowed us to progressively and safely increase the use of laparoscopic liver and pancreatic surgery. We now perform more than 50% of our hepatobiliary and pancreatic resections with minimally invasive approaches. Our adult LT program began in 1999, and to date we have performed over 1,000 liver transplants.

Our pediatric LT program started in 2003, and to date we have performed 160 procedures. With this background, we progressively introduced miniinvasive surgery in organ procurement from living donors, initially for kidney transplantation and later for pediatric LT.

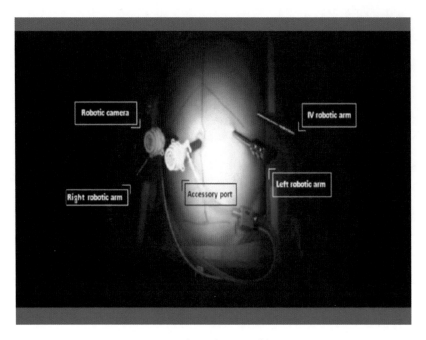

Figure 2. Trocar positioning for robotic and laparoscopic instruments.

Over the last 3 years, we have performed LLLS in pediatric LDLT. Eleven of 15 LDLT donors (five male, six female) underwent LLLS at a mean age of 30 ± 7 years, with no mortality.

The average length of hospitalization was 6 days, with no major complications. Only three minor complications were detected: wound hematoma, abdominal collection, and pleural effusion. The average recipient age was 5.1 ± 5.1 years (range 2 months–17 years). The most common etiology of liver disease was cholestatic liver disease (45.6%) caused primarily by biliary atresia (36.2%), followed by metabolic disorders (13.1%) and acute liver failure (9.3%). Neoplasms (hepatoblastoma, hepatocellular carcinoma, hemangioendothelioma) were indications for transplantation in 6.9% of the patients.

Mean PELD/MELD score at the time of transplant was 15 ± 10. Overall patient and graft survivals at 1 year, 5 years, and 10 years were 85%, 79%, and 79%, respectively.

5.1. Surgical notes

The donor is placed in the lithotomy position, with optional degree of reverse Trendelenburg. The surgeon stands between the donor legs and, depending on liver graft type, the procurement procedure is conducted with the first and second assistants set by the left or right side [39].

Cholecystectomy, when indicated, can be performed at the end of the procedure using the gallbladder to safely mobilize the liver. Most of the time, routine intraoperative cholangiography is performed [40]. However, high quality magnetic resonance cholangiography can help surgeons to feel safe without intraoperative cholangiography in left-lateral grafts or left lobe procurement.

The method used to define the transection plane ultimately depends on the surgeon's approach. Intraoperative ultrasound can be very helpful to localize intrahepatic vascular structures, such as the middle hepatic vein [41]. The bile duct(s) can be identified and sectioned prior to, or during, the parenchymal transection, but sectioning must be performed sharply in order to not jeopardize bile duct vascularization.

Due to the lack of randomized trials, it is difficult to recommend the mandatory devices and the best techniques. Preparation for the Pringle maneuver is necessary to prevent unexpected hemorrhages and ensure prompt surgical hemostasis. The surgical procedure should be based on transsection techniques that fall within the expertise of the surgical team, particularly in the use of suitable tools, in order to minimize the risk of severe vascular and/or biliary lesions during the parenchymal resection [42]. Approach to the hepatic veins (HVs) is tailored according to anatomy. A careful dissection of the anatomic area between the inferior vena cava (IVC) and the left HV or the common trunk of left and middle HV, above the caudate lobe, is very helpful in procurement maneuvers during LLLS and LLH.

The tunnel developed between the HVs and the IVC skeletonization guarantees the performance of the hanging maneuver, which can be helpful for a safe parenchymal transection of the deepest part of the liver graft (Figure 3) [43]. Vessel division can be accomplished with unilateral linear staplers or cut-and-sew articulating staplers. With the latter, the staple line must be removed from the vessels' stumps on the back table, shortening them slightly [44].

There is no agreement on what should be considered an absolute contraindication for a minimally invasive approach to liver resection in living donors: some surgeons consider it should be an unfavorable anatomy, such as the presence of short left or right bile duct, or multiple portal and arterial branches, which lead to indications to perform an open procedure. However, we used the laparoscopic approach in the presence of variances of the HV

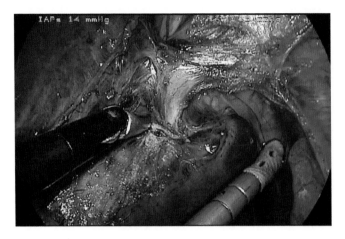

Figure 3. Extraparenchymal isolation of the left hepatic vein: the tunnel development between left hepatic vein and inferior vena cava skeletonization guarantees that the hanging maneuver for a safe hepatic transaction can be performed.

and/or hepatic artery, and the presence of multiple bile ducts. The improved three-dimensional view offered by the robot can be very helpful during parenchymal transection. It also allows an optimal visualization of the biliary duct anatomy that can be further improved using a near-infrared light modality with Indocyanine Green [18]. The robot's fourth arm, and the articulating instruments potentially offer better control of bleeding, without the need for conversion, but this is likely to be counterbalanced by the greater difficulty of conversion, if this is required [45].

In addition to the learning curve, it should be noted that the limited availability of dissection and sealing devices lengthens the parenchymal transection [46–49].

6. Conclusions

Laparoscopic donor hepatectomy has been proposed as a strategy to enhance donor acceptance and recovery, thus expanding the donor pool. A recent meta-analysis by Berardi, which compared minimally invasive living-donor hepatectomy with the open approach in LDLT, showed the many advantages of laparoscopy: a substantial reduction in bleeding, shorter operative times, a shorter hospital length of stay, less use of analgesia, and overall less donor morbidity, thus confirming what we already known about minimally invasive surgery [50].

The second international consensus on laparoscopic liver resection, held in Morioka, Japan, in October 2014, dedicated a question to LLDH and concluded that LLLS for adult-to-pediatric LDLT exhibited the advantages of scarless procedures, and that safety was not different from that of open surgery [51]. The two reported cases of robotic living-donor right hepatectomy clearly demonstrate the feasibility and safety of the procedure for both donor and recipient. Robotic right hepatectomy for liver donation can potentially help the diffusion of a laparoscopic approach to living-donor liver donation for adults, provided this technique is further developed and standardized by centers with extended experience in both robotic liver surgery and LDLT.

Although the preliminary data are very promising, current experience with LLDH is very limited. Surgeons who used this approach in reference centers still had no specific technical skills. This is especially important in living donation, where the learning curve is not acceptable because the death of a single donor can cause serious setbacks in the LDLT program. Referral centers interested in these procedures should develop well-structured training programs for surgeons who want to offer this promising new therapeutic option to their patients. Moreover, the creation of an international registry to better evaluate the benefit/risk ratio for LLLS and LDH and certify short- and long-term outcomes in both donors and recipients, is strongly recommended.

References

1. Ciria R, Cherqui D, Geller DA, Briceno J, and Wakabayashi G. Comparative short-term benefits of laparoscopic liver resection: 9000 cases and climbing. *Ann Surg* 2016;263(4):761–77.
2. Lo CM. Expanding living donor liver transplantation. *Liver Transpl* 2016. doi: 10.1002/lt.24618.
3. Bekheit M, Khafagy PA, Bucur P, *et al*. Donor safety in live donor laparoscopic liver procurement: systematic review and meta-analysis. *Surg Endosc* 2015;29(11):3047–64.
4. Soubrane O, Perdigao Cotta F, and Scatton O. Pure laparoscopic right hepatectomy in a living donor. *Am J Transplant* 2013;13:2467–71.
5. Takahara T, Wakabayashi G, Hasegawa Y, and Nitta H. Minimally invasive donor hepatectomy: evolution from hybrid to pure laparoscopic techniques. *Ann Surg* 2015;261:e3–4.
6. Nguyen KT, Gamblin TC, and Geller DA. World review of laparoscopic liver resection-2,804 patients. *Ann Surg* 2009;250(5):831–41.

7. Buell JF, Cherqui D, Geller DA, *et al*. World Consensus Conference on Laparoscopic Surgery. The international position on laparoscopic liver surgery: the Louisville Statement, 2008. *Ann Surg* 2009;250(5):825–30.

8. Soubrane O, Cherqui D, Scatton O, *et al*. Laparoscopic left lateral sectionectomy in living donors: safety and reproducibility of the technique in a single center. *Ann Surg* 2006;244(5):815–20.

9. Soubrane O, de Rougemont O, Kim KH, *et al*. Laparoscopic living donor left lateral sectionectomy: a new standard practice for donor hepatectomy. *Ann Surg* 2015;262(5):757–6.

10. Han HS, Cho JY, Yoon YS, Hwang DW, Kim YK, Shin HK, *et al*. Total laparoscopic living donor right hepatectomy. *Surg Endosc* 2015;29:184.

11. Cherqui D, Soubrane O, Husson E, *et al*. Laparoscopic living donor hepatectomy for liver transplantation in children. *Lancet* 2002;359(9304):392–6.

12. Abood GJ and Tsung A. Robot-assisted surgery: improved tool for major liver resections? *J Hepatobiliary Pancreat Sci* 2013;20(2):151–6.

13. Kim KH, Jung DH, Park KM, *et al*. Comparison of open and laparoscopic live donor left lateral sectionectomy. *Br J Surg* 2011;98(9):1302–08.

14. Yu YD, Kim KH, Jung DH, Lee SG, Kim YG, and Hwang GS. Laparoscopic live donor left lateral sectionectomy is safe and feasible for pediatric living donor liver transplantation. *Hepatogastroenterology* 2012;59(120):2445–49.

15. Reddy SK, Tsung A, and Geller DA. Laparoscopic liver resection. *World J Surg* 2011;35(7):1478–86.

16. Scatton O, Katsanos G, Boillot O, *et al*. Pure laparoscopic left lateral sectionectomy in living donors: from innovation to development in France. *Ann Surg* 2015;261(3):506–12.

17. Samstein B, Griesemer A, Cherqui D, *et al*. Fully laparoscopic left-sided donor hepatectomy is safe and associated with shorter hospital stay and earlier return to work: a comparative study. *Liver Transpl* 2015;21(6):768–73.

18. Suh KS, Hong SK, Yi NJ, *et al*. Pure 3-dimensional laparoscopic extended right hepatectomy in a living donor. *Liver Transpl* 2016;22(10):1431–6.

19. Kim SH, Lee SD, Kim YK, and Park SJ. Pushing the frontiers of living donor right hepatectomy. *World J Gastroenterol* 2014;20(48):18061–9.

20. Cauchy F, Schwarz L, Scatton O, and Soubrane O. Laparoscopic liver resection for living donation: where do we stand? *World J Gastroenterol* 2014; 20(42):15590–8.

21. Koffron AJ, Kung R, Baker T, *et al*. Laparoscopic-assisted right lobe donor hepatectomy. *Am J Transplant* 2006;6(10):2522–5.

22. Kurosaki I, Yamamoto S, Kitami C, *et al*. Video-assisted living donor hemihepatectomy through a 12-cm incision for adult-to-adult liver transplantation. *Surgery* 2006;139(5):695–703.

23. Baker TB, Jay CL, Ladner DP, *et al*. Laparoscopy-assisted and open living donor right hepatectomy: a comparative study of outcomes. *Surgery* 2009;146(4):817–23.

24. Ha TY, Hwang S, Ahn CS, *et al*. Role of hand-assisted laparoscopic surgery in living-donor right liver harvest. *Transplant Proc* 2013;45(8):2997–9.

25. Zhang X, Yang J, Yan L, *et al*. Comparison of laparoscopy-assisted and open donor right hepatectomy: a prospective case-matched study from China. *J Gastrointest Surg* 2014;18(4):744–50.

26. Makki K, Chorasiya VK, Sood G, *et al*. Laparoscopy-assisted hepatectomy versus conventional (open) hepatectomy for living donors: when you know better, you do better. *Liver Transpl* 2014;20(10):1229–36.

27. Rotellar F, Pardo F, Benito A, *et al*. Totally laparoscopic right-lobe hepatectomy for adult living donor liver transplantation: useful strategies to enhance safety. *Am J Transplant* 2013;13(12):3269–73.

28. Han HS, Cho JY, Yoon YS, *et al*. Total laparoscopic living donor right hepatectomy. *Surg Endosc* 2015;29(1):184.

29. Kim JH, Ryu DH, Jang LC, and Choi JW. Lateral approach liver hanging maneuver in laparoscopic anatomical liver resections. *Surg Endosc* 2016;30(8):3611–7.

30. Chan SC, Fan ST, Chok KS, Sharr WW, Dai WC, Fung JY, *et al*. Increasing the recipient benefit/donor risk ratio by lowering the graft size requirement for living donor liver transplantation. *Liver Transplant* 2012;18(9):1078–82.

31. Marubashi S, Wada H, Kawamoto K, *et al*. Laparoscopy-assisted hybrid left-side donor hepatectomy. *World J Surg* 2013;37(9):2202–10.

32. Soyama A, Takatsuki M, Hidaka M, *et al*. Hybrid procedure in living donor liver transplantation. *Transplant Proc* 2015;47(3):679–82.

33. Halazun KJ, Przybyszewski EM, Griesemer AD, *et al*. Leaning to the left: increasing the donor pool by using the left lobe, outcomes of the largest single-center North American experience of left lobe adult-to-adult living donor liver transplantation. *Ann Surg* 2016;264(3):448–56.

34. Ogura Y, Hori T, El Moghazy WM, Yoshizawa A, Oike F, Mori A, Kaido T, Takada Y, and Uemoto S. Portal pressure <15 mm Hg is a key for successful adult living donor liver transplantation utilizing smaller grafts than before. *Liver Transplant* 2010;16(6):718–28.

35. Tzvetanov I, Bejarano-Pineda L, Giulianotti PC, *et al*. State of the art of robotic surgery in organ transplantation. *World J Surg* 2013;37(12):2791–9.

36. Ocuin LM and Tsung A. Minimally invasive hepatic surgery. *Surg Clin North Am* 2016;96(2):299–313.

37. Giulianotti PC, Tzvetanov I, Jeon H, *et al*. Robot-assisted right lobe donor hepatectomy. *Transpl Int* 2012;25(1):e5–9.

38. Martucci G, Burgio G, Spada M, and Arcadipane AF. Anesthetic management of totally robotic right lobe living-donor hepatectomy: new tools ask for perioperative care. *Eur Rev Med Pharmacol Sci* 2013;17(14):1974–7.

39. Gruttadauria S, Pagano D, Cintorino D, *et al*. Right hepatic lobe living donation: a 12 years single Italian center experience. *World J Gastroenterol* 2013;19(38):6353–9.

40. Pagano D, Spada M, Cintorino D, *et al*. Evolution of surgical technique in conventional open hepatectomy for living liver donation over a 12-year period in a single center. *Transplant Proc* 2014;46(7):2269–71.

41. Gruttadauria S, di Francesco F, Pagano D, *et al*. Liver resections for liver transplantations. *World J Gastrointest Surg* 2010;2(3):51–6.

42. Gruttadauria S, di Francesco F, Li Petri S, *et al*. Technical aspects of living-related liver donation: single-center experience. *Transplant Proc* 2009; 41(4):1273–4.

43. Gruttadauria S, Pagano D, Liotta R, *et al*. Liver volume restoration and hepatic microarchitecture in small-for-size syndrome. *Ann Transplant* 2015;20:381–9.

44. Gruttadauria S, di Francesco F, Spada M, *et al*. Different modalities of arterial reconstruction in hepatic retransplantation using right partial graft. *World J Gastroenterol* 2009;15(26):3322–3.

45. Coelho FF, Kruger JA, Fonseca GM, *et al*. Laparoscopic liver resection: experience based guidelines. *World J Gastrointest Surg* 2016;8(1):5–26.

46. Cheek SM, Sucandy I, Tsung A, Marsh JW, and Geller DA. Evidence supporting laparoscopic major hepatectomy. *J Hepatobiliary Pancreat Sci* 2016;23(5):257–9.

47. Brown KM and Geller DA. What is the learning curve for laparoscopic major hepatectomy? *J Gastrointest Surg* 2016;20(5):1065–71.

48. Cheek SM and Geller DA. The learning curve in laparoscopic major hepatectomy: what is the magic number? *JAMA Surg* 2016. doi: 10.1001/jamasurg. 2016.1698.

49. van der Poel MJ, Besselink MG, Cipriani F, *et al*. Outcome and learning curve in 159 consecutive patients undergoing total laparoscopic hemihepatectomy. *JAMA Surg*. doi:10.1001/jamasurg.2016.1655.

50. Berardi G, Tomassini F, and Troisi RI. Comparison between minimally invasive and open living donor hepatectomy: a systematic review and meta-analysis. *Liver Transpl* 2015;21(6):738–52.

51. Wakabayashi G, Cherqui D, Geller DA, Buell JF, Kaneko H, Han HS, *et al*. Recommendations for laparoscopic liver resection: a report from the second international consensus conference held in Morioka. *Ann Surg* 2015;261:619–29.

6. Adult Living-Donor Liver Transplantation: Right Lobe

Young-In Yoon and Dong-Sik Kim

Korea University College of Medicine, 73 Inchon-Ro,
Seongbuk-Gu, Seoul, Korea 136-705

1. Introduction

The disparity between supply and demand for donor organs has led to the development of living-donor liver transplantation (LDLT). Extension of LDLT from pediatric recipients to adult patients has created the problem of determining an appropriate graft size in order to avoid the small-for-size syndrome (SFSS). When adult-to-adult LDLT was attempted using a left-lobe graft, the functionally impaired small-for-size graft could not provide adequate hepatic function for a relatively large recipient.

In contrast, the use of the right lobe, whose size is sufficient to satisfy the metabolic demands of most adult recipients, has improved clinical outcomes at many transplantation centers [1–3]. The adult right-lobe LDLT procedure has improved markedly since the first successful transplantation of an extended right-lobe graft from a living donor to a 90-kg man with fulminant Wilson's disease, performed in Hong Kong in May 1996. The development of right-lobe LDLT has increased graft supply and contributed to increasing efficiency of adult-to-adult LDLT procedures worldwide [1]. Despite significant progress, the achievement of adequate graft volume, ensuring the safety of the donor as well as a good engraftment by the recipient, and comprehensive understanding of the dynamic nature of posttransplant allograft regeneration have remained major challenges [4]. This chapter focuses on the efficient selection of the right-lobe donor and the surgical techniques of right-lobe LDLT that ensure sufficient inflow and outflow.

129

2. Donor evaluation

Selection of a suitable donor is very important for successful LDLT. Donor evaluation is essential not only for reducing the risks of complications for the donor but also for increasing the survival of both the graft and recipient. Tanaka has stated that routine use of the right lobe for LDLT "would significantly increase the risks" to the donor [5]. Although the lack of an international registry complicates the determination of mortality risk, it has been estimated to be approximately 0.2%, on an average [6]. Although donor safety is an absolute prerequisite in the LDLT program, the morbidity rate of donors is not sufficiently low. The maximal effort should be applied in donor selection and operation for donor safety.

The voluntary intent of the donor should be confirmed first. Physical examination and retrospective analysis of the donor's medical records relative to medical disorders that would significantly increase perioperative risks, such as thromboembolic disorder, are performed before beginning a full-scale study. Once deemed suitable, the donors proceed through a series of investigations that include detailed blood tests, viral serology, and imaging. The indocyanine green retention test is instrumental in assessing the remaining liver function after donation in most Asian centers. Potential donors for right-lobe hepatectomy are generally confined to healthy volunteers below 55 years of age. Older donors (>50 years) have an increased risk of occult medical diseases, and their livers have reduced regenerative capacity [7]. The total liver volume and right hemiliver volume are determined using computed tomography (CT) volumetry. For donor safety, many LDLT programs limit the minimum remnant liver volume to 30–35% of the total liver volume for right liver graft donation, even in young healthy donors. A graft-to-recipient weight ratio (GRWR) of 0.8% is currently recognized as the safe limit to avoid SFSS. Previous studies, however, have suggested a minimal graft volume of 40% of the standard liver volume (SLV) or a GRWR of 0.6–0.8%, depending on the recipient and graft conditions [8–10]. Percutaneous liver biopsy can be performed if fatty liver is suspected in the donor because steatosis affects hepatocyte function and impairs regeneration after major hepatectomy and transplantation [11]. Recently, noninvasive imaging methods, including dual-echo magnetic resonance (MR) imaging and MR spectroscopy, have gradually replaced percutaneous liver biopsy. There are no universal guidelines for the acceptable range of steatosis in LDLT, but in many centers, moderate-to-severe (≥30%) macrovesicular steatosis represents an absolute contraindication for LDLT, while a mild degree (<30%) of steatosis is considered acceptable [12–13].

Preoperative three-dimensional reconstruction of the hepatic blood vessels and the biliary system is recommended. Dynamic CT with three-dimensional reconstruction usually provides detailed information on the branching patterns of the hepatic veins (HVs), the portal vein (PV), and the hepatic arteries of the donor in addition to the distribution of large short HVs. Whether the middle hepatic vein (MHV) should be included in the graft depends on venous tributaries of the MHV, the right hepatic vein (RHV), and the drainage vein from segment 4b, as well as their drainage areas. The decision to remove the MHV with the graft or to leave it in place should be tailored to the vascular anatomy and remnant liver volume of the donor as well as the metabolic demands of the recipient. MR cholangiography is useful for evaluating the biliary anatomy.

3. Surgical technique

There are some essential requirements for successful LDLT. First, a proper graft mass providing sufficient metabolic capacity while ensuring donor safety is necessary. Second, adequate inflow and outflow to avoid injury from ischemia or congestion must be ensured. Successful management of the MHV and/or reconstruction of MHV tributaries, combined with various refinements of the anastomotic technique in right-lobe LDLT, provides functional liver mass, which eliminates the problem of congestion in the right anterior sector and improves the results. Third, rapid liver graft regeneration requires optimal portal inflow. A good understanding of portal hemodynamics, careful intraoperative portal pressure and flow measurement with modulation of the portal inflow of the graft, including splenic artery ligation or embolization, splenectomy, and partial portosystemic shunting, can prevent portal hyperperfusion or steal and reduce instances of early graft failure.

4. Donor operation

Right subcostal and reverse L-shaped incision has been the most widespread approach for many years. This conventional incision facilitates adequate exposure of all segments of the liver and provides easy access for dissection of the short HVs. However, since these incisions are associated with prolonged hospital stay and poorer cosmetic outcome, a mini-incision open technique has been developed [14]. The upper midline incision without any laparoscopic assistance, can be used safely for donor hepatectomy regardless of the graft type in donors with favorable body habitus, and improved cosmetic outcomes can be achieved. To facilitate mobilization of right liver, laparoscopic approach with or without hand port through upper midline can be used. When using a mini-incision open technique, the use of a Kent tractor is recommended to provide sufficient exposure. The bilateral edge of the wound is moved upward and laterally with the use of retractors. Intermittent adjustment of traction power between each retractor blades is helpful to achieve an optimized view for the dissection of the hilum and liver parenchyma. Moreover, the use of hand-held retractors such as malleable Deaver rather than assistant's hand is helpful to obtain more space for surgeon to work. A minimal incision enhances the cosmetic aspects of abdominal skin incisions, but it can be a very demanding procedure for surgeons in some instances, even in experienced hands. It must be kept in mind that donor safety is the utmost priority; thus, if necessary, there should be no hesitation in extending the incision. Over the last decade, various approaches using minimal incision have been developed for use in living-donor surgery, including totally laparoscopic right hepatectomy, although careful candidate selection is mandatory [15, 16].

After exposure, the donor liver should be further assessed for suitability via thorough examination of the morphology, size, and consistency.

After inspection of the abdominal cavity, the ligamentum teres, the falciform, coronary and right triangular ligaments are divided. The MHV and RHV are exposed, with dissection being minimized in the vicinity of the left hepatic vein (LHV). After cholecystectomy, intraoperative cholangiography using a catheter through the cystic duct stump is frequently used for anatomic assessment of bile ducts. MR cholangiography has been advocated, but it may miss small ductal anomalies [17]. Hilar dissection is performed to define the right hepatic artery and the right PV (RPV). Precise knowledge of the anatomy and meticulous hilar dissection is mandatory. If a segment 4 hepatic artery is present on preoperative imaging or during hilar dissection, it is recommended to be preserved to prevent potential ischemic necrosis of segment 4. If any branches to segment 4 need to be sacrificed, the artery is temporarily occluded and a Doppler scan is performed to ascertain the existence of good collateral supply from the left hepatic artery. This method is useful when the presence of an artery to segment 4 is uncertain. Ischemia due to excessive dissection of the right hepatic artery is likely responsible for biliary stricture in the donor. To avoid this complication, the tissue around the common hepatic duct (CHD) is preserved to prevent devascularization, while limiting dissection to isolation of artery only. Careful use of cautery is essential to avoid diathermic injury to bile duct. To avoid bleeding during encircling of the PV and to acquire sufficient length on both graft and recipient sides, the caudate branches can be ligated and then divided. The transection line is demarcated on the liver surface by temporary occlusion of the right hepatic artery and the PV. The posterior vena cava ligament and short HVs are ligated, and inferior HVs larger than 5 mm are preserved for reconstruction. After separation of the right lobe from the inferior vena cava (IVC), the RHV is encircled.

Parenchymal transection is performed with a cavitron ultrasonic aspirator. Inflow and outflow vascular occlusion is not advised unless necessary. One of the most controversial issues during the procedure is whether to remove the MHV with the graft. Currently, most transplant centers routinely ligate the MHV tributaries from segments 5 and 8 during procurement of the right lobe and use interposition vein grafts to drain the anteromedial aspect of the right-lobe graft. Alternatively, the MHV can remain with the right-lobe grafts in selected donors if the remnant liver volume is sufficient or the large segment 4 venous tributaries draining close to MHV–LHV junction can be identified preoperatively. In general, to prevent donor morbidity, preservation of the MHV on the donor side is recommended when the anterior segment of the remnant liver (segment 4b) lacks a separate drainage vein.

Following parenchymal transection, the field of view is sufficient to enable dissection of the hilar plate. A small amount of liver tissue should be left around the RHD to prevent devascularization. Particular attention should be paid to retaining the surrounding tissue of the hilar plate without exposing the bile duct, and the right hilar plate should be fully exposed along the anticipated bile duct resection plane. Before transection of the bile duct, another cholangiogram should be obtained to confirm the accurate cutting line. Metal clips or radio-opaque rubber band markers can be used as markers; two radio-opaque rubber band markers are placed parallel to each other and fixed with 6.0 polypropylene sutures over the sheath covering the RHD. The left marker is placed just to the right of the RHD–CHD junction, while the right marker is placed along the transection surface. To avoid damaging the bile duct, a clean transection must be performed at least 2 mm away from the bifurcation using sharp scissors.

The timing of the actual graft procurement is probably the most stressful moment. To avoid any mishaps or delays, it is mandatory for the surgeon to communicate with all other members in the room including the anesthesiology and recipient team. Vascular clamps for PV and RHV should be selected beforehand, and adequate exposure has to be securely obtained. Intravenous heparin is administered at a dose of 5000 IU prior to ligation of the right artery. The graft is removed after sequentially transecting the right hepatic artery, the right portal trunk, and the RHV, whose stumps are then secured. 50 mg of protamine sulfate is injected slowly starting immediately after removal of graft. The RPV stump and orifice of the RHD on the donor side are closed with 6.0 polypropylene running sutures. Before removing the catheter from the cystic duct stump, a final cholangiogram should be obtained to confirm the absence of leakage or stricture in the remnant biliary structure. The falciform ligament of the remnant liver is fixed to the anterior abdominal wall to maintain its anatomical position. A drain is then placed in the right subphrenic space.

5. Back-table procedure

After procurement of the graft liver, it is placed in an ice basin and perfused with histidine-tryptophan-ketoglutarate (HTK) solution or University of Wisconsin solution via the RPV until clear perfusate can be identified from the HV. The RHD is flushed with cold HTK solution in order to remove the bile.

All the venous orifices on the cut surface and the inferior RHV orifices, if any, are assessed. Diameters of the branches are determined using dilators and ruler, and back-table venoplasty is planned accordingly. Inclusion of the MHV in the graft could simplify the reconstruction of the outflow. The walls of the RHV and the MHV can be joined together to form a triangular cuff for a single anastomosis (Figure 1). When the graft does not include the MHV, reconstruction of the MHV should be performed to prevent possible congestion at segments 5 and 8. Although the most commonly used grafts consist of the cryopreserved iliac vein or arteries, polytetrafluoroethylene (PTFE) grafts or even sizable vessels procured from the recipient explanted liver can be used [18–20]. A cryopreserved iliac vein is often utilized owing to its excellent early patency rate (>90%) and simplicity of the procedure [17].

It is essential in order to avoid congestion and serious graft dysfunction that HV reconstruction achieves optimal venous outflow in the right-lobe graft [21, 22]. The various methods available for MHV reconstruction can be broadly divided in two types: those utilizing a separate opening of the graft RHV and reconstructed MHV tributaries and those employing a one-orifice venoplasty of the graft RHV and reconstructed MHV tributaries.

Anatomical variations, such as early branching of the right posterior section, may result in a graft with two PV openings. Even though the two

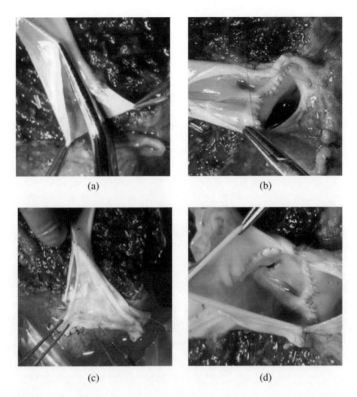

(a)   (b)

(c)   (d)

Figure 1. Modified diamond patch plasty using a cryopreserved iliac vein. (a) After reconstruction of the MHV tributaries, the anterior wall of the reconstructed MHV is cut approximately 2 cm along the long axis. (b) Posterior wall of the reconstructed MHV and anterior wall of the RHV sutured together to form a posterior wall of common outflow orifice. (c) Cryopreserved vein patch is roofed over the triangular gap to form a redundant anterior wall of the MHV. (d) After the completion of bench work; equilateral triangular venoplasty providing the largest cross-sectional area.

separate graft PVs can be anastomosed to the corresponding right anterior and posterior PV branches for the recipient, creating a single orifice at the back table makes reconstruction in the recipient technically easier and prevents complications derived from redundancy such as PV thrombosis and PV stenosis. The Y-graft interposition technique using the recipient's portal confluence or great saphenous vein can be successfully applied (Figure 2).

At the back table, the number of hepatic duct openings should be re-examined. When double ducts are close to each other and share a common septum, they can be anastomosed as a single orifice. Otherwise, if there are two separate openings, albeit adjacent to each other, ducts can be unified into a single orifice with ductoplasty. Although there are several ways to

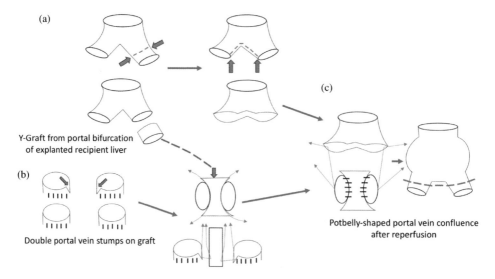

Figure 2. Schematic illustration of the conjoined unification venoplasty technique [23]. (a) A 5-mm-long segment of the sectional portal vein branch limb is excised from the explanted Y-graft for a central patch, and the remnant explanted Y-graft is crutch-opened. (b) Two 3–4 mm-deep niches are made at each PV orifice, and a central patch is inserted between the widely separated graft PV orifices. (c) The crutch-opened Y-graft is anastomosed to the unified graft portal vein orifice, and this makes a potbelly-shaped PV confluence.

perform ductoplasty, the most common method is to divide the septum between the reconstituted ducts vertically and then to suture the gap by using a 6-0 polydioxanone (PDS) to create a larger single opening.

6. Recipient operation

The abdomen is entered through an inverted T incision or a Mercedes-Benz incision. Unlike in deceased-donor liver transplantation (DDLT), special modifications toward preservation of a sufficient length of inflow and out-flow vessels are required for successful surgery to facilitate vascular anastomosis. Hilar dissection should be performed meticulously to isolate and divide branches of the hepatic artery and PV. The individual hepatic arteries are dissected free at the level of its entry to liver parenchyma, and the separation of the right hepatic artery from the posterior wall of CHD should not be performed for preservation of collaterals to bile duct. The distal end of the hepatic artery is determined based on the size of the donor's right hepatic artery. The usual position is at the bifurcation of the right anterior and posterior arteries. Compared to deceased donor liver grafts, partial living donor liver grafts have smaller, shorter arterial stumps, and sometimes multiple arteries. Small and multiple arteries from graft may require extensive dissection of the recipient hepatic arteries for size matching. Since the main PV is usually used for anastomosis, further dissection along an extended portion of the RPV and left PV (LPV) is not mandatory as is for the hepatic arteries. However, when a temporary portocaval shunt is planned, to preserve the maximal length of the RPV, the RPV and the transverse portion of the LPV are isolated. The bile duct should be dissected above the point of bifurcation to obtain right and left bile duct opening separately. To preserve adequate blood supply to the native bile duct, there should be no excessive removal of surrounding tissue. Dissection around the common bile duct should be restricted to preserve the "3 o'clock" and "9 o'clock" vessels and the right hepatic artery placed either behind or in front of the CHD. The liver is mobilized by dividing the coronary and triangular ligaments, and the RHV and the common trunk of the LHV and MHV are encircled respectively. If the separation of the caudate lobe from the IVC is difficult because of a large caudate lobe or severe inflammation and adhesion, transaction of the artery and portal vein prior to dissection of liver from the IVC is often easier and safer. However, in this case, in order to reduce the duration of functional anhepatic phase, communication with the donor team regarding the precise timing for transaction of the artery and the portal vein of the recipient and the actual graft procurement of the donor is necessary. For the removal of the recipient liver, the HVs are cut following the application of vascular clamps on the RHV, the inferior HV, if present, and on the common trunk of the LHV, respectively. The acquisition of an adequate length and strength of the resulting HV stump is important for easy and secure anastomosis. If the stump is too friable, reinforcement or lengthening can be achieved using the recipient's greater saphenous vein.

Following control of bleeding points, the implantation starts with anastomosis of the RHV. The techniques for RHV anastomosis can differ, depending on the method of back-table venoplasty applied. The first is to separate the anastomoses of the graft RHV and the reconstructed MHV to their corresponding locations of recipient. The second is a single anastomosis between the one-orifice venoplasty of graft HVs and recipient RHV with transverse extension (Figure 3). In the former case, the recipient's RHV stump can be extended caudally, and the size of this opening is made approximately 20–30% wider than the longitudinal dimension of the graft outflow by means of venoplasty. The graft RHV is anastomosed to the open-

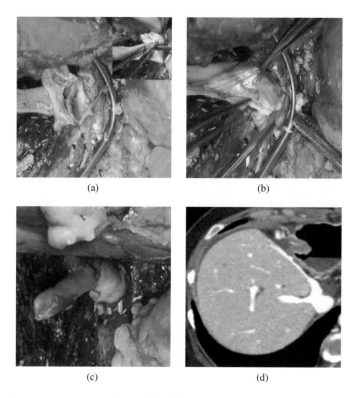

(a) (b)

(c) (d)

Figure 3. HV reconstruction with modified diamond patch plasty using cryopreserved iliac vein. (a) The anterior wall of the recipient IVC is cut approximately 2 cm under partial clamping of IVC. (b) Anastomosis is being performed between the anterior wall of IVC and common outflow orifice with continuous sutures starting from lateral edge. (c) After reperfusion, the reconstructed outflow is bulging and shows its optimal outflow capacity from the right liver graft. (d) Follow-up computed tomography imaging showing wide outflow tract from both right and middle HVs.

ing of the recipient RHV. The reconstructed MHV graft is then anastomosed to the MHV–LHV stump, which is usually performed after reperfusion. In the latter case, a sufficiently large opening is needed. The IVC is partially clamped together with the RHV (sufficiently to provide space for subsequent transverse extension) and is incised longitudinally first from the caudal corner of the RHV to widen its diameter by 20–30% with respect to the graft RHV, and a transverse extension of the RHV stump is made across the anterior wall of the IVC to form the triangular orifice. The reconstructed common outflow of the graft is anastomosed to this triangular orifice. The LHV and MHV stumps are closed by continuous suture. Once the anastomosis is completed, the larger vascular clamp, used for the anastomosis, can be replaced by a smaller one that is more suitable for RHV occlusion during the remaining anastomoses. If either the Inferior RHV or Middle RHV is preserved in the graft, it is anastomosed directly to the IVC in an end-to-side fashion.

After hepatic venous reconstruction, the PV is anastomosed to the trunk of the recipient's PV in an end-to-end fashion either directly or via an inter-position of the vascular graft in case of a dual opening on the graft. Elimination of redundancy and anastomosis tailored to the correct axis are important to avoid kinking after reperfusion. Because the portal vein of the graft is usually extremely thin, even a thin-layered portal vein thrombus on the recipient portal vein needs to be cleared before anastomosis is made in order to avoid any unexpected tearing or folding of the anastomosis line. Growth factor, loosening of the tie length by 30–50% of the diameter of the anastomosis, is recommended to avoid narrowing and to maximize the caliber of the anastomosis. The graft is reperfused after completion of the PV anastomosis and before the microsurgical reconstruction of the hepatic artery.

Although a wide consensus or recommendation regarding the optimal range of portal flow or pressure or the method for inflow modulation is lacking yet, an excessive portal flow and pressure are detrimental for the adequate regeneration of the graft and outcome of LDLT [24, 25]. Intraoperative modulation of the PV flow (PVF) with real-time PV pressure (PVP) monitoring may be necessary [26, 27]. PVP can be easily measured intraoperatively using a thin butterfly needle inserted directly into the PV. The difference between PVP and central venous pressure (CVP) can be calculated, and can be regarded as the hepatic venous pressure gradient. In our institution, inflow modulation is considered in cases where the PVP is above 20 mmHg or the pressure gradient between the PVP and CVP is above 10 mmHg [28]. Portal inflow modulation can be achieved through splenic artery ligation, splenectomy, or portocaval shunt. A combination of CT and Doppler ultrasonography helps in the localization of the large collateral vessels and determination of flow direction as either hepatofetal or hepatofugal. Those collateral vessels may be left *in situ* or ligated, depending on the portal pressure and flow following reperfusion to augment the portal flow in case of portal flow steal, or to decrease the portal flow in presence of excessive portal flow. A direct portogram may be used for evaluation of and intervention on collaterals through the inferior mesenteric vein or the small mesenteric veins. After localizing the steal by studying the flow direction on the portogram, the route of the steal can be abolished by embolization alone or in conjunction with surgical ligation.

The hepatic artery is usually reconstructed using microvascular techniques, with either 9-0 or 10-0 nylon sutures in an end-to-end fashion to one of the stumps of the recipient hepatic artery. To avoid size mismatch and kinking after biliary anastomosis, careful selection of the candidate recipient artery and anastomosis level is important. Careful inspection of the condition of the intima and pulsatile flow is important especially in patients with a history of repeated transarterial chemoembolization. Alternative recipient arterial sources include the right gastroepiploic artery (RGEA), the splenic artery, the left gastric artery, the middle colic artery, and various interposition grafts [29–31]. The RGEA is used largely owing to two definite advantages. The first is because its dissection is simple and safe, and bleeding can be avoided because the RGEA is surrounded by soft tissue. Secondly, its length is usually sufficient for anastomosis with graft arterial stumps. Immediately after the completion of all vascular reconstructions, an intraoperative Doppler ultrasonography is performed to confirm triphasic hepatic venous outflow, sufficient portal flow, and excellent intrahepatic arterial flow.

Either a duct-to-duct (D-D) or hepaticojejunostomy (H-J) biliary anastomosis can be performed. The choice of biliary reconstruction is influenced by multiple factors, such as underlying liver disease, graft type, and the number and size of donor and recipient bile ducts. H-J was the standard biliary reconstruction technique applied after the first reports on right liver graft adult-to-adult LDLT. However, it has disadvantages including longer operative time, increased infection risk, and delay in return of gastrointestinal functions. Recently, the use of D-D anastomosis in LDLT has been advocated [32]. H-J is usually limited to cases with multiple separate bile duct orifices in the graft or underlying liver disease prohibiting D-D reconstruction. Adequate blood supply should be ensured for performing a D-D reconstruction. When the ends of the recipient's ducts are debrided, substantial arterial bleeding from the cut ends is a positive sign; in the absence of such bleeding, the bile duct needs to be shortened. Surgical options for the management of a double bile duct include double reconstruction and reconstruction as a single orifice with or without ductoplasty. Either a short internal or long external biliary stent or even no stent can be used depending on individual cases and preferences.

7. Portal vein thrombosis

End-stage liver cirrhosis is often associated with concomitant portal vein thrombosis (PVT) caused by portal hypertension, escape of blood to collateral vessels, and coagulopathy [34, 35]. Pre-existing PVT is no longer a contraindication for DDLT at most centers because of recent surgical innovations [36–40]. Unlike DDLT, LDLT is associated with additional challenges in acquiring appropriate vein grafts, obtaining adequate portal flow, and releasing portal hypertension. This has led to a careful reassessment of some recipient selection criteria. Although advanced PVTs such as Yerdel grades III and IV is no longer considered as absolute contraindication for LDLT, transplant surgeons have to develop precise technical strategies preoperatively to acquire sufficient portal flow and proper portal pressure to the graft as well as appropriate vascular graft to be used [41]. Surgical procedures such as thrombectomy, jump graft implantation from superior mesenteric vein, and renoportal anastomosis have been developed with various success rates [37–40] to ensure sufficient portal flow to liver grafts. The choice of the surgical technique for re-establishing portal flow in recipients with PVT depends on the extent of the thrombosis and the experience of the transplantation team. Partial PVT of less than 25% is usually local and has no clinical repercussions because it can be treated with resection, whereas partial PVT above 25% requires extensive thrombectomy [41].

For thrombectomy, the PV should be exposed to the level of the splenic vein confluence. The coronary vein and the superior pancreaticoduodenal vein should be carefully divided at both sides. After the PV is carefully clamped at the level of the splenic vein confluence, low grade PVT with complete patency of superior mesenteric vein (SMV) can be managed by low dissection and simple and easy eversion thrombectomy with an end-to-end donor–recipient portal anastomosis. Sometimes a longitudinal incision in the PV allows removal of the thrombus. If the closure of the incision narrows the PV, venoplasty using a venous patch should be considered. When the PV is small, stiff, or damaged by thrombectomy, PV replacement using a vein graft should be considered.

In patients with PVT and proximal occlusion of the SMV, a jump graft between the SMV and the donor's PV, using the cryopreserved cadaveric iliac or jugular vein, is often used. If the thrombus obstructs the SMV and the PV trunk, and all the portal blood flows into the left renal vein through splenorenal shunts, a renoportal anastomosis, using an interposed vein graft or artificial graft between the recipient's left renal vein and the PV of the donor graft, can be used [42].

LDLT in patients with PVT is complicated by the need for distal dissection of the hilum and by restricted availability of a vein graft. Despite the current development in surgical techniques, LDLT in patients with extensive PVT should be performed only in specialized centers.

8. Common complications

8.1. *Small-for-size graft*

When a small graft cannot meet the functional demands of a large recipient, the recipient may experience SFSS. The corresponding clinical findings range from mild hepatic dysfunction with isolated laboratory abnormalities to irreversible fatal graft failure. Although right lobe grafting is the standard strategy for avoiding SFSS, the use of grafts smaller than the native liver is unavoidable in adult LDLT. Graft volume and recipient prognosis are thought to be correlated, and the minimal graft volume required for partial liver transplantation is considered to be 40–50% of the SLV [42, 44, 45] or 0.8–1% of the graft weight to patient weight ratio [46, 47]. However, it has recently been suggested that the right-lobe graft size in patients with low Model for End-stage Liver Disease (MELD) score can be decreased to 35% of the SLV or a graft weight to patient weight ratio of 0.7 [48, 49]. Although the development of SFSS in left-lobe LDLT has caused debate, increasing utilization of right-lobe LDLT has led to increasing controversy regarding the pathogenesis, clinical manifestations and management of SFSS in recent years [50]. This means that graft size is not the only critical factor for SFSS and graft quality and perioperative recipient-related factors, including the MELD score and the portal venous circulation, should be considered.

Over the last decade, the role of portal hyperperfusion as a critical factor in the development of SFSS has been emphasized. Because excessive portal flow through a graft leads to graft dysfunction and failure, successful clinical application of portal inflow modulation by surgical means has led to improved survival of smaller grafts and prevention of SFSS. The relationship between PVP and flow volume is important for graft function after LDLT [51]. A PVP of 20 mmHg early after LT is associated with graft dysfunction and poor outcome. Troisi and de Hemptinne [52] emphasized that the recipient's PVF should be modulated to prevent SFSS and improve outcomes since SFS grafts are often associated with graft hyperperfusion. The best way to modulate portal inflow is still a matter of debate. Perioperative splenic artery ligation, embolization, splenectomy, and shunt ligation with PVP or PVF monitoring have been used to relieve portal hypertension. There is currently no consensus on the optimal target value of PVP, PVF, or hepatic venous portal pressure gradient (PVP–CVP). A typical target of portal inflow modulation is currently PVP of <15–20 mmHg or PVF of <250 mL/minute per 100 g of liver graft [53–56]. Even in right-lobe LDLT, because portal hyperperfusion, graft congestion, and small functional liver mass have been considered as the possible causes of SFSS, graft inflow regulation guided by flowmeter and portal manometry is sometimes useful; intraoperative modulation of the PVF with real-time PVP monitoring is essential especially when recipients are at risk of SFSS.

Venous outflow should not be compromised while graft inflow abnormalities are being addressed. The optimal outflow capacity of a right liver graft is a product of MHV inclusion, recruitment of the largest number of right anterior sector HVs, equilateral triangular venoplasty providing the largest cross-sectional area, and a measure-to-fit anastomosis with the IVC.

Overall, the focus is now shifting from obtaining a larger graft from the living donor to using a smaller graft efficiently in the recipient. Proper prevention and management of SFSS would allow transplantation of smaller grafts, making LDLT safer for both the donor and the recipient.

8.2. Biliary complications

Despite advances in surgical techniques, biliary complications due to anatomical and technical factors constitute the most common morbidities after LT. They include biliary leaks, strictures, and cast formation and occur in both the recipient and the donor. Moreover, the small diameter of the bile duct at the level of anastomosis leads to more biliary complications after LDLT than after DDLT. A variety of factors related to the recipient, graft, operative procedure, and postoperative course are associated with anastomotic biliary stricture and biliary leakage. The presence of multiple duct orifices is one of the risk factors for the development of biliary complications. Moreover, the presence of multiple biliary orifices is an issue that is almost specific for right-lobe grafts. Placement of an indwelling biliary stent is a matter of debate, but our previous study has demonstrated that the use of the internal stent may be helpful to decrease the biliary complication rate [57], and we prefer to use a short silastic internal stent secured with absorbable suture. Particularly in cases where there is a high risk for biliary complications, a biliary stent is thought be more helpful. In some cases, a long external stent can be used. It may allow easier access to the biliary tree, with the possibility of performing a quick and noninvasive cholangiography and obtaining bile cultures, as well as protecting the anastomosis from leakage by lowering biliary pressure.

MR cholangiopancreatography is the first-choice examination for suspected biliary complications following liver transplantation. A multidisciplinary approach involving surgery, endoscopic and radiologic intervention is used for successful management. Endoscopic retrograde cholangiopancreatography (ERCP) is commonly regarded as the first-choice treatment modality in most cases of anastomosis stricture. Repeated aggressive endoscopic treatment with balloon dilation and temporary placement of multiple plastic stents is considered the first-line treatment for biliary stricture. The success rate of endoscopic treatment varies between 53% and 88%, depending on series. Percutaneous and surgical treatments are now reserved for patients in whom endoscopic management fails and for those with multiple, inaccessible intrahepatic strictures or Roux-en-Y anastomoses. Rendezvous techniques can be considered when the endoscopic treatment of biliary stricture is unfeasible. Biliary sphincterotomy and transpapillary stenting are the standard approaches for biliary leak treatment, which results in leak resolution in >85% of patients.

In LDLT, donors are also at risk of developing biliary complications. The overall incidence of biliary complications in living liver donors ranges from 6% to 18%. In contrast to the recipient, bile leaks and biliary fistulas rather than strictures are more common in the donor. Although interventions for biliary complication in donors, including ERCP, are similar to those in recipients, strictures can be more difficult to manage after right-lobe donation as they develop as the liver regenerates, complicating endoscopic and percutaneous access to the remaining left-lobe biliary tree. Surgical revision may be required in rare cases.

8.3. *Vascular complications*

LDLT recipients have a higher risk of postoperative vascular complications compared to DDLT recipients because of the complex vascular reconstruction that involves slender vessels.

Hepatic artery thrombosis and PVT are the most severe complications, which may lead to graft dysfunction and failure.

Outflow obstruction of the HVs may induce congestion in the draining area, which may lead to functional SFSS and graft loss. When obstruction occurs within 28 days of the early postoperative period, it is usually caused by technical factors such as a tight suture line, donor–recipient size discrepancy, kinking of a redundant HV, or caval compression from a large graft. In particular, a modified right-lobe graft with reconstruction of the MHV tributaries presents with higher potential risks due to the complex and multiple anastomoses.

When the recipient is suspected of having hepatic venous outflow obstruction on the basis of clinical findings, confirmatory imaging including Doppler ultrasound and CT scan should promptly be performed. Primary

HV stenting has been accepted as a useful treatment method for hepatic venous outflow obstruction after LDLT, with acceptable patency observed, although balloon angioplasty can be tried [58].

In LDLT recipients, early posttransplant vascular complications may induce deterioration in liver function, graft failure, or death. Therefore, early detection and timely treatment of vascular complications are critical for the survival of the graft and recipient.

9. Conclusion

LDLT using a right-lobe graft is believed to be effective in patients who cannot undergo timely DDLT, and it can alleviate the pressure of organ shortage. Despite the innovations in surgical techniques and improvement in outcomes, concerns with donor safety has not been completely resolved. Therefore, careful preoperative assessment and sound surgical performance is mandatory. Comprehensive understanding of the dynamic nature of a regenerating partial liver graft and of surgical techniques is essential for improving the results of adult-to-adult LDLT using the right hepatic lobe.

References

1. Adcock L, Macleod C, Dubay D, *et al.* Adult living liver donors have excellent long-term medical outcomes: the University of Toronto liver transplant experience. *Am J Transplant* 2010;10:364–71.
2. Shah SA, Grant DR, Greig PD, *et al.* Analysis and outcomes of right lobe hepatectomy in 101 consecutive living donors. *Am J Transplant* 2005;5:2764–9.
3. Lo CM, Fan ST, Liu CL, *et al.* Lessons learned from one hundred right lobe living donor liver transplants. *Ann Surg* 2004;240:151–8.
4. Lee SG. A complete treatment of adult living donor liver transplantation: a review of surgical technique and current challenges to expand indication of patients. *Am J Transplant* 2015;15:17–38.
5. Habib N and Tanaka K. Living-related liver transplantation in adult recipients: a hypothesis. *Clin Transplant* 1995;9:31–4.
6. Cheah YL, Simpson MA, Pomposelli JJ, and Pomfret EA. Incidence of death and life-threatening near-miss events in living donor hepatic lobectomy: a world-wide survey. *Liver Transplant* 2013;19:499–506.
7. Akamatsu N, Sugawara Y, Tamura S, *et al.* Impact of live donor age (>50) on liver transplantation. *Transplant Proc* 2007;39:3189–93.
8. Ben-Haim M, Emre S, Fishbein TM, *et al.* Critical graft size in adult-to-adult living donor liver transplantation: impact of the recipient's disease. *Liver Transpl* 2001;7:948–53.

9. Sugawara Y, Makuuchi M, Takayama T, *et al*. Small-for-size grafts in living-related liver transplantation. *J Am Coll Surg* 2001;192:510–3.

10. Kiuchi T, Kasahara M, Uryuhara K, *et al*. Impact of graft size mismatching on graft prognosis in liver transplantation from living donors. *Transplantation* 1999;67:321–7.

11. Reddy SK, Marsh JW, Varley PR, *et al*. Underlying steatohepatitis, but not simple hepatic steatosis, increases morbidity after liver resection: a case-control study. *Hepatology* 2012;56:2221–30.

12. Fan ST, Lo CM, Liu CL, Yong BH, Chan JK, and Ng IO. Safety of donors in live donor liver transplantation using right lobe grafts. *Arch Surg* 2000;135:336–40.

13. Soejima Y, Shimada M, Suehiro T, *et al*. Use of steatotic graft in living-donor liver transplantation. *Transplantation* 2003;76:344–8.

14. Kim SH, Cho SY, Lee KW *et al*. Upper midline incision for living donor right hepatectomy. *Liver Transpl* 2009;15:193–8.

15. Takahara T, Wakabayashi G, Hasegawa Y, *et al*. Minimally invasive donor hepatectomy: evolution from hybrid to pure laparoscopic techniques. *Ann Surg* 2015;261:e3–4.

16. Suh SW, Lee KW, Lee JM, *et al*. Clinical outcomes of and patient satisfaction with different incision methods for donor hepatectomy in living donor liver transplantation. *Liver Transpl* 2015;21:72–8.

17. Ragab A, Lopez-Soler RI, Oto A, and Testa G. Correlation between 3D-MRCP and intraoperative findings in right liver donors. *Hepatobiliary Surg Nutr* 2013;2:7–13.

18. Hwang S, Jung DH, Ha TY, *et al*. Usability of ringed polytetrafluoroethylene grafts for middle hepatic vein reconstruction during living donor liver transplantation. *Liver Transpl* 2012;18:955–65.

19. Yaprak O, Balci NC, Dayangac M, *et al*. Cryopreserved aortic quilt plasty for one-step reconstruction of multiple hepatic venous drainage in right lobe living donor liver transplantation. *Transplant Proc* 2011;43:2817–9.

20. Guan Z, Ren X, Xu G, *et al*. Cryopreserved iliac vein for reconstruction of middle hepatic vein in living donor right liver transplantation. *Zhongguo Xiu Fu Chong Jian Wai Ke Za Zhi* 2011;25:1393–6.

21. Gyu Lee S, Min Park K, Hwang S, *et al*. Modified right liver graft from a living donor to prevent congestion. *Transplantation* 2002;74:54–9.

22. Sugawara Y, Makuuchi M, Sano K, *et al*. Vein reconstruction in modified right liver graft for living donor liver transplantation. *Ann Surg* 2003;237:180–5.

23. Ha T-Y, Hwang S, Moon D-B, *et al*. Conjoined unification venoplasty for graft double portal vein branches as a modification of autologous Y-graft interposition. *Liver Transpl* 2015;21:707–10.

24. Chan SC, Lo CM, Ng KK, *et al*. Portal inflow and pressure changes in right liver living donor liver transplantation including the middle hepatic vein. *Liver Transpl* 2011;17:115–21.

25. Man K, Fan ST, Lo CM, *et al.* Graft injury in relation to graft size in right lobe live donor liver transplantation: a study of hepatic sinusoidal injury in correlation with portal hemodynamics and intragraft gene expression. *Ann Surg* 2003;237:256–64.

26. Troisi R, Cammu G, Militerno G, *et al.* Modulation of portal graft inflow: a necessity in adult living-donor liver transplantation? *Ann Surg* 2003;237:429–36.

27. Troisi R, Ricciardi S, Smeets P, *et al.* Effects of hemi-portocaval shunts for inflow modulation on the outcome of small-for-size grafts in living donor liver transplantation. *Am J Transplant* 2005;5:1397–404.

28. Yagi S, Iida T, Hori T, *et al.* Optimal portal venous circulation for liver graft function after living-donor liver transplantation. *Transplantation* 2006;81:373–8.

29. Ikegami T, Kawasaki S, Hashikura Y, *et al.* An alternative method of arterial reconstruction after hepatic arterial thrombosis following living-related liver transplantation. *Transplantation* 2000;69:1953–5.

30. Katz E, Fukuzawa K, Schwartz M, Mor E, Miller C. The splenic artery as the inflow in arterial revascularization of the liver graft in clinical liver transplantation. *Transplantation* 1992;53:1373–4.

31. Asakura T, Ohkohchi N, Orii T, Koyamada N, Satomi S. Arterial reconstruction using vein graft from the common iliac artery after hepatic artery thrombosis in living-related liver transplantation. *Transplant Proc* 2000;32:2250–1.

32. Lo CM, Fan ST, Liu CL, *et al.* Adult-to-adult living donor liver transplantation using extended right lobe grafts. *Ann Surg* 1997;226:261–9.

33. Gondolesi GE, Varotti G, Florman SS, *et al.* Biliary complications in 96 consecutive right lobe living donor transplant recipients. *Transplantation* 2004;77:1842–8.

34. Nonami T, Yokoyama I, Iwatsuki S, and Starzl TE. The incidence of portal vein thrombosis at liver transplantation. *Hepatology* 1992;16:1195–8.

35. Davidson BR, Gibson M, Dick R, Burroughs A, Rolles K. Incidence, risk factors, management, and outcome of portal vein abnormalities at orthotopic liver transplantation. *Transplantation* 1994;57:1174–7.

36. Seu P, Shackleton CR, Shaked A, *et al.* Improved results of liver transplantation in patients with portal vein thrombosis. *Arch Surg* 1996;131:840–4; discussion 844–5.

37. Dumortier J, Czyglik O, Poncet G, *et al.* Eversion thrombectomy for portal vein thrombosis during liver transplantation. *Am J Transplant* 2002;2:934–8.

38. Manzanet G, Sanjuán F, Orbis P, *et al.* Liver transplantation in patients with portal vein thrombosis. *Liver Transpl* 2001;7:125–31.

39. Molmenti EP, Roodhouse TW, Molmenti H, *et al.* Thrombendvenectomy for organized portal vein thrombosis at the time of liver transplantation. *Ann Surg* 2002;235:292–6.

40. Yerdel MA, Gunson B, Mirza D, *et al*. Portal vein thrombosis in adults undergoing liver transplantation: risk factors, screening, management, and outcome. *Transplantation* 2000;69:1873–81.

41. Cho JY, Suh KS, Shin WY, *et al*. Thrombosis confined to the portal vein is not a contraindication for living donor liver transplantation. *World J Surg* 2008;32:1731–7.

42. Moon DB, Lee SG, Ahn CS, *et al*. Management of extensive nontumorous portal vein thrombosis in adult living donor liver transplantation. *Transplantation* 2014; 27:97.

43. Lee S, Park K, Hwang S, *et al*. Congestion of right liver graft in living donor liver transplantation. *Transplantation* 2001;71:812–4.

44. Lo CM, Fan ST, Liu CL, *et al*. Minimum graft size for successful living donor liver transplantation. *Transplantation* 1999;68:1112–6.

45. Sugawara Y, Makuuchi M, Takayama T, *et al*. Small-for-size grafts in living-related liver transplantation. *J Am Coll Surg* 2001;192:510–3.

46. Kiuchi T, Kasahara M, Uryuhara K, *et al*. Impact of graft size mismatching on graft prognosis in liver transplantation from living donors. *Transplantation* 1999;67:321–7.

47. Ben-Haim M, Emre S, Fishbein TM, *et al*. Critical graft size in adult-to-adult living donor liver transplantation: impact of the recipient's disease. *Liver Transpl* 2001;7:948–53.

48. Ito T, Kiuchi T, Yamamoto H, *et al*. Efficacy of anterior segment drainage reconstruction in right-lobe liver grafts from living donors. *Transplantation* 2004;77:865–8.

49. Shirouzu Y, Ohya Y, Suda H, Asonuma K, and Inomata Y. Massive ascites after living donor liver transplantation with a right lobe graft larger than 0.8% of the recipient's body weight. *Clin Transplant* 2010;24:520–7.

50. Kiuchi T, Tanaka K, Ito T, *et al*. Small-for-size graft in living donor liver transplantation: how far should we go? *Liver Transpl* 2003;9:S29–35.

51. Yagi S, Iida T, Taniguchi K, *et al*. Impact of portal venous pressure on regeneration and graft damage after living-donor liver transplantation. *Liver Transpl* 2005;11:68–75.

52. Troisi R and de Hemptinne B. Clinical relevance of adapting portal vein flow in living donor liver transplantation in adult patients. *Liver Transpl* 2003;9:S36–41.

53. Wu TJ, Dahiya D, Lee CS, *et al*. Impact of portal venous hemodynamics on indices of liver function and graft regeneration after right lobe living donor liver transplantation. *Liver Transpl* 2011;17:1035–45.

54. Lo CM, Liu CL, and Fan ST. Portal hyperperfusion injury as the cause of primary nonfunction in a small-for-size liver graft-successful treatment with splenic artery ligation. *Liver Transpl* 2003;9:626–8.

55. Troisi R and de Hemptinne B. Clinical relevance of adapting portal vein flow in living donor liver transplantation in adult patients. *Liver Transpl* 2003;9:S36–41.

56. Feng AC, Fan HL, and Chen TW. Hepatic hemodynamic changes during liver transplantation: a review. *World J Gastroenterol* 2014;20:11131–41.
57. Jung SW, Kim DS, Yu YD, Suh SO. Clinical outcome of internal stent for biliary anastomosis in liver transplantation. *Transplant Proc* 2014;46:856–60.
58. Ko GY, Sung KB, Yoon HK, *et al*. Early posttransplant hepatic venous outflow obstruction: long-term efficacy of primary stent placement. *Liver Transpl* 2008;14:1505–11.

7. Adult Living-Donor Liver Transplantation: Left Lobe

Hillary J. Braun*, Garrett R. Roll[†], and John Paul Roberts[‡]

*Department of Surgery, University of California
San Francisco, 513 Parnassus Avenue, Room S-321,
San Francisco, CA 94143-0470, USA
[†]Department of Surgery, Division of Transplant, University of
California San Francisco, 505 Parnassus Ave., Room M896,
San Francisco, CA 94143-0780, USA
[‡]Division of Transplant Surgery, University of California
San Francisco, 400 Parnassus Ave., 7th Floor, San Francisco,
CA 94143, USA

1. Living donor and graft selection

1.1. Background

Over the past two decades, the use of living donors in liver transplant(ation) (LT) has expanded worldwide and more than 10,000 living-donor liver transplants (LDLTs) have been performed [1]. Compared with deceased donor organs, living donor grafts offer recipients shorter time-to-transplant and improved waiting-list mortality [2] with similar five-year survival rates after transplant (83%) [3]. LDLT can reduce the mortality burden on patients with end stage liver disease who have long projected waiting times, high MELD scores, or live in areas where deceased-donor liver transplant (DDLT) is not culturally acceptable. The first successful adult-to-adult LDLT was performed in 1993 in Japan using a left-lobe (LL) graft [4] from a male donor to a female recipient. The LL graft comprised 45% of the recipient's ideal liver volume. In Asia, the use of adult-to-adult LDLT began to increase, but centers quickly realized that the majority of their transplant candidates were men with hepatitis B, and the LL graft was not enough liver tissue to meet the metabolic demands of the recipient, so LDLT using right-lobe (RL) grafts become more commonplace [5, 6].

The ethical grounds for LDLT were proposed in 2001, and the concept of double equipoise was introduced [7]. LDLT is a relatively unique situation, because the risk to the donor and the risk to the recipient can be seen as competing. Therefore, LDLT requires balancing donor and recipient risk. The risk of donor death is very low and is decreasing as surgeon and center experiences grow. Many feel that donating a LL graft has a lower complication rate for the donor, and concerns about the safety of RL donors began in the early 2000s after several groups reported increased morbidity in RL donors [8–10]. In the current era the estimated donor mortality rate is 0.1% for LL donors and 0.5% for RL donors [11], however, the safety of RL donation vs. LL donation is controversial. A recent worldwide survey of donor morbidity and near miss events in LDLT programs reported no significant difference in mortality between RL and LL donors [12]. If the risk of death is lower with LL grafts, LL grafts are one potential way to increase the number of donor organs at lower donor risk. Recently, a metric was introduced to quantify recipient benefit measured as recipient lives saved at 1 year per donor death (RS/DD) [13]. That analysis suggested LL is more efficient than RL donor hepatectomy in converting donor risk into recipient benefit depending on the relative risk of death of the two procedures. The shifting of preference toward LL grafts underscores the increased value placed on the health and security of the living donor [8–11].

LDLT with a LL graft is an option for most patients awaiting LT. The percentage of patients who would be eligible for LDLT using a LL has been estimated to be 29.1% if the lower limit of graft weight (GW)/standard liver volume (SLV) is ≥30%, and 62.3% if the GW/SLV is reduced to ≥25% (Figure 1) [14]. Patients expected to require full vena caval replacement are not ideal candidates for LDLT grafts, as this would require replacement of the vena cava with a vascular graft. Finally, there has been concern over the use of LDLT for patients with high MELD scores after the observation of poor outcomes after transplantation in patients with MELD ≥25 [15]. However, recent evidence has suggested that recipients with a high MELD can safely receive either DDLT or LDLT, and single-center data has shown that even recipients with a high MELD who receive a small graft have comparable 1-year survival rates [16]. Notably, the relatively smaller LL grafts can be subject to graft hyperperfusion, and animal studies suggest this can

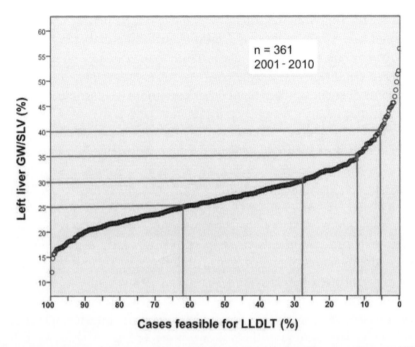

Figure 1. Percentages of cases in which left-lobe LDLT is feasible according to GW/SLV ratio. (Reprinted with permission from Ref. [14]. Copyright © 2012 American Association for the Study of Liver Diseases (AASLD).)

cause significant graft dysfunction which can be overcome by reducing portal flow [17, 18]. Graft inflow modification in the recipient, discussed later, is a strategy to mitigate the risk of graft congestion [19]. The evolution of LDLT has been hampered by significant variation in center practices, and the literature is composed of almost entirely of retrospective single-center reports, making conclusions difficult to apply broadly.

1.2. Donor evaluation

Donor safety is paramount in LDLT, so the donor evaluation process is crucial to ensuring the donor can makes an educated decision about donation. The specifics of the donor evaluation vary by institution, but in general all potential donors will be evaluated for both medical and psychological conditions, and graft suitability for the given recipient [1]. The evaluation process is staged, and typically initiated by the donor, who contacts the transplant center to provide basic demographic and medical details. Exclusion criteria are center specific, but in general donors may be excluded at any point in the process for the following reasons: age <18 or >60, BMI >30, significant prior abdominal surgery, medical comorbidities including diabetes, hypertension, history of malignancy, obesity, cardiopulmonary disease, poorly controlled psychiatric conditions, and concerns over liver anatomy. Once the donor candidate is deemed suitable from a medical and psychiatric perspective, the liver is evaluated in greater detail. At the University of California San Francisco (UCSF), donors undergo high-resolution abdominal computed tomography (CT) scan to delineate arterial and venous anatomy and calculate graft volumes, contrast enhanced magnetic resonance imaging of the liver to examine the biliary tree, and abdominal ultrasound to evaluate liver parenchyma. Liver biopsy may be indicated in potential donors with BMI 25–30, suggestion of fatty liver on imaging or first-degree relatives of patients with autoimmune diseases. Many centers have begun to use donors between the ages 50–60 years old in recent years. A graft from an older donor may lead to a higher complication rate in the donor and/or the recipient, although this is controversial in the literature [20–24]. Therefore, donor age should be considered when use of a small graft is planned, or if the remnant liver volume in the donor will be <35%.

Approximately 40% of donors are accepted after complete evaluation [25]. Factors associated with an increased likelihood of approval include younger age, biological relationship to recipient, and lower BMI [25]. ABO-compatible donors are most often rejected due to medical history, or anatomical contraindications [25].

1.3. *Donor complications*

Discussion of donor complications is complicated by significant variation in graft preference (LL vs. RL) and surgeon experience between centers. While donor mortality is low (0.1–0.5%) [11], the rate of complications is relatively high; the overall complication rate in liver donors is approximately 20% [26], although individual studies have reported rates as high as 50% [27, 28]. The majority of complications ultimately resolve without the need for reoperation, but an estimated 1–2% of complications become chronic problems [29]. Unfortunately, most studies have focused on the overall complication rate following living donor hepatectomy without stratifying by graft laterality. A review of 12 years of donor data at our institution revealed a 20% donor complication rate, with no significant difference in the incidence of complications between LL and RL donors [30]. However, a recent review of the world's literature concluded that donor morbidity was increased in RL donors compared with LL donors [2], and an analysis of 5,202 living donors revealed that major complications (≥Clavien grade III) were twice as a high in RL donors [31]. Continued investigations will better delineate the relationship between graft type and postoperative complication type and severity.

Complications from the donor evaluation are rare, but occur in the setting of contrast imaging with CT or MRI and with liver biopsy [1]. The bulk of donor complications occur postoperatively, with infection and biliary complications such as wound infection, biloma/leak and stricture are the most frequently reported [26]. Other common complications include incisional hernia and prolonged ileus. According to data from the Adult-to-Adult Living-Donor Liver Transplantation (A2ALL) cohort [28] and individual institutions [30], the majority of complications are minor (Clavien grade 1–2) and occur within the first 3 months of donation. Approximately 95% of complications have resolved within 1 year of donation [28]. It is suggested that RL donation including the middle hepatic vein (MHV), especially if this yields a remnant liver volume less than 35%, should be avoided in donors over 50 years old due to a higher rate of severe complications and the need for reoperation [24]. Older donors may also have a higher risk of bile duct stricture [21].

1.4. *Graft selection, balancing donor and recipient risk*

Graft selection is determined by the recipient's standard liver volume (SLV), which can be calculated using one of several equations, all of which rely on the recipient's body surface area or weight [32]. Smaller LL grafts leave the donor with more residual liver volume but may place the recipient at risk for graft hyperperfusion. It is generally accepted that the functional graft size should be between at least 30–40% of the recipient's SLV and that no more than 70% of the donor's liver should be removed [33]. An alternative to the SLV calculations is one based on the graft-to-recipient weight ratio (GRWR). Although there is not consensus, a rule of thumb is that GRWR >0.8%, or a GW/SLV >0.4 is enough liver mass to avoid complications in the recipient related to early graft dysfunction and small-for-size syndrome (SFSS) [2, 34]. One criticism of these approaches to graft selection is that recipient weight, and consequently SLV or GRWR calculations, may be altered in the setting of recipient deconditioning, fluid retention and obesity and may not accurately reflect the appropriate graft size required by the recipient.

Recent data from the United States suggested that GW does not predict early graft dysfunction [35], and also demonstrated that early graft dysfunction does not correlate with graft loss or recipient mortality [30]. It is generally believed, however, that if both lobes offer at least 30–40% of the SLV the left lobe should be used to minimize donor risk [2]. The caudate lobe can be included with the LL graft to increase size [36]. Though the caudate may seem relatively small, it can add up to 10% to the total graft volume [37], and may augment venous drainage [37, 38].

2. Living donor

2.1. *Preoperative issues and anesthesia*

The specific anesthetic and perioperative management of living liver donors will vary according to institution, however there are three main objectives in regard to living donor anesthesia and perioperative management: (1) minimization of blood loss, (2) prevention of deep vein thrombosis, and (3) and safe and effective postoperative analgesia [1].

Limiting fluid administration throughout the case minimizes blood loss. At UCSF, donors will receive less than 1 L of fluid during the dissection phase to maintain central venous pressure (CVP). Once the graft is removed from the field and any bleeding is addressed, volume resuscitation begins. Donors typically donate one unit of autologous blood prior to donation, and this unit is available for use. Cell saver is also routinely used to minimize the need for donated packed red cells.

Venous thrombosis is addressed with the use of sequential compression devices perioperatively and early ambulation postoperatively. Donors are not routinely anticoagulated with heparin or enoxaparin due to the expected mild postoperative coagulopathy that occurs with LL, and is more pronounced with RL donation. Although, several groups have implemented anticoagulation with low-dose heparin in RL donors with good outcomes [39, 40].

The LL graft is generally procured via a vertical midline incision. Analgesia poses a challenge in balancing the comfort of the patient with the vasodilatory, ileus prolonging and respiratory depressive side effects of opiate medications. LL donors are offered epidural analgesia, which usually remains in place through postoperative day 3 or 4, at which time the INR has normalized and removal is safe. RL donors are not offered an epidural out of concern for epidural hematoma formation. Donors are given intravenous (IV) narcotics, frequently delivered via patient-controlled analgesia before transitioning to oral medications. Thoughtful administration of narcotics with vigilant monitoring for over sedation is paramount in living donor safety.

One major limiting factor in discharge after donor hepatectomy is return of bowel function [30]. Nonopioid agents such as ketorolac, acetaminophen (2 g/day) and tramadol should be used to decrease the need for narcotics. While opioid medications are required, patients should be on an aggressive bowel regimen. In extreme refractory cases of opioid-induced constipation, methylnaltrexone injections may be warranted.

3. Surgical considerations for the left-lobe (LL) donor

Slightly larger than a left-lateral segment (LLS) graft is the LL graft (segments 2–4 with or without the left portion of segment 1), which generally entails removing about 40% of the donor liver. Typically, temporary clamping of the left hepatic artery and portal vein (PV) demonstrates the area supplied by the left structures. The donor operation from a technical standpoint is similar to procuring an LLS, but the resection plane is along Cantlie's line (from the gallbladder fossa to the space between the middle and right hepatic veins (HVs)). Obtaining a LL graft requires removal of the gallbladder. LLS and LL grafts share similar points of division of the hepatic artery, PV, and bile duct. Inclusion of the caudate with the LL graft leaves the pedicle branches to this segment and requires division of the branches entering the cava.

The donor operation starts with a general assessment of the liver and the foregut for evidence of unexpected pathology. The gallbladder is then removed. The hilum is dissected with care to avoid injury to the biliary or vascular structures, and specifically, dissection around the bile duct is limited to prevent future ischemia. The left hepatic artery and the artery to segment 4 are identified and traced proximally to identify the origin of the right hepatic artery. The left portal vein (LPV) is identified, and caudate branches to the right (paracaval portion of the caudate lobe) are ligated while branches to the left (Spigelian lobe) are persevered. With the arterial and portal supply to the LL isolated, a brief period of vascular occlusion identifies the transection plane on the surface of the liver along the Rex line.

Generally, parenchymal transection occurs at this time. Some use intermittent inflow occlusion, which has been shown to be safe for the donor and the graft [41, 42]. The dissection proceeds to the right of the MHV, so the

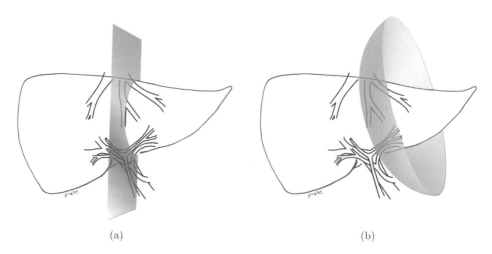

(a)   (b)

Figure 2. Plane of transection. (a) A strictly vertical anterior to posterior plane will not keep the MHV with the LL graft. (b) The curvilinear plane of transection is required to take the majority of the MHV with the LL, while preserving the portal pedicle to the RL, and ensuring the proper location of transection of the left bile duct without skeletonizing either the left or right portal pedicle.

vein is included in the graft. Leaving some parenchyma between the MHV and the cut surface of the graft may prevent thrombosis in the vein [43].

The surgeon's hand is placed under the liver, and lifting up this hand slows or stops parenchymal bleeding when it occurs. Some centers use the Pringle maneuver to help with blood loss. This resection plane is the same as that for a right hepatectomy, crossing the branches of the MHV that extend to the right of the plane. The plane of transection is not strictly vertical (Figure 2(a)), rather it is curvilinear (Figure 2(b)), aiming to include the majority of the MHV with the left lobe. This plane leaves only the distal MHV branches with the right lobe. Care is taken not to encroach on the right anterior portal pedicle before the plane turns back to the right to approach the left portal pedicle. The transection plane becomes vertical for division of the caudate.

3.1. Arterial anatomy

There is significant variability in the arterial blood supply of the LL of the liver, so the incidence of multiple hepatic artery orifices is much higher for LL grafts than for RL grafts (48% vs. 2%, $p < 0.01$). The variable arterial anatomy to segment 4 is the source of most of the variant arterial anatomy to the LL graft. Despite the common variations in arterial anatomy, complex reconstruction is not often required for LL grafts, similar to reconstruction of LLS grafts, because the arteries often communicate within the liver [44]. The presence of communication is determined by looking for arterial back bleeding from the smaller branch. The artery to segment 4 can be independent in about 50% of patients, and this must be accounted for in the reconstruction [45, 46]. The use of a branch patch in the planned arterial reconstruction is important; therefore the dissection in the donor should include potential branch patches when possible. Approximately 20% of the time, the left hepatic artery arises in an aberrant location, from the left gastric artery [45–47]. The disadvantage when using aberrant arterial vessels for transplant is that they can have a small diameter or be thin walled. The stomach has redundant blood supply, so the advantage of an aberrant left hepatic artery is the freedom to take the artery with the first gastric branch(es) off the left gastric artery. The orifices of the donor gastric branch(es) and the aberrant left hepatic artery off the left gastric artery can be used to create a branch patch during the arterial reconstruction. Another common variation is a replaced right hepatic artery originating from the superior mesenteric artery, whose circulation is isolated from a left hepatic artery in the conventional location, occurring about 7% of the time [46]. The branch patch most commonly used in this situation includes the origin of the donor gastroduodenal artery.

3.2. *Biliary anatomy (anatomy, hilar dissection, bile duct transection)*

Bile leak and stricture are recognized complications of LDLT, so thoughtful assessment, as well as temperate and precise handling of biliary tissue is important. A preoperative MRI cholangiogram is required to plan the site of bile duct transection [48]. A right posterior duct drains into the left duct approximately 12% of the time [46] and has to be accounted for with the left bile duct transection. Interestingly, variant biliary anatomy is seen more commonly in patients who have variant portal venous anatomy, and approximately one-third of patients with a trifurcation of the PV will also have a right posterior bile duct that drains into the left duct.

Once the dissection is carried down to the hilar plate, the plate must be sutured to prevent bile leak. The base of the left bile duct is identified. Some advocate intraoperative cholangiogram with fluoroscopy (via the cystic duct stump) at the time of duct transection to decrease biliary complications, ensuring a safe margin of duct remains in the donor to be closed without stricture [49].

3.3. *Portal vein (PV) anatomy*

The extrahepatic portion of the LPV is usually longer and more horizontally oriented compared to the right portal vein (RPV). Anatomic variation in portal anatomy is relatively rare, and is not a contraindication to use of a left lobe graft except with Type 3 anatomy where the anterior right pedicle arises a great distance from the right posterior pedicle. Approximately 90% of patients have conventional portal venous anatomy, and 10% have a trifurcation of the PV, and approximately 1% have this Type 3 variation [46]. In patients with this anatomic variant it can be difficult to obtain length on the LPV prior to division because it is located deep to segment 4. The presence of two PVs to the left lobe is exceedingly rare, but is not a contraindication to use of a LL graft, although reconstruction is required on the back table.

3.4. *Hepatic venous and caudate vein anatomy*

The left and middle HVs most frequently have a common trunk, and the right hepatic vein (RHV) enters the vena cava separately [50]. In all patients the MHV drains both the left and right liver, so in essence, the donor and recipient would both benefit from the MHV. Therefore, management of the MHV is an important consideration in LDLT. In approximately a quarter of patients the MHV is the dominant drainage of the RL of the liver [51]. Taking this vein with the LL graft ensures the recipient receives enough functional liver mass because it drains segment 4, but leaves behind an area of congested RL of the donor [52]. Some advocate leaving the MHV with the right liver when a significant vein draining the right liver via the MHV is identified [52]. Reconstruction of the MHV in the LL graft must be considered in these cases [52, 53]. For donors with separate MHV and LHV orifices, reconstruction with a vein patch maybe required.

Approximately 65% of people have a significant vein draining the Spigelian lobe of the caudate into the vena cava. To ensure optimal graft function in larger recipients, significant veins draining the caudate lobe can be reconstructed end-to-side to the IVC or combined with the nearby left and middle HVs to generate a common trunk [54].

3.5. *Graft preparation*

The graft is devascularized and removed when the recipient hepatectomy is almost complete. Any remaining short HVs draining the caudate are divided, and the LPV is divided. A fine arterial clamp is placed proximally and the left hepatic artery(ies) are divided. The confluence of the left and middle HVs is controlled and divided. The graft is immersed in slush and the artery, PV and HVs are flushed with preservative. The hepatic artery cannulation should be done with great care to prevent injury leading to an intimal flap, and some actually advocate not flushing the artery [55]. Venous congestion can significantly inhibit graft function, so management of the HVs is important [56]. The orifice of the confluence of the left and middle HV is widened with hepatic venoplasty, with or without a quilted patch venoplasty. These alterations are designed to configure a uniform outflow orifice that is easily anastomosed to the recipient left and middle HVs, preventing distortion from fibrous septae or mechanical torsion. If there is a significant size mismatch, hepatic venoplasty incorporating the recipient's RHV, in addition to the middle and left veins, can be created. Alternatively, the outflow orifice of the graft can be sewn directly to the vena cava.

If there is a short HV orifice close to the cranial aspect of the graft, it can be directly incorporated with the middle and left HVs at this time with a venoplasty [57]. Alternatively, significant veins draining the graft can be reconstructed with a venous conduit that will be anastomosed directly to the vena cava separately in end-to-side fashion.

If the graft offers two arteries, the surgeon tests for interarterial communication to decide of both arteries are required. This is done by flushing the dominant artery and looking for back flow out the smaller artery orifice. If significant black flow occurs, only the dominant artery requires reconstruction and the smaller artery can be ligated.

4. Surgical considerations for the recipient

4.1. *Hilar dissection (minimizing the anhepatic phase)*

Infusion of octreotide may reduce blood loss during the hepatectomy in the recipient and has minimal side effects. Laparotomy and exploration of the recipient usually begin once the donor anatomy has been confirmed and parenchymal transection has commenced. The goal is to retain length of hilar structures, leaving as many reconstruction options as possible, following the "waste not, want not" methodology. Therefore, hilar dissection involves mobilizing the bile duct and hepatic artery as they enter the liver, much more distal compared to a hepatectomy being done in preparation for a whole liver deceased donor graft. The bile duct is identified and divided at the level of the bifurcation into the left and right. The cystic duct is divided where it enters the gallbladder, leaving a long cystic duct stump that may be used later. There is no need to dissect the hepatic artery proximally to the gastroduodenal artery, rather careful dissection of the left and right hepatic artery is carried up the hilum, often past the first branches of the right hepatic artery so they can be used as branch patches. Similarly, dissection of the PV is carried past the bifurcation of left and RPVs, and these branches are individually ligated and divided. The LPV is long, and excess vein can be useful in back table venoplasty of the HV outflow. Carefully identifying and dividing the short HVs prevents bleeding as the liver is mobilized off the cava because caval preservation is required. Careful synchronization of graft availability with completion of the recipient hepatectomy, requiring preoperative planning and frequent communication between teams minimizes the anhepatic phase. Continuity of the recipient hepatic artery and PV should be maintained until the last stage of the hepatectomy, when the liver graft is available. Implantation commences along the same sequence as when a whole liver graft is implanted, with the addition of graft inflow modification, when indicated, prior to reconstruction of the bile duct.

4.2. Hepatic veins (HVs)

The middle and left HVs of the recipient are controlled with a Satinski clamp and divided, and the RHV is stapled with a vascular stapler, and the diseased liver is removed. The graft is brought into the field after back-table work is complete and reconstruction of the HVs commences. Venous congestion of a LL graft can occur as the graft regenerates, rotating to the graft to the right, therefore a wide orifice that is properly positioned is critical. Most commonly, the donor middle and left HVs are anastomosed to vena cava at the level of the orifice of the middle and left HVs of the recipient. It is not often necessary to carry the recipient venotomy over to include the RHV, as is typically done for whole liver grafts. Separate reconstruction of caudate lobe veins should be considered if they are significant to ensure optimal early graft function.

4.3. Portal vein (PV)

The LL graft most commonly offers a single PV for reconstruction. The LPV of the recipient is anastomosed to the LPV on the graft. Regeneration and rotation must be considered when creating the PV anastomosis. As the graft enlarges, all the portal structures will need to lengthen a bit, so a small amount of redundancy in the PV at the time of reconstruction avoids untoward tension on the PV as the graft regenerates. The recipient's RPV stump is available for use if a portocaval shunt is required later in the procedure. Significant PV branches to the caudate that previously originated from the RPV can be reconstructed individually to ensure optimal early graft function in selected cases. These reconstructions are probably most important when the graft volume is small and approaches 40% of the recipient's SLV.

4.4. Hepatic artery

The risk of hepatic artery thrombosis is higher than the risk of hepatic artery thrombosis after orthotopic LT. This risk is most likely due to the small caliber of the arteries being reconstructed, but the hepatic artery buffer response may also play a role if PV flow is high. Clearly, technical precision during the arterial reconstruction is paramount. Some advocate arterial reconstruction under the microscope [55, 58, 59].

4.5. Graft inflow modification

After PV and hepatic artery reconstructions are complete, and hemostasis is achieved, octreotide infusion is stopped, and portal venous pressure and flow to the graft are assessed. Our understanding of portal hyperperfusion continues to evolve, but it is thought that too much flow to the graft is detrimental to the graft's ability to effectively regenerate. The disorganized regeneration that leads to significantly elevated bilirubin, renal dysfunction and persistent ascites has been termed small-for-size syndrome (SFSS) [60]. SFSS was seen 29% of recipients of LL grafts in the A2ALL study, although it was also seen in 15% of recipients of RL grafts in the same cohort [61]. Reducing portal inflow improves survival of recipients with small grafts (graft-to-recipient body ratio ≤0.8) [19]. Specifically, keeping portal venous pressure <15 mmHg seems to improve survival [62]. The relationship between pressure and flow is not completely understood, but it has been suggested that reduction of graft inflow is required if portal venous flow is >360 Ml/minute 100 g/LW, if the HV pressure gradient is >15 mmHg, or if hepatic artery flow is <100 Ml/minute [63]. Various modifications can achieve a reduction in portal flow, including splenic artery ligation, portocaval shunting and splenectomy. Splenectomy carries a significant risk of PV thrombosis and pancreatic fistula, so it is generally avoided. Ligation of the splenic artery will achieve a modest reduction of portal venous flow. The splenic artery is accessed at its most superficial location in the body of the pancreas. If a larger reduction in flow is required, a hemiportocaval shunt is created. Graft inflow modification should be performed prior to reconstruction of the bile duct to allow proper access to the PV and vena cava. SFSS is seen more commonly in grafts with a low GW/RW ratio, but there are more variables than just graft size at play, and a similar syndrome can be seen in recipients of larger grafts.

4.6. *Biliary reconstruction*

Late surgical biliary revision of the LL graft for biliary stricture is fraught with difficulty, and should be avoided. The goal is to minimize biliary complications, although this is difficult due to the size of the duct(s) offered by a LL graft. Duct-to-duct biliary reconstruction, termed choledocholcholedochostomy, has a significant advantage over Roux-en-Y hepaticjejunostomy because it allows postoperative access to the biliary tree via an endoscopic approach. Many have moved to using choledocholcholedochostomy whenever possible for this reason. Some surgeons leave a biliary tube for decompression and access to the biliary tree. Our practice in recent years has been to place a straight biliary tube into the cystic duct and up into the liver, with the other end coming through the skin. The tube is secured with a small rubber band around the cystic duct. Six weeks after transplant, a tube cholangiogram is performed. If the cholangiogram is normal the tube is removed, and the rubber band closes the cystic duct stump. This does not require an additional ductotomy for tube placement.

References

1. Fan ST. *Living Donor Liver Transplantation,* 2nd ed. Singapore: World Scientific Publishing Co, 2011.
2. Roll GR, Parekh JR, Parker WF, *et al*. Left hepatectomy versus right hepatectomy for living donor liver transplantation: shifting the risk from the donor to the recipient. *Liver Transplant* 2013;19(5):472–81.
3. Berg CL, Merion RM, Shearon TH, *et al*. Liver transplant recipient survival benefit with living donation in the model for endstage liver disease allocation era. *Hepatology* 2011;54(4):1313–21.
4. Ichida T, Matsunami H, Kawasaki S, *et al*. Living related-donor liver transplantation from adult to adult for primary biliary cirrhosis. *Ann Internal Med* 1995;122(4):275–6.
5. Fan ST, Lo CM, and Liu CL. Transplantation of the right hepatic lobe. *N Engl J Med* 2002;347(8):615–18; author reply 615–18.

6. Lo CM, Fan ST, Liu CL, *et al*. Extending the limit on the size of adult recipient in living donor liver transplantation using extended right lobe graft. *Transplantation* 1997;63(10):1524–8.

7. Cronin DC, 2nd, Millis JM, and Siegler M. Transplantation of liver grafts from living donors into adults — too much, too soon. *N Engl J Med* 2001;344(21):1633–7.

8. Middleton PF, Duffield M, Lynch SV, *et al*. Living donor liver transplantation — adult donor outcomes: a systematic review. *Liver Transplant* 2006;12(1):24–30.

9. Salame E, Goldstein MJ, Kinkhabwala M, *et al*. Analysis of donor risk in living-donor hepatectomy: the impact of resection type on clinical outcome. *Am J Transplant* 2002;2(8):780–8.

10. Umeshita K, Fujiwara K, Kiyosawa K, *et al*. Operative morbidity of living liver donors in Japan. *Lancet* 2003;362(9385):687–90.

11. Barr ML, Belghiti J, Villamil FG, *et al*. A report of the Vancouver Forum on the care of the live organ donor: lung, liver, pancreas, and intestine data and medical guidelines. *Transplantation* 2006;81(10):1373–85.

12. Cheah YL, Simpson MA, Pomposelli JJ, and Pomfret EA. Incidence of death and potentially life-threatening near-miss events in living donor hepatic lobectomy: a world-wide survey. *Liver Transplant* 2013;19(5):499–506.

13. Roll GR, Parekh JR, Parker WF, *et al*. Left hepatectomy versus right hepatectomy for living donor liver transplantation: shifting the risk from the donor to the recipient. *Liver Transpl*19(5):472–81.

14. Chan SC, Fan ST, Chok KS, *et al*. Increasing the recipient benefit/donor risk ratio by lowering the graft size requirement for living donor liver transplantation. *Liver Transplant* 2012;18(9):1078–82.

15. Suzuki H, Bartlett AS, Muiesan P, Jassem W, Rela M, and Heaton N. High model for end-stage liver disease score as a predictor of survival during long-term follow-up after liver transplantation. *Transplant Proc* 2012;44(2):384–88.

16. Yi NJ, Suh KS, Lee HW, *et al*. Improved outcome of adult recipients with a high model for end-stage liver disease score and a small-for-size graft. *Liver Transplant* 2009;15(5):496–503.

17. Boillot O, Delafosse B, Mechet I, Boucaud C, and Pouyet M. Small-for-size partial liver graft in an adult recipient; a new transplant technique. *Lancet* 2002;359(9304):406–7.

18. Wang HS, Ohkohchi N, Enomoto Y, *et al*. Excessive portal flow causes graft failure in extremely small-for-size liver transplantation in pigs. *World J Gastroenterol* 2005;11(44):6954–9.

19. Troisi R, Ricciardi S, Smeets P, *et al*. Effects of hemi-portocaval shunts for inflow modulation on the outcome of small-for-size grafts in living donor liver transplantation. *Am J Transplant* 2005;5(6):1397–1404.

20. Goldaracena N, Sapisochin G, Spetzler V, *et al*. Live donor liver transplantation with older (≥50 years) versus younger (<50 years) donors: does age matter? *Ann Surg* 2016;263(5):979–85.

21. Shah SA, Cattral MS, McGilvray ID, *et al.* Selective use of older adults in right lobe living donor liver transplantation. *Am J Transplant* 2007;7(1):142–50.

22. Akamatsu N, Sugawara Y, Tamura S, *et al.* Impact of live donor age (≥50) on liver transplantation. *Transplant Proc* 2007;39(10):3189–93.

23. Han JH, You YK, Na GH, *et al.* Outcomes of living donor liver transplantation using elderly donors. *Ann Surg Treat Res* 2014;86(4):184–91.

24. Dayangac M, Taner CB, Yaprak O, *et al.* Utilization of elderly donors in living donor liver transplantation: when more is less? *Liver Transplant* 2011;17(5):548–55.

25. Trotter JF, Wisniewski KA, Terrault NA, *et al.* Outcomes of donor evaluation in adult-to-adult living donor liver transplantation. *Hepatology* 2007;46(5):1476–84.

26. Braun HJ, Ascher NL, Roll GR, and Roberts JP. Biliary complications following living donor hepatectomy. *Transplant Rev* 2015;30(4):247–52.

27. Kamel E, Abdullah M, Hassanin A, *et al.* Live donor hepatectomy for liver transplantation in Egypt: lessons learned. *Saudi J Anaesth* 2012;6(3):234–41.

28. Abecassis MM, Fisher RA, Olthoff KM, *et al.* Complications of living donor hepatic lobectomy — a comprehensive report. *Am J Transplant* 2012;12(5): 1208–17.

29. Olthoff KM, Abecassis MM, Emond JC, *et al.* Outcomes of adult living donor liver transplantation: comparison of the adult-to-adult living donor liver transplantation cohort study and the national experience. *Liver Transplant* 2011;17(7):789–97.

30. Braun HJ, Dodje JL, Roll GR, Freise CE, Ascher NL, and Roberts JP. Impact of graft selection on donor and recipient outcomes following living donor liver transplantation. *Transplantation* 2016;100(6):1244–50.

31. Rössler F, Sapisochin G, Song G, *et al.* Defining benchmarks for major liver surgery: a multicenter analysis of 5202 living liver donors. 2016; Abstract. Submitted. American Surgical Association. Ann Surg. 2016;264(3):492–500.

32. Kokudo T, Hasegawa K, Uldry E, *et al.* A new formula for calculating standard liver volume for living donor liver transplantation without using body weight. *J Hepatol* 2015;63(4):848–54.

33. Kokudo N, Sugawara Y, Imamura H, Sano K, and Makuuchi M. Tailoring the type of donor hepatectomy for adult living donor liver transplantation. *Am J Transplant* 2005;5(7):1694–703.

34. Kiuchi T, Kasahara M, Uryuhara K, *et al.* Impact of graft size mismatching on graft prognosis in liver transplantation from living donors. *Transplantation* 1999;67(2):321–7.

35. Pomposelli JJ, Goodrich JP, Emond JC, *et al.* Patterns of Early Allograft Dysfunction in Adult Live Donor Liver Transplantation: The A2ALL Experience. *Transplantation* 2016;100(7):1490–1499.

36. Miyagawa S, Hashikura Y, Miwa S, *et al.* Concomitant caudate lobe resection as an option for donor hepatectomy in adult living related liver transplantation. *Transplantation* 1998;66(5):661–3.

37. Takayama T, Makuuchi M, Kubota K, Sano K, Harihara Y, and Kawarasaki H. Living-related transplantation of left liver plus caudate lobe. *J Am Coll Surg* 2000;190(5):635–8.
38. Sugawara Y, Makuuchi M, and Takayama T. Left liver plus caudate lobe graft with complete revascularization. *Surgery* 2002;132(5):904–5; author reply 905–6.
39. Sapisochin G, Goldaracena N, Laurence JM, Levy GA, Grant DR, and Cattral MS. Right lobe living-donor hepatectomy-the Toronto approach, tips and tricks. *Hepatobiliary Surg Nutr* 2016;5(2):118–26.
40. Yoo T, Kim SH, Kim YK, Cho SY, and Park SJ. Low-dose heparin therapy during living donor right hepatectomy is associated with few side effects and does not increase vascular thrombosis in liver transplantation. *Transplant Proc* 2013;45(1):222–4.
41. Imamura H, Kokudo N, Sugawara Y, *et al*. Pringle's maneuver and selective inflow occlusion in living donor liver hepatectomy. *Liver Transplant* 2004;10(6):771–8.
42. Imamura H, Takayama T, Sugawara Y, *et al*. Pringle's manoeuvre in living donors. *Lancet* 2002;360(9350):2049–50.
43. Arita J, Kokudo N, Hasegawa K, *et al*. Hepatic venous thrombus formation during liver transection exposing major hepatic vein. *Surgery* 2007;141(2):283–4.
44. Takatsuki M, Chiang YC, Lin TS, *et al*. Anatomical and technical aspects of hepatic artery reconstruction in living donor liver transplantation. *Surgery* 2006;140(5):824–8; discussion 829.
45. Hiatt JR, Gabbay J, and Busuttil RW. Surgical anatomy of the hepatic arteries in 1000 cases. *Ann Surg* 1994;220(1):50–52.
46. Kishi Y, Imamura H, Sugawara Y, *et al*. Evaluation of donor vasculobiliary anatomic variations in liver graft procurements. *Surgery* 2010;147(1):30–39.
47. Takayama T, Makuuchi M, Kawarasaki H, *et al*. Hepatic transplantation using living donors with aberrant hepatic artery. *J Am Coll Surg* 1997;184(5):5 25–28.
48. Goldman J, Florman S, Varotti G, *et al*. Noninvasive preoperative evaluation of biliary anatomy in right-lobe living donors with mangafodipir trisodium-enhanced MR cholangiography. *Transplant Proc* 2003;35(4):1421–22.
49. Sultan AM, Salah T, Elshobary MM, *et al*. Biliary complications in living donor right hepatectomy are affected by the method of bile duct division. *Liver Transplant* 2014;20(11):1393–401.
50. Nakamura S and Tsuzuki T. Surgical anatomy of the hepatic veins and the inferior vena cava. *Surg Gynecol Obstet* 1981;152(1):43–50.
51. Couinaud C. Liver lobes and segments: notes on the anatomical architecture and surgery of the liver. *La Presse Medicale* 1954;62(33):709–12.
52. Sano K, Makuuchi M, Takayama T, Sugawara Y, Imamura H, and Kawarasaki H. Technical dilemma in living-donor or split-liver transplant. *Hepatogastroenterology* 2000;47(35):1208–9.

53. Makuuchi M and Sugawara Y. Living-donor liver transplantation using the left liver, with special reference to vein reconstruction. *Transplantation* 2003;75 (3 Suppl):S23–24.

54. Hashimoto T, Sugawara Y, Tamura S, *et al.* One orifice vein reconstruction in left liver plus caudate lobe grafts. *Transplantation* 2007;83(2):225–7.

55. Uchiyama H, Hashimoto K, Hiroshige S, *et al.* Hepatic artery reconstruction in living-donor liver transplantation: a review of its techniques and complications. *Surgery* 2002;131(1):S200–4.

56. Emond JC, Heffron TG, Whitington PF, and Broelsch CE. Reconstruction of the hepatic vein in reduced size hepatic transplantation. *Surg Gynecol Obstet* 1993;176(1):11–17.

57. Sugawara Y, Makuuchi M, Kaneko J, Ohkubo T, Matsui Y, and Imamura H. New venoplasty technique for the left liver plus caudate lobe in living donor liver transplantation. *Liver Transplant* 2002;8(1):76–77.

58. Mori K, Nagata I, Yamagata S, *et al.* The introduction of microvascular surgery to hepatic artery reconstruction in living-donor liver transplantation — its surgical advantages compared with conventional procedures. *Transplantation* 1992;54(2):263–8.

59. Inomoto T, Nishizawa F, Sasaki H, *et al.* Experiences of 120 microsurgical reconstructions of hepatic artery in living related liver transplantation. *Surgery* 1996;119(1):20–26.

60. Dahm F, Georgiev P, and Clavien PA. Small-for-size syndrome after partial liver transplantation: definition, mechanisms of disease and clinical implications. *Am J Transplant* 2005;5(11):2605–10.

61. Olthoff KM, Emond JC, Shearon TH, *et al.* Liver regeneration after living donor transplantation: adult-to-adult living donor liver transplantation cohort study. *Liver Transplant* 2015;21(1):79–88.

62. Ogura Y, Hori T, El Moghazy WM, *et al.* Portal pressure <15 mm Hg is a key for successful adult living donor liver transplantation utilizing smaller grafts than before. *Liver Transplant* 2010;16(6):718–28.

63. Sainz-Barriga M, Scudeller L, Costa MG, de Hemptinne B, and Troisi RI. Lack of a correlation between portal vein flow and pressure: toward a shared interpretation of hemodynamic stress governing inflow modulation in liver transplantation. *Liver Transplant* 2011;17(7):836–48.

8. Pediatric Liver Transplantation with Technical Variant Allografts

Kyle Soltys, Geoff Bond, Rakesh Sindhi, and George Mazariegos

*Department of Surgery, University of Pittsburgh,
Pittsburgh, PA 15213, USA*

1. Introduction

Liver transplant(ation) (LT) offers children with end-stage liver disease a chance at long-term survival and greatly diminishes the morbidity associated with severe metabolic diseases. Unfortunately, due to the overwhelming success of transplant, the number of children awaiting LT exceeds the number of suitable pediatric deceased donors, particularly in small children. This shortage has resulted in a large body of work describing ways to safely increase the number of hepatic allografts for children. Some of this work has focused on the improved management of potential pediatric donors, which is critical to meet the need for whole pediatric livers, especially those prospectively allocated for use as part of combined liver and intestinal or multivisceral grafts. By nature of their size and anatomic needs, children waiting for these composite allografts require the use of organs from children of similar size. In addition to the highly morbid diseases processes that require composite liver and intestinal transplantation, the paucity of physiologically stable pediatric donors in the United States contributes to the exceedingly high waiting-list mortality in this population. In an effort to alleviate this mortality rate, current allocation schemes favor the utilization of whole pediatric livers donors for children awaiting combined liver and intestine transplants.

Although helpful for this group of candidates, this has not significantly changed the annual pediatric liver waiting-list mortality in the United States, which has ranged from 7% to 12% since 2010. This has led to the development of techniques to allow the use of portions of larger livers for transplant into children waiting for isolated LTs. The technique of orthotopic LT was first reported by Dr. Starzl [1] in 1963 and again in 1968 [2], however the techniques that would allow the utilization of portions of adult livers in children were not developed until the waiting list began to exhaust the number of available donors. The anatomic aspects of left-lateral segment (LLS) living liver donation were initially described by Dr. Blanca Smith [3], a Pediatric Surgeon from Ohio, in 1968 and rely on the segmental nature of the human liver as described by Couniaud and Bismuth. Although the initial anatomic descriptions suggested that segmental transplant was feasible, the first reports of partial LT did not emerge for two decades.

The pediatric portion of *technical variant allografts* generally consists of the LLS (Couniaud segments 2 and 3) or the left-lobe (segments 2–4) of a whole liver, from either a deceased or living donor. Several early pioneering reports highlighted the possibility of using technical variant allografts in pediatric recipients. The first reports were of *reduced* left-sided allografts, in which the right side of the liver was discarded. Two centers reported the initial experience with *reduced liver transplantation (RLT)* in the early 1980s [4, 5]. A combination of techniques were used to remove the right side of the donor liver on the back table, however the first cases had excessive technical morbidity associated with allograft reduction. As the procedure allowed the increased utilization of livers in the pediatric age group, experience rapidly grew and as expected, results of RLT improved, with survival eventually becoming equivalent to whole pediatric LT [6–9].

Although liver reduction increased the number of allografts available to children awaiting LT, the procedure did nothing to increase the total number organs available for candidates awaiting LT. This disparity fostered the development of split liver transplantation (SLT), in which both portions of the liver are utilized — traditionally with the LLS (segment 2/3) being transplanted into a child and the extended right-lobe (segments 1, 4–8) into an adult recipient [10, 11]. This experience also furthered the development of *living-donor liver transplant (LDLT)*, with the first adult-to-child case reported in 1990 [12].

Early series of SLT from the Unites States had low patient and graft survivals when compared to whole organ transplant. In addition, there was an increased risk of technical complications and a higher need for urgent retransplantation [13, 14]. Pediatric transplant groups quickly learned that avoidance, and prompt treatment of technical complications of technical variant transplants can impact short and long-term patient and graft survival. Indeed, the utility of transplanting technical variant allografts to decrease an individual child's time on the waiting list can only be measured on the success of each individual transplant and as graft failure frequently requires retransplant, from a system standpoint, any increases in graft loss associated with the use of technical variant grafts can be viewed as a failure to decrease the number of children on the list over time. Taken one step further, "failure to rescue" as a quality metric in pediatric transplant supports the importance of the rapid treatment of any graft-threatening complications, while balancing the often extraordinary measures required to salvage the allograft with the ultimate individual goal of preserving the life of the child [15]. Need for retransplantation is not only met with increased short- and long-term morbidity and mortality [16], but it also requires a second liver to be used from an already contracted population of donors. In addition, early technical complications continue to have a negative impact on long-term graft survival well after the first posttransplant year [17].

European centers led the way in reporting the results of large numbers of patients undergoing SLT. Despite high graft losses (20%) due to technical complications, survival amongst recipients undergoing elective LT were comparable to results in the European Liver Transplant Registry. Common technical complications included an 11% incidence of hepatic arterial thrombosis and a 19% incidence of biliary complications [18].

Several methods exist to successfully divide the liver for transplantation and due to relatively small numbers of patients undergoing SLT, little well controlled data exists to compare the procedures. From a developmental standpoint, surgeons began splitting the liver into the classical LLS and extended right allografts as an *ex vivo* technique. As this procedure occurs on the back table, it allows for a controlled and bloodless division of the liver and minimizes the time and resources needed at the donor institution. In addition, concern for operative stress in hemodynamically labile brain-dead donors is eliminated with the *ex vivo* technique. Disadvantages of the *ex vivo* technique are logistic and potentially physiologic. *Ex vivo* division generally occurs at the recipient institution, potentially necessitating the transport of the whole deceased-donor organ to the recipient site. This transport causes geographic issues with allocation of the "other" side of the liver, in that it would greatly increase the cold-ischemic time if shared with a distant site. Extended cold-ischemia times were felt to contribute to the increased morbidity seen in the *ex vivo* technique in one large study [19]. In addition, *ex vivo* separation of the liver can take a significant amount of time (often greater than 2 hours) and during this time, the graft is exposed to variable amounts of physiologic stress resulting from "rewarming", a product of physical manipulation of the allograft out of the protective ice bath. The *ex vivo* technique may also lead to increased hemorrhage along the cut surface of the hepatic parenchyma on reperfusion [20].

As experience with splitting donor livers for two recipients accumulated throughout the transplant community, centers began to publish reports of complete *in situ* splitting, in which the liver parenchyma is divided before circulatory arrest in the donor. As the technique is similar to that used in LLS living donation, surgeons require technical proficiency in hepatobiliary surgery as parenchymal transection should be performed without inflow occlusion and intraoperative cholangiograms are needed to identify the biliary anatomy of the LLS and remnant extended right lobe. *The in situ* technique results in shorter cold-ischemia times for the two allografts and also eliminates the risk of significant rewarming injury. As vessels are readily identified during transection, cut surface bleeding on reperfusion is minimized. Although the *in situ* technique can increase donor operative times by 1–2 hours, this is generally not an issue with thoracic or abdominal teams, as long as the need for a delay is known in advance. Preoperative communication should also occur between the teams recovering the two sides of the liver with clear plans made for division of the hilar vessels, as well as the allocation of donor arterial and vein grafts for potential reconstruction. Hosting organ procurement organizations should also have alternative recipients in case the splitting procedure is not able to be done due to variant anatomy or physiologic instability. Obviously candidates waiting for the two sides of the liver should be advised of the possibility that the procedure may not be possible.

In the case of hemodynamic instability or unexpected hemorrhage, the *in situ* procedure can be quickly aborted and the organs flushed, with completion of the liver transection performed on the back table. Indeed, it should be well understood that brain death causes a significant amount of physiologic stress on visceral organs, including the liver and regardless of otherwise favorable characteristics, deceased donors are *NOT* living donors. Operative times should therefore not be indefinitely extended, nor should significant blood loss be allowed. It is our general practice to perform the majority of the dissection *in situ*, with completion of the liver division on the donor back table after cross-clamp. This technique offers the possibility of reaping the benefits of both techniques, with short cold-ischemia times, minimal cut surface hemorrhage. This also allows for a controlled division of the hilar and outflow structures, reduced operative times minimal physiologic stress and for the donor.

Conflicting data exists regarding the outcomes of both sides of split liver allografts which has likely contributed to some of the reluctance to use these grafts [21–34]. Early reports of these grafts, as mentioned prior, were fraught with increased morbidity and mortality from technical complications. Larger single-center studies from Europe and the United States contradicted these findings, with patient and graft survival of both sides of the split equivalent to, if not better than that achieved with deceased-donor organs [25–27, 32–34]. In addition, patient and graft survival of the extended right allograft has also been shown to be equivalent to that in whole organ transplant [33, 34]. However, it should be noted that despite equivalent survival rates, most studies do continue to show some increased rates of technical complications, especially biliary strictures and leaks, in patients who have received technical variant allografts [37].

Interestingly, despite encouraging results from high volume centers adept at performing SLTs, when one looks at pooled data from multicenter trials, use of split liver allografts continues to be associated with decreased patient and graft survival. This difference is not surprising as multicenter trials include results from smaller centers who do not have a large experience with the technical aspects of SLT and more importantly, may not be adept at handling the increased complications seen with these grafts. In addition, centers that do not primarily utilize split liver allografts may be using these only as "last resorts" in highly acute patients, who represent a high-risk population.

2. Donor selection for pediatric split liver transplantation (SLT)

Standards for consideration of a donor for potential splitting were developed in an attempt to eliminate the high rate of primary nonfunction in early studies of SLT. In addition, a working group of the American Society of Transplant Surgeons and the American Society of Transplant helped establish national policy to increase the number of potential donors allocated to be split into LLS and extended right allografts. Since 2007, the Organ Procurement Transplantation Network has used four characteristics to identify donors that should be considered for splitting.

1. Donor is less than 40 years old
2. Donor is on a single vasopressor or less
3. Donor transaminases are no greater than three times the normal level
4. Donor body mass index (BMI) is 28 or less.

OPTN data shows that 10% of all deceased donors and more than 20% of donors less than 35 years old meet the minimal criteria for splitting. Unfortunately, early results after institution of this policy revealed that only 1% of those meeting criteria are actually split [35].

The UK has similar donor criteria, with the sole addition of an ICU stay of less than 5 days. It should also be stressed that the four criteria above are certainly not absolute and can be modified to fit the clinical scenario of the potential candidates. Livers from donors older than 45 have been split and utilized in children, though were found to be potentially associated with biliary strictures and prolonged cholestasis [35–37]. Communication amongst the teams is of utmost importance in these scenarios, as is open communication with the candidates and their families. In cases where a team is extending these criteria for a split liver, liberal use of liver biopsy and close attention to predonation imaging and donor history is important. Significant fibrosis, steatosis, prolonged use of alcohol or calcification of hilar vessels on planar imaging should discourage the team from splitting the liver. The results of these should obviously be reviewed prior to parenchymal transection, so that prompt allocation of the whole liver can be accomplished. Utilization of an intention to split policy at one combined pediatric/adult center in Birmingham, UK eliminated waiting-list mortality on the pediatric list without compromising outcomes.

3. Technical aspects of pediatric split liver transplantation (SLT) — donor

A great amount of information regarding the donor anatomy can be ascertained from a review of premortem imaging performed on the donor as part of their medical admission. Most victims of blunt trauma will have undergone contrast enhanced CT imaging as part of their secondary screening. Careful review of this imaging can reveal potential anatomic barriers to successful splitting and can also factor into the selection of potential recipients, based on size and acuity. Although several formulas exist to estimate the weight of adult livers, the volume of the LLS can vary considerably.

1. Always isolate the aorta (and IMV if a portal flush is planned) early in the operation to allow for rapid heparinization and cold perfusion in the event of catastrophic instability.
2. Evaluate the liver size and quality and, if biopsy is needed to determine the potential for splitting, perform the biopsy early in the procedure. An onsite pathologist should be arranged prior to arrival at the donor hospital.
3. Evaluate for potential anatomic variants.

   a. The *surgical anatomy of the left hepatic vein* (HV) should be assessed early in the procedure, especially if not known based on predonation imaging. The most common variant of the LHV, seen in 73% of cases is one in which the individual segment 2/3 veins form a confluent left HV before joining the middle vein and the vena cava. In another 13% of cases, a single large left hepatic vein (LHV) is present, with segment 2/3 veins joining well in the parenchyma. In the final 14%, special care must be taken, as the segment 2 and 3 veins join outside the parenchyma and drain into the vena cava. Rare variants of the segment 2 and 3 veins and the entire LHV have been described, with varied points of connection to the middle hepatic vein (MHV) [38, 39]. Without the benefit of preoperative imaging, a high index of suspicion should be held if the LHV above the umbilical fissure is smaller than expected, or if the MHV cannot be well defined. Early suspicion of this anatomy should prompt the donor team to complete the transaction of the liver on the back table. In these cases, vein grafts have been utilized to preserve outflow from the MHV tributary of the right sided graft.
   b. *Hepatic arterial and portal vein* (PV) dissection should then be undertaken with attention to the hepatic arterial branch to segment 4. Although this is often sacrificed when it originates from the left hepatic artery without apparent morbidity, it should be preserved when possible. PV dissection above the bifurcation can be performed to allow the passage of an umbilical tape from the LHV, along the sinus venosus and through the bifurcation to serve as a guide for parenchymal transection. This step, though often performed, is not particularly necessary and if dissection of the portal or left HV is difficult, can be skipped. Replaced or accessory left hepatic arteries arising from the left gastric artery are found in roughly 5% of cases [40, 41]. Totally replaced left hepatic arteries are handled by utilization of either the left

branch, left gastric artery or the celiac as inflow. In general, LLS allografts with accessory left hepatic arteries can be arterialized with the anatomic left hepatic artery, if there is pulsatile flow in the accessory artery after reperfusion. However, if there is any question in the flow, performance of a second hepatic arterial anastomosis is suggested [41].

   c. *Cholangiography* is very helpful in defining biliary variants that could impact either side of the split allograft. The most frequent encountered anatomy consists of segment 2 and 3 ducts joining before the umbilical fissure to form the left-lateral duct, which is then joined by a single duct draining segment 4 just medial to the fissure, giving rise to the left hepatic duct. The second most common variant includes a second segment 4 duct joining a LLS duct. These variants will be found in 85% of donors. The most concerning variant observed consists of a segment 4 duct draining into the segment 3 duct, joining the segment 2 duct close to the hilum. This variant occurs in roughly 10% of patients and requires the ligation of the segment 4 duct and often, the creation of two orifices for biliary anastomoses [38, 39, 41]. Though this does statistically increase the risk of biliary stricture on the LLS (by a factor of 2), as long as the anatomy is identified, inadvertent injury or ligation of the duct can be avoided. Back-table transection of the biliary system may be facilitated in cases of variant anatomy with the introduction of coronary dilators or dilute methylene blue to delineate the exact point of segment 4 bile ducts.

4. *Parenchymal transection* can be accomplished by a number of techniques. The division can occur either through or immediately adjacent to the umbilical fissure [42]. The most common process utilized in deceased-donor split liver is simple clamp fracture and electrocautery with hemoclips and/or ligatures for larger vessels and biliary radicals. Preoperative preparation should be made for cases in which large vessels are encountered and vascular clamps and vascular suture should be readily available. A clear understanding of hepatic venous anatomy is needed to safely divide the parenchyma, with careful attention to the path of the HV from segment 3. If there is no preoperative imaging and large veins are unexpectedly encountered during transection, the process should be halted for clarification of the anatomy on the back table. Intraoperative ultrasound is also an option, depending on the technical ability at the donor institution. Ultrasonic dissection, harmonic scalpels, bipolar

coagulation and staplers have all been described to assist in parenchymal transection and their use is highly dependent on the experience of the operative team recovering the organ.

5. *Back-table preparation.* Once the liver is properly flushed and is brought to the back table, final division of the hilar vessels and bile duct can occur and any remaining parenchyma can be divided between multiple silk ties, reducing bleeding and leaks from small biliary radicals. The cut surface should also be tested for leaks by injecting cold preservative solution into the vasculature and into the bile duct. Hepatic venous division can also occur in a controlled fashion, with careful inspection of the intrahepatic anatomy through the open upper vena cava.

4. Technical aspects of pediatric split liver transplantation (SLT) — recipient

Although not specifically addressed, operative concepts described in this section are applicable to implantation of any LLS allograft, regardless of whether the donor was deceased or living.

1. *Preoperative phase.* The recipient operation begins with comprehensive preoperative planning, involving all members of a multidisciplinary team.

    a. *Cardiac evaluation.* Several indications for LT in children are associated with cardiac structural (biliary atresia, Alagille's syndrome) and functional (organic acidemias, glycogen storage diseases and Portopulmonary hypertension) pathology. Careful preoperative evaluation in these children should include cardiac catheterization and monitoring for a response to treatment (e.g., 100% FiO_2 challenges, nitric oxide infusion). Structural defects should prompt intraoperative venting of the allograft at reperfusion to reduce the risk of paradoxical embolization of air and debris across the defect into the systemic circulation.

    b. *Pulmonary evaluation.* Two liver diseases are generally associated with significant pulmonary pathology. As a result of portal-systemic shunting, patients with hepatopulmonary syndrome have significant intrapulmonary shunts, which result in significant hypoxia. This shunting worsens in the upright position (orthodoxia), but can also worsen with increased cardiac output and hypoxia. Chronic pulmonary hypoxia also can lead to the development of pulmonary hypertension. Strategies to improve oxygenation in these patients include use of inhaled nitric oxide and use of pulmonary vasodilators should be tested for efficacy preoperatively. The well-described pulmonary disease, cystic fibrosis, causes frequent intrapulmonary infections, loss of pulmonary reserve, and fibrosis. Functional testing of the lungs should be utilized to ensure that the patient will tolerate LT. In addition, deep suction cultures should be obtained with intubation to guide perioperative antibiotic therapy.

   c. *Metabolic disease.* Careful perioperative metabolic control should be obtained with protocolized intraoperative and early postoperative monitoring. Communication between the anesthesia and metabolic/genetics team is imperative. In addition, timing of organ recovery is important with every effort made to decrease the amount of time the child is fasted. Use of iso-osmotic dextrose infusions, including the utilization of specific parenteral nutrition products (e.g., BCAA free amino acid preparations) may be necessary to gain the best metabolic control in the immediate preoperative period.

   d. *Acute liver failure (ALF).* Children with ALF represent some of the most challenging patients to manage in the perioperative period. Once again, direct communication between the critical care, transplant and anesthetic teams is required for an optimal outcome. In cases of ALF, the organ recovery needs to be timed around the supportive treatments often required to stabilize these children; hemodialysis, plasmapheresis and transfusions should be carefully orchestrated to afford the most benefit in the perioperative period. Careful monitoring of cerebral perfusion pressures with invasive monitors, transcutaneous Doppler's and other imaging should also be considered, as well as the potential management decisions that would be based on the information gained from their use.

2. *Intraoperative phase.* A detailed discussion of all intraoperative techniques used in pediatric LT is beyond the scope of this text, however a few salient points are important in the use of LLS grafts in children. In the preanhepatic phase, the liver is carefully dissected from its attachments to the retroperitoneum and the diaphragm. Hilar dissection involves the skeletonization of the hepatic artery and the PV. The native biliary system (if existent) is generally not utilized with LLS transplantation. The hepatic arteries are identified and divided above the bifurcation and dissection of the proper hepatic artery is performed below the level of the gastroduodenal artery. Arterial dissection in children should generally include the

common hepatic artery and when technically possible, circumferential dissection of the splenic artery. In cases of poor arterial flow, augmentation of hepatic flow can often be accomplished with ligation of the splenic artery at its origin, just proximal to the common hepatic artery. If flow still appears inadequate, allograft iliac or carotid arteries can be anastomosed to the infra renal aorta and tunneled through the transverse mesocolon to the hepatic hilum. Dissection and division of the GDA affords excellent exposure of the proximal PV, just above the confluence of the splenic and superior mesenteric veins. Dissection of the PV to this level allows for greater mobilization of the vein in cases of size mismatch and in cases of SLT. It also allows more proximal occlusion of the vein during the anhepatic phase, making anastomosis easier. Assessment of portal flow and the caliber of the vein should be made prior to the anhepatic phase and if the PV is diminutive or has inadequate flow, allograft veins, or the recipient's left internal jugular vein, can be used as a jump graft — either from the level the confluence of the splenic an superior mesenteric veins or from the superior mesenteric vein itself. Preservation of the native **inferior vena cava** (when present) is required for transplantation of allografts that do not include a donor vena cava. This "piggyback technique" allows preservation of caval and portal flow during the entire preanhepatic phase and also shortens warm-ischemia times during the anhepatic phase. Although children tend to tolerate a short periods of caval clamping, minimization of portal occlusion times is essential in patients without chronic liver disease (metabolic disorders and acute liver failure), as lack of portal collateral flow in this population leads to visceral engorgement with occlusion of the portal flow. Serial ligation of short HVs separates the caudate from the vena cava. The right hepatic vein (RHV) can be encircled, as can the confluence of the left and middle veins. Dissection in technical variant livers should also free the cava and the HVs from the diaphragmatic hiatus with careful division of the phrenic veins (Figure 1). This allows a more direct clamping of the suprahepatic cava ABOVE the level of the HVs and is also vital in the performance of domino LT (vide infra). Controlled circumferential dissection of the retrohepatic cava above the level of the right adrenal vein allows for occlusion with a clamp for implantation. Occlusion of the PV inflow allows the relatively bloodless removal of the liver after control of the HVs with individual clamps. This technique allows the creation of long hepatic venous cuffs, often needed for the successful implantation of technical variant allografts.

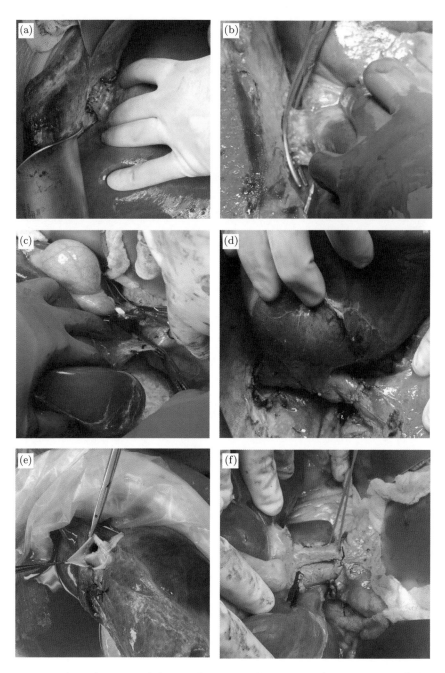

Figure 1. Technical aspects of domino liver transplantation. Safe preparation of the liver from the domino donor begins with extensive dissection of the suprahepatic vena cave with ligation and division of phrenic and posterior caval branches, completely freeing the vena cava from the diaphragmatic hiatus (a). This dissection continues inferiorly, frequently requiring ligation and division of the right adrenal vein. Proper skeletonization of the cava

←──

Figure 1. (*Continued*)   allows the controlled camping and division of the vena cava above the entrance of the hepatic venous orifices (b) and proper division of the retrohepatic vena cava (c) for easier implantation of the deceased donor liver (d). In cases where the hepatic orifices cannot be safely included in one patch, reconstruction can be accomplished utilizing the infrahepatic vena cava of the deceased-liver donor (e). Hilar dissection in the domino donor involves careful circumferential dissection of the vessels and delayed division of the hepatic artery until just prior to completion of the hepatectomy (f).

Vascular reconstruction begins with an end-to-end anastomosis of the outflow vessel of the allograft. In cases of LLS transplant, this is the LHV. The outflow of a left-lobe graft is the confluence of the left and middle veins and the outflow of a whole "domino" allograft is generally the entire supra-hepatic cava. The outflow of the allograft should be anastomosed to the largest possible cuff of the recipient. In general, this is accomplished by creating a common cuff of all three HVs. At the completion of this anasto-mosis, flow through the native vena cava can be restored by careful reposi-tioning of a vascular clamp onto the *allograft* cava (or LHV), *above* the anastomosis and subsequent release of the supra and infrahepatic clamps. An end-to-end allograft to native portal (or jump graft) anastomosis is then fashioned. Careful consideration to the position of the liver once the abdo-men is closed (with placement of cold laparotomy pads above and behind the liver) often leads to considerable shortening of the allograft PV and to the reorientation of the vein along its axis. The PV should be carefully flushed prior to completion of the anastomosis by temporarily releasing the clamp and filling the allograft with heparinized saline. This technique avoids distal of embolization of clot if any is present in the occluded native portal and mesenteric systems. The portal anastomosis should be completed with a "growth factor" approximating the diameter of the PV and some bleeding should be appreciated from it after reperfusion.

Reperfusion of the allograft occurs with the release of the PV. The allo-graft should be aggressively warmed during this phase and surgical hemo-stasis is obtained. In children, arterialization should be performed with optimal inflow, utilizing any potential arterial branch orifices for creation of branch patches. In the majority of cases, end-to-end anastomoses are achieved with interrupted 7-0 or 8-0 monofilament suture. Doppler inter-rogation of the intrahepatic artery should be performed in all cases and any concerns should be immediately addressed. As mentioned previously, arte-rial inflow can be augmented by occluding the splenic artery. If this is unsuc-cessful or if there is any concern regarding the anastomosis, revision should be performed and an arterial conduit can be used from the abdominal aorta. **Biliary reconstruction** is then performed as an end-to-side hepaticojejunostomy to a roux limb tunneled behind the colon and lays in a straight line with the cut surface [43]. The distal ends of the bile duct should be carefully trimmed prior to reconstruction, to ensure adequate vascularity. The anastomosis is generally accomplished with nine well-placed absorbable monofilament sutures in an interrupted fashion over a small indwelling biliary stent which can be carefully removed prior to the completion of the anastomosis. If there is any question regarding intrahepatic biliary anatomy, an on-table cholangiogram can verify segment 2 and 3 ducts within the parenchyma, even if a common left hepatic duct has not been preserved.

Immediate **abdominal closure** is not possible in all cases and is often limited by allograft size mismatches and visceral edema during portal occlusion. Post closure, transabdominal ultrasound and Doppler interrogation of the allograft should be performed in all cases and the abdomen immediately reopened if there are any changes in vessel waveforms. Temporary mesh closure with silastic sheeting should be liberally employed, with delayed fascial closure after edema subsides (usually within 3–5 days). Skin closure over a deliberate ventral hernia is frequently required with large graft:recipient ratios, with abdominal wall reconstruction performed after 6–12 months. Doppler ultrasonographic interrogation of the allograft vessels is useful to evaluate the patency of the vasculature and to evaluate any changes with abdominal closure. Protocol Doppler exams assist in the rapid diagnosis and treatment hepatic arterial thrombosis in the early postoperative period [44].

5. Pediatric living-donor liver transplant (LDLT)

The number of pediatric brain-dead liver donors (donors under 18) has steadily decreased from over 1,000 in 1995 to 729 in 2015 (Figure 2). This decrease, coupled with the number of children being listed for LT has led to a corresponding shortage in pediatric organs available for use in children and has, in addition to increasing the utilization of split livers, furthered the utilization of adult living donors for transplantation into children. The results of pediatric living donor liver are excellent with long and short term patient and graft survival equal to those of deceased-donor liver transplantation [44–47]. The techniques utilized in the recovery of a LLS allograft from a healthy adult donor is beyond the scope of this text, but have been reviewed extensively in other texts [48, 49]. Donor selection in children is extremely important and careful attention should be paid to the potential hazards in utilization of

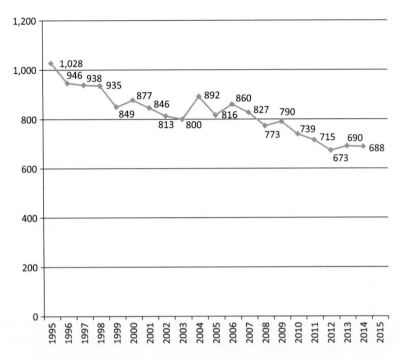

Figure 2. Pediatric liver donation in the United States. The graph demonstrates the gradual decrease in the number of liver donors under 18 years of age in the United States from 1995 to 2015.

heterozygous parental or familial donors in children with inherited metabolic diseases. Recipient techniques are very similar to those with split liver segments from deceased donors, however careful attention to preoperative imaging of the recipient is required as living donation does not generally afford vascular conduits. In cases of known preoperative portal thrombosis or variant recipient arterial anatomy, the team should attempt to plan to perform the transplant when deceased-donor vessels are available from other recoveries. Allogenic saphenous vein, autologous inferior mesenteric and internal jugular veins offer other potential options for reconstruction in these challenging cases. PTFE grafts have been used for hepatic venous and arterial reconstruction in adults, however there are no large reports describing their use in children.

6. Domino liver transplantation (LT)

The sequential transplant of livers, first from a deceased or living donor into a primary recipient with a metabolic disease (the domino donor — DD) with the subsequent transplantation of that patient's liver into a second recipient (the domino recipient — DR), is referred to as domino LT. The first domino transplantation was performed in Portugal in 1995 with a patient with familial amyloid polyneuropathy (FAP) acting as the domino donor. Since that time, the Domino Liver Transplant Registry has logged over 1,000 domino LTs in more than 20 countries around the world. Most these domino transplant have been performed using DD with FAP and although these livers are certainly appropriate for well selected adult patients, their utility in children is limited by the potential for de novo development of FAP-linked diseases in the domino recipients after a prolonged period [50].

Over the ensuing decade, the results of domino transplantation using liver allografts from patients with a variety of metabolic diseases have been reported from around the world. One of the larger experiences is utilizing patients receiving LT for Maple Syrup Urine Disease (MSUD) as the domino donors [51, 52]. MSUD is a disease characterized by a defect in the branched-chain ketoacid dehydrogenase complex (BCKDH) with resulting elevations in plasma branched chain amino acids. As the whole body BCKDH activity is primarily located in nonhepatic tissues (only 10% of the activity is found in the liver), domino transplantation using these livers will result in only a 10% reduction in whole body BCKDH activity in the domino recipient. Fortunately, the utility of LT in obtaining long-lasting control of branched-chain amino acid metabolism has been well described in patients with Classical MSUD [51, 52].

Experience utilizing livers from small children with MSUD for domino donation is building with two separate case reports, totaling three domino transplants from patients aged 22–38 months of age without reported technical complications [53]. In addition, our center has experience with use of LLS allografts from a domino donor with classical MSUD, as well as the use of these liver explants for hepatocyte isolation for both research and clinical use [54]. There have also been reports of living related liver donation in MSUD, however this should be done with some degree of caution, as posttransplant metabolic control may be inadequate due to reduced enzyme expression in heterozygous donors [55–58].

Operative principles for domino transplantation are similar to those in all technical variant transplants, however the *domino donor* operation requires additional circumferential dissection of the hilar and outflow vessels and planned sites of vessel division for optimal results for both recipients (Figure 1). Recovery of the *deceased-donor* allograft should also be performed by an experienced recovery surgeon with careful attention to the adequacy of length of hilar and caval lengths. Use of deceased-donor iliac vein or infrahepatic caval grafts from the deceased donor may be necessary if there is inadequate length above the confluence of the domino donor's HVs below the suprahepatic vena caval clamp. Systemic heparinization should be considered in domino donors prior to clamping the inflow and should be promptly reversed with signs of bleeding. In addition, patients with MSUD should only be utilized as domino donors if they have controlled BCAA at the time of donation. Both patients should undergo extensive pretransplant education at the time of evaluation regarding the technical risks of domino donation and transplantation, as well as those associated with receiving the allograft from the "diseased" domino donor. Technical aspects of the procedure for *recipient* of the domino liver allograft is similar to those described for recipients of technical variant allografts. Careful attention should be paid to the preservation of vascular cuff length and the potential for choledochocholedochotomy for biliary reconstruction when recipient characteristics allow it.

Results of domino LTs are excellent and have been extensively reported by several centers. The risk–benefit ratio for the DR hinges on the additional technical risks of caval reconstruction and other grafts often needed [59, 60]. The operative techniques utilized in the DD are no different than those in a standard LT, however careful skeletonization and preservation of vessel length may prolong the operation. As the variety of metabolic diseases amenable to LT expands, there will need to be careful analysis of disease specific risk factors before these recipients are utilized as domino donor [61]. Transplant of livers from DD with methylmalonic aciduria [62], familial amyloid [59], and oxaluria [63] may have short and long-term consequences that need to be factored into the overall risk–benefit algorithm and discussed carefully with the potential recipients and their families.

References

1. Starzl TE, Marchioro TL, Von Kaulla KN, *et al*. Homotransplantation of the liver in humans. *Surg Gynecol Obstet* 1963;117:659–76.
2. Starzl TE, *et al*. Orthotopic homotransplantations of the human liver. *Ann Surg* 1968;168:392.
3. Smith B. Segmental liver transplantation from a living donor. *J Ped Surg* 1969;4(1):126–32.
4. Broelsch CE, Emond JC, Thistlethwaite JR, *et al*. Liver transplantation with reduced size donor organs. *Transplantation* 1988;45:519–24.

5. Bismuth H and Houssin D. Reduced-sized orthotopic liver graft in hepatic transplantation in children. *Surgery* 1984;95:367–70.

6. DeHemptinne B, Salizzoni M, Yandza TC, *et al*. Indication, technique and results of liver graft reduction before orthotopic transplantation in children. *Transplant Proc* 1987;19:3549–51.

7. Emond JC, Whitington PF, Thistlethwaite JR, *et al*. Reduced-size orthotopic liver transplantation: use in the management of children with chronic liver disease. *Hepatology* 1989;10:867–72.

8. Otte JB, de Ville de Goyet J, and Sokal E. Size reduction of the donor liver is a safe way to alleviate the shortage of size matched organs in pediatric liver transplantation. *Ann Surg* 1990;211;146–57.

9. Ringe B, Burdelski M, Rodeck B, *et al*. Experience with partial liver transplantation in Hannover. *Clin Transplant* 1990;135–44.

10. Bismuth H, Morino M, Castaing D, *et al*. Emergency orthotopic liver transplantation in two patients using one donor. *Br J Surg* 1989;76:722–4.

11. Pichlmayr R, Ringe B, and Gubernatis G. Transplantation of a donor liver to two recipients (splitting transplantation) — a new method in the further development of segmental liver transplantation. *Langenbecks Archiv Chir* 1989;373:127–30.

12. Strong RW, Lynch SV, Ong TH, *et al*. Successful liver transplantation from a living donor to her son. *N Engl J Med* 1990;322:1505–7.

13. Emond JC, Whitington PF, Thistlewaite JJ, *et al*. Transplantation of two patients with one liver. Analysis of preliminary experience with split liver grafting. *Ann Surg* 1990;212:14–22.

14. Emond JC, Heffron T, Thistlewaite JJ, *et al*. Innovative approaches to donor scarcity: a critical comparison between split liver and living related liver transplantation. *Hepatology* 1991;14:92A.

15. Cramm SL, Waits SA, Englesbe MJ, *et al*. Failure to rescue as a quality improvement approach in transplantation: a first effort to evaluate this tool in pediatric liver transplantation. *Transplantation* 2016;100(4):801–7.

16. Dreyzin A, Lunz J, Venkat V, *et al*. Long-term outcomes and predictors in pediatric liver retransplantation. *Pediatr Transplant* 2015;19(8):866–74.

17. Soltys KA, Mazariegos GV, Squires RH, *et al*. Late graft loss or death in pediatric liver transplantation: an analysis of the SPLIT database. *Am J Transplant* 2007;7:2165–71.

18. de Ville de Goyet J. Split liver transplantation on Europe — 1988 to 1993. *Transplantation* 1995;59:1371–6.

19. Reyes J, Gerber D, Mazariegos GV, *et al*. Split-liver transplantation: a comparison of ex vivo and in situ techniques. *J Pediatr Surg* 2000;35(2):283–9.

20. Salzedas-Netto AA, Amadei HL, Castro CCL, *et al*. Impact of ex-situ transection on pediatric liver transplantation. *Transplant Proc* 2010;42:507–10.

21. Renz JF, Yersiz H, Reichert PR, *et al*. Split-liver transplantation: a review. *Am J Transplant* 2003;3:1323–35.

22. Ye H, Wang Y, Wang D, *et al*. Outcomes of technical variant liver transplantation versus whole liver transplantation for pediatric patients: a meta-analysis. *PLoS ONE* 2015;14;10(9):e0138202.

23. Diamond IR, Fecteau A, Millis MJ, *et al*. Impact of graft type on outcome in pediatric liver transplantation. A report from Studies of Pediatric Liver Transplantation (SPLIT). *Ann Surg* 2007;246:301–10.

24. Bordeaux C, Darwish A, Jamart J, *et al*. Living-related versus deceased donor pediatric liver transplantation: a multivariate analysis of technical and immunological complications in 235 recipients. *Am J Transplant* 2007;7:440–7.

25. Doyle MBM, Maynard E, Lin Y, *et al*. Outcomes with split liver transplantation are equivalent to those with whole organ transplantation. *J Am Coll Surg* 2013;217:102–14.

26. Farmer DG, Venick RS, McDiarmid SV, *et al*. Predictors of outcomes after pediatric liver transplantation: an analysis of more than 800 cases performed at a single institution. *J Am Coll Surg* 2007;204:904–16.

27. Yersiz H, Renz J, Farmer DG, *et al*. One hundred in situ split liver transplantations. A single-center experience. *Ann Surg* 2003;238:496–507.

28. Ng V, Anand R, Martz K, and Fecteau A. Liver re-transplantation in children: a SPLIT database analysis of outcome and predictive factors for survival. *Am J Transplant* 2008;8:386–95.

29. McDiarmid SV, Anand R, Martz BS, *et al*. A multivariate analysis of pre-, peri- and post-transplant factors affecting outcome after pediatric liver transplantation. *Ann Surg* 2011;254:145–54.

30. Rana A, Pallister ZS, Guiteau JJ, *et al*. Survival outcomes following pediatric liver transplantation (Pedi-SOFT) Score: a novel predictive index. *Am J Transplant* 2015;15:1855–63.

31. Lauterio A, Di Sandro S, Concone G, *et al*. Current status and perspectives in split liver transplantation. *World J Gastroenterol* 2015;21(39):11003–15.

32. Becker NS, Barshes NR, Aloia TA, *et al*. Analysis of recent pediatric orthotopic liver transplantation outcomes indicates that allograft type is no longer a predictor of survivals. *Liver Transpl* 2008;14:1125–32.

33. Hong JC, Yersiz H, Farmer DG, *et al*. Longterm outcomes for whole and segmental liver grafts in adult and pediatric liver transplant recipients: a 10-year comparative analysis of 2,988 cases. *J Am Coll Surg* 2009;208(5): 682–9.

34. Moussaoui D, Toso C, Nowacka A, *et al*. Early complications after liver transplantation in children and adults: are split grafts equal to each other and equal to whole livers? *Pediatr Transplant* 2017;21(4):e12908.

35. OPTN/UNOS Ethics committee. Split versus whole liver transplantation. August 2016.

36. Hsu EK and Mazariegos GV. Global lessons in graft type and pediatric liver allocation: a path toward improving outcomes and eliminating wait-list mortality. *Liver Transpl* 2017;23(1):86–95.

37. Battula NR, Platto M, Anbarasan R, *et al.* Intention to split policy: a successful strategy in a combined pediatric and adult liver transplant center. *Ann Surg* 2017;265(5):1009–15.

38. Reichert PR, Renz JF, D'Albuquerque LA, *et al.* Surgical anatomy of the left lateral segment as applied to living-donor and split-liver transplantation: a clinicopathologic study. *Ann Surg* 2000;232(5):658–64.

39. Chaib E, Ribeiro MAF, Saad WA, *et al.* The main hepatic anatomic variations for the purpose of split-liver transplantation. *Transplant Proc* 2005;37:1063–6.

40. Seda-Neto J, da Fonseca EA, Pugliese R, *et al.* Twenty years of experience in pediatric living donor liver transplantation: focus on hepatic artery reconstruction, complications and outcomes. *Transplantation* 2016;100:1066–72.

41. Renz JF, Reichert PR, and Emond JC. Biliary anatomy as applied to pediatric living donor and split-liver transplantation. *Liver Transpl* 2000;6(6):801–4.

42. De Ville de Goyet J, di Francesco F, Sottani V, *et al.* Splitting livers: trans-hilar or trans-umbilical division? Technical aspects and comparative outcomes. *Pediatr Transplant* 2015;19:517–26.

43. Nadalin S, Monti L, Grimaldi C, *et al.* Roux-en-Y hepatico-jejunostomy for a left segmental graft: do not twist the loop, stick it! *Pediatr Transplant* 2015;19(4):358–65.

44. Nishida S, Kata T, Levi D, *et al.* Effect of protocol Doppler ultrasonography and urgent revascularization on early hepatic artery thrombosis after pediatric liver tranaplantation. *Arch Surg* 2002;137:1279–83.

45. Seda Neto J, Pugielese R, Fonseca EA, *et al.* Four hundred thirty consecutive pediatric living donor liver transplants: variables associated with posttransplant patients and graft survival. *Liver Transpl* 2012;18:577–84.

46. Yankol Y, Fernandez LA, Kanmaz T, *et al.* Results of pediatric living donor compared to deceased donor liver transplantation in the PELD/MELD era: experience from two centers on two different continents. *Pediatr Transplant* 2016;20(1):72–82.

47. Hong JC, Yersiz H, Farmer DG, *et al.* Longterm outcomes for whole and segmental liver grafts in adult and pediatric liver transplant recipients: a 10-year comparative analysis of 2,988 cases. *J Am Coll Surg* 2009;208(5):682–9.

48. Humar A and Sturdevent M. *Atlas of Organ Transplantation.* Heidelberg: Springer, 2016.

49. Sharma V, Tan HP, Marsh JW, and Marcos A. Technical aspects of live-donor hepatectomy. In: Tan H, Marcos A, and Shapiro R, Eds. *Living Donor Transplantation.* New York: Informa Healthcare, 2007, pp. 169–83.

50. Wilczek HE, Larsson M, and Ericzon BG. Report from the Domino Liver Transplant Registry. In: Gruessner RWG and Benedetti E, Eds. *Living Donor Organ Transplantation.* New York: McGraw-Hill Medical, 2008, pp. 637–43.

51. Mazariegos GV, Morton DH, Sindhi R, *et al*. Liver transplantation for classical maple syrup urine disease: long-term follow-up in 37 patients and comparative united network for organ sharing experience. *J Pediatr* 2012;160:116–21.

52. Khanna A, Hart M, Nyhan WL, *et al*. Domino liver transplantation in maple syrup urine disease. *Liver Transpl* 2006;12(5):876–82.

53. Mohan N, Karkra S, Rastogi A, *et al*. Living donor liver transplantation in maple syrup urine disease — Case series and world's youngest domino liver donor and recipient. *Pediatr Transplant* 2016;20(3):395–400.

54. Gramignoli R, Tahan V, Dorko K, *et al*. New potential cell source for hepatocyte transplantation: discarded livers from metabolic disease liver transplants. *Stem Cell Res* 2013;11:563–73.

55. Matsunami M, Fukuda A, Sasaki K, *et al*. Living donor domino liver transplantation using a maple syrup urine disease donor: a case series of three children — the first report from Japan. *Pediatr Transplant* 2016;20:633–9.

56. Pham TA, Enns GM, and Esquivel CO. Living donor liver transplantation for inborn errors of metabolism — An underutilized resource in the United States. *Pediatr Transplant* 2016;20:770–3.

57. Soltys KA, Mazariegos GV, and Strauss KA. Living related transplantation for MSUD-caution, or a new path forward? *Pediatr Transplant* 2015;19:247–8.

58. Al-Shamsi A, Baker A, Dhawan A, *et al*. Acute metabolic crises in maple syrup urine disease after liver transplantation from a related heterozygous living donor. *JIMD Rep* 2016;30:59–62.

59. Tincani G, Hoti E, Andreani P, *et al*. Operative risks of domino liver transplantation for the familial amyloid polyneuropathy liver donor and recipient: a double analysis. *Am J Transplant* 2011;11:759–66.

60. Ericzon BG, Larsson M, and Wilczek HE. Domino liver transplantation: risks and benefits. *Transplant Proc* 2008;40(4):1130–1.

61. McKiernan PJ. Recent advances in liver transplantation for metabolic disease. *J Inherit Metab Dis* 2017;40(4):491–5. doi: 10.100

62. Khanna A, Gish R, Winter SC, *et al*. Successful domino liver transplantation from a patient with methylmalonic acidemia. *JIMD Rep* 2016;25:87–94.

63. Saner FH, Treckmann J, Pratschke J, *et al*. Early renal failure after domino liver transplantation using organs from donors with primary hyperoxaluria type 1. *Transplantation* 2010;90(7):782–5.

9. ABO-Incompatible Liver Transplantation

Abhideep Chaudhary, Prashant Pandey, and Sunil Taneja

Department of Surgery, Jaypee Hospital, Noida, India

1. Introduction

Liver transplant(ation) (LT) is a time-honored treatment for end-stage liver disease (ESLD); however, availability of deceased donors still remains a task to be accomplished for LT. The deceased-donor liver transplantation (DDLT) is an established method of transplantation in the West; however, living-donor liver transplantation (LDLT) is now gaining acceptability particularly in the East to overcome the shortage of deceased donors. Despite introduction of LDLT worldwide, organ shortage is still present and transplant waiting-list mortality is high. Hence to overcome this issue of organ shortage and reduce the waiting-list mortality crossing the ABO blood type barrier has become the only option.

The ABO barrier was first crossed during 1970s; however, initial results were poor in terms of both short-term graft loss and the long-term survival [1–8]. In the current era of LT, with the use of Rituximab and plasma exchange therapy for desensitization, ABO-incompatible (ABO-I) transplantation has become an acceptable method of transplantation in a select group of patients [8–13]. ABO-I LT is also the only option in LDLT if only one suitable blood group unmatched donor is available. In this chapter, we will try to review major aspects of ABO-I LT.

2. History and milestones

The Human beings have two important transplantation antigen systems, ABO blood group and human leukocyte antigen (HLA) antigen system.

Landsteiner in 1945 first proposed the ABO blood group systems and their importance. He proposed the Landsteiner law that implied that persons with ABO blood group have these antigens expressed in almost all body cells while corresponding antibodies are present in them. ABO antigens are expressed in almost all organs of body and are imperative for solid organ transplantation like kidney, heart, liver, and lungs.

Liver is believed to be an immunotolerogenic organ. In spite of its unusual location in body by which it is continuously exposed to outside antigens in gut it exerts only a minimal immune response. This unique property of liver first came to notice in early 1970s about 50 years back when Thomas E. Starzl performed the first human LT.

In 1985, kidney was the first ABO-I organ to be transplanted when Alexandre *et al.* proposed a method to avoid the phenomenon of graft failure due to reaction between isoagglutinin antibody (IA) present in recipient and the corresponding antigen present on graft [14]. This protocol consisted of removal of IAs by plasmapheresis and suppression of antibody production by splenectomy combined with intensive immunosuppression with calcineurin inhibitors, steroids and cyclophosphamide. This protocol revolutionized ABO-I transplants and based on this protocol Takahashi *et al.* performed the first successful ABO-I kidney transplantation. Between 1989 and 1994, most of the ABO-I kidney transplantations were carried out according to this protocol and showed a dramatic improvement in 1-year graft survival from 33% to 81%. Thereafter, in Japan where cadaveric organs were in extremely short supply, ABO-I kidney transplantation spread rapidly, and 1,025 were performed in 92 institutions by the year 2006. During this period, ABO-I LT were also tried but failed due to increased risk of serious infections because of intense immunosuppression [8, 15, 16].

The first successful ABO-I LDLT was performed in the year 2000 where the antirejection therapy included multiple perioperative plasmapheresis, splenectomy, systemic triple immunosuppressive regimen with tacrolimus, methylprednisolone, and cyclophosphamide or azathioprine. In addition to these conventional approaches intraportal infusion therapy with methylprednisolone, prostaglandin E1, and gabexate mesilate were used after transplantation [17]. With these protocols, antidonor blood group antibody titers remained low without any evidence of rejection, vascular or biliary complications throughout the postoperative course. Since then several protocols have been proposed with the aim of avoiding acute graft necrosis and chronic biliary damage, both of which are recognized as major causes of poor outcome.

The three most important developments in the history of ABO-I transplants were the antirejection protocol developed and used by

Tanabe *et al.*, introduction and administration of intrahepatic arterial infusion of prostaglandin (PG) E1 with standard antirejection therapy by the Kyoto group and use of Rituximab (a monoclonal chimeric human-murine anti-CD20 antibody) by Monteiro *et al.* and Tohoku group in 2002 and 2003 [10, 18, 19]. Since then, several protocols have been developed for ABO-I LT with the aim of avoiding antibody-mediated rejection (AMR), acute graft necrosis, and chronic biliary damage, which are recognized as major causes of poor outcome.

3. Mechanism of hyperacute rejection in ABO-I LT

In ABO-I LT, the basic underlying pathology believed for the early graft failure is severe hyper acute rejection due to antibody–antigen reaction and the response triggered by this event. The ABO antigen present on graft endothelium and the corresponding antibody present in patient blood reacts and causes damage to endothelium. This reaction triggers production of chemotactic factors, cytokines, free radicals that further causes complement and platelet activation and thrombus formation (Figure 1). High anti-A/anti-B titer, during perioperative period closely associated with hepatic necrosis and intrahepatic biliary complications [6]. Hence the basic effort of desensitization protocol in ABO-I transplants is to remove the preformed antibodies and stop production of new antibodies. This strategy to reduce the ABO antibody titers plays the fundamental role in ABO-I transplants [20, 21]. During the initial posttransplant phase, there is no rise in ABO titers as the trace of antibodies present is adsorbed on graft endothelium. In fact, titers sometimes decrease to zero several days post transplant as long as the antibodies remain attached to the endothelial cell surface. In some cases, as a result of reperfusion, injury, subclinical rejection and microvascular thrombus may develop which can either lead to complete vascular blockage or may get reversed by fibrinolysis. However, in surviving grafts, in spite of the presence of ABO blood group antigens on vascular endothelial cells in the graft and presence of anti-A/anti-B antibodies, AMR does not occur. This resistance that develops to antibody-mediated injury has been studied and has been described as "accommodation" representing the endothelial resistance to antibody-mediated injury [22].

4. Principle and modalities of desensitization

The basic principle of desensitization in ABO-I transplant is both the removal of preformed IA and cessation of its production. In addition, local

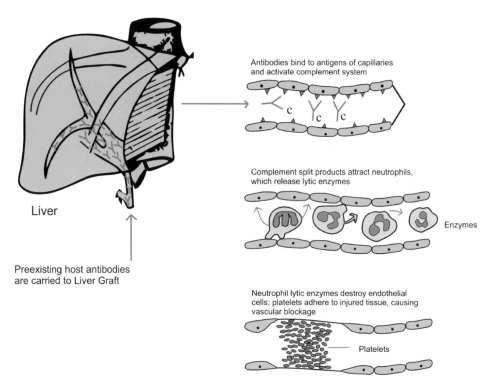

Figure 1. Mechanism of hyperacute rejection in ABO-I LT.

Table 1. Desensitization modalities used for ABO-I LT.

Cessation of antibody production	Removal of existing antibodies	Prevention of Intrahepatic DIC
✓ Rituximab ✓ Intravenous immunoglobulin G ✓ Splenectomy ✓ Immunosuppression • Tacrolimus (IL-2 by T cells) • MMF — mycophenolate mofetil (lymphocyte proliferation and activation) Steroids — IV and oral	✓ Total plasma exchange ✓ Antigen-specific immunoadsorption ✓ Double filtration plasma exchange (DFPP)	✓ Local infusion therapy • Portal vein infusion therapy (PVIT) • Hepatic artery infusion therapy (HAIT)

infusion therapy (LIT) is used with the aim to prevent intrahepatic vascular thrombosis. Desensitization is one of the most evolving aspects of ABO-I transplantation. Table 1 summarizes different methods of desensitization modalities used for ABO-I LT.

4.1. *Various agents used for desensitization by cessation of antibody production*

4.1.1. *Rituximab*

It is a chimeric monoclonal, human-murine anti-CD20 antibody. It causes depletion of B cells by complement dependent cytotoxicity, induces apoptotic death and causes antibody dependent cytotoxicity [10, 11, 19]. Rituximab can suppress all stages of B lymphocyte differentiation except stem cells and long-lived plasma cells. The majority of pharmacokinetic and pharmacodynamic studies have been performed in patients with B-cell lymphoma. However, no pharmacokinetic or pharmacodynamics data on rituximab are available in subjects with ESLD. Therefore, we do not know how much, how often or when rituximab should be administered for desensitization in ABO-I LT. Rituximab was first used for LT in 2003 by Monteiro *et al.* and was later found to be effective against AMR also [19, 23, 24]. According to the Japanese registry, optimum results are achieved if Rituximab was used 7–15 days preoperatively [11]. To deplete normal B cells in ABO-I recipient, single dose of Rituximab is sufficient. Doses <300 mg/body surface area (BSA) were found to be associated with increased incidence of AMR as compared to 500 mg/BSA as per the Japanese registry. Most programs have adopted the original dosage used in malignant lymphoma, i.e., 375 mg/BSA. Administration is done 1 to 3 weeks prior to transplantation, and the frequency of dosing was titrated from multiple to single dosing after there was found to be significantly higher rates of infectious complications and profound long-standing leukopenia with multiple dosing. An incidence of 1.6% of adverse effects was seen with rituximab but all patients recovered and underwent transplantation [25]. Bacterial infections were same as non-rituximab group but fungal infections were significantly lower in rituximab group.

4.1.2. *Intravenous immunoglobulins (IVIGs)*

Immunoglobulins block Fc receptors on mononuclear phagocytes and directly neutralize alloantibodies. They also inhibit expression of CD19 on activated B cells, reactive T cells and the complement system [26]. IVIG can be used in cases of severe AMR, when there isn't enough time for rituximab to exert its effect [27]. Graft survival is enhanced to above 87% when IVIG is used in treatment protocol [28–30]. Due to passive transfer of anti A/B after IVIG administration, it should not be administered before ABO-I LT.

4.1.3. Splenectomy

Spleen being the major organ for antibody production, splenectomy was performed in both renal and liver ABO-I transplantations initially. However, nowadays performing splenectomy before ABO-I transplantation is becoming controversial. In Asian countries, along with splenectomy, other immunosuppressive measures were being used in past [31]. However, Raut *et al.* observed no significant statistical difference in the titers between splenectomised and non-splenectomised patients [32]. However due to a low threshold for splenectomy and its reliability regarding antibody reduction splenectomy is still being carried out in many centers across Asia.

4.2. Methods used for desensitization by antibodies' removal

4.2.1. Total plasma exchange (TPE)

Total plasma exchange (TPE) is the simplest method for reducing IA titer and is generally used for desensitization. It takes 3–4 hours per session and uses fresh frozen blood type AB plasma. In one session of TPE one can filter 1.5 plasma volumes. This approach can be used for lowering elevated IA titers by 63–72% during the posttransplant period, as well as pretransplant period [12]. Plasma exchange is performed three or more times until the titer of the antibody becomes ≤16. The disadvantages of TPE are hypersensitivity, citrate toxicity, hemodynamic stress and relatively low efficiency and selectivity. To overcome the drawbacks of TPE, a Japanese group has developed double-filtration plasmapheresis, which permits selective removal of the plasma fraction containing the immunoglobulins [33]. It consists of two systems, plasma separator and fractionator. Removal of coagulation factors can be avoided and only small amounts of replacement fluids are needed. American society of apheresis guidelines designate perioperative use of TPE in ABO-I LT as category I recommendation [34].

4.2.2. Immunoadsorption

Immunoadsorption depletes large number of circulating antibodies without considerable loss of essential plasma constituents. Two methods of Immunoadsorption have been described. The first method is the blood group antigen-specific immunoadsorption column that is used preferentially to reduce IA titer. This column is highly selective for anti-A/B antibodies, hence rest of the antibodies are not affected and no replacement fluid is required. IgG titers are reduced by 59% and IgM titers are reduced by 30% compared to baseline. The second method is the semi selective antibody removal. These columns mostly remove IgG and to a lesser extent IgM, regardless of their specificity which is beneficial for transplant patients. Immunoadsorption is commonly used in Europe but Asian countries still prefer to use conventional TPE or semiselective double filtration plasmapheresis [35].

4.2.3. *Local infusion therapy (LIT)*

The pathologic findings of failed ABO-I liver grafts showed the features of intrahepatic disseminated intravascular coagulation [6]. Portal vein (PV) infusion therapy was developed by Keio university in 1998 with the aim to reduce local inflammation, inhibition of platelet aggregation and vasodilatation to improve microcirculation and hence reduce chances of AMR [17]. PGE1, Gabexate mesylate and methylprednisolone are infused through the catheter into the PV. To prevent thrombosis of PV, they suggested that catheter be inserted from middle colic vein and tip placed peripheral to superior mesenteric vein [17, 36]. Another approach from Kyoto group suggested plasmapheresis, splenectomy, treatment with tacrolimus, methylprednisolone and cyclophosphamide and intra-arterial infusion with PGE1 alone and catheter placed in one branch of hepatic artery after anastomosis led to decreased incidence of PV thrombosis and improved 1-year survival [18]. LIT was once regarded as an essential component of the desensitization protocol. However, the increasing use of rituximab to prevent AMR has raised questions on the role of local graft infusion therapy as it does not prevent AMR. In fact, the technique often causes complications such as bleeding and vascular thrombosis. Egawa *et al.* reported LIT-related complications in 16–37% of patients [9]. The majority of LIT-related complications in cases of PV infusion are due to PV thrombosis and catheter dislocation often causes intra-abdominal bleeding. The complication rate associated with hepatic artery (HA) infusion is slightly lower, HA injury, thrombosis, and catheter dislocation, are potentially lethal. Although there is still some controversy about the clinical usefulness of LIT, recent clinical studies have obtained success without LIT [37–39].

5. ABO-Incompatible liver transplantation (LT): desensitization protocols

The basic rule of compatibility of graft remains similar to blood transfusion compatibility wherein O group individual is universal donor and AB group individual is universal recipient. Most of the recipients in ABO-I solid organ transplant are group O individuals. The immunosuppressive therapy for

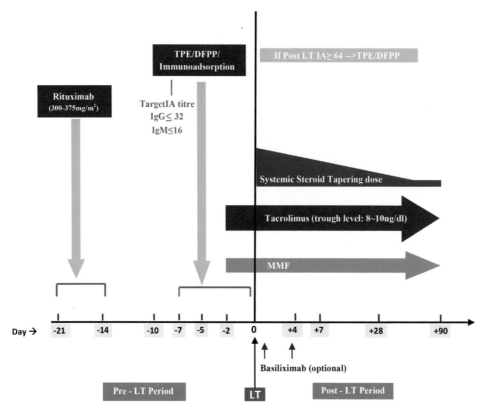

Figure 2. Desensitization protocol for ABO-I liver transplantation. LT, liver transplant; MMF, mycophenolate mofetil; IA, isoagglutinin antibody.

ABO-I LT is same as ABO-C LT; only difference is the desensitization protocols. Most episodes of AMR occur within first week after transplantation. That is the reason why first 2 weeks after ABO-I LT are considered to be the critical period. The titer of antidonor blood group antibody does not disappear in the recipient's blood, even then AMR does not occur after one month. This phenomenon is termed accommodation and is usually induced by 7–15 days after transplantation. The various desensitization protocols to prevent immunologic injury to graft are described below (Figure 2).

5.1. *Preoperative desensitization*

The aim of preoperative desensitization is to stop immunoagglutinins production and remove as much IA as possible before transplantation to prevent AMR during the critical period until accommodation is established. Most centers use rituximab and plasma exchange or immunoadsorption to reduce IA

Table 2. Principles of blood product transfusion in ABO-I LT.

Recipient	Donor	Packed red cells	Plasma products FFP	Platelets
O	A	O	AB/A	AB/A
O	B	O	AB/B	AB/B
O	AB	O	AB	AB
A	B	O or A	AB	AB
A	AB	O or A	AB	AB
B	A	O or B	AB	AB
B	AB	O or B	AB	AB

titers to 16 or less. To get an optimal benefit rituximab should be given at least 7–21 days before the transplant. If it is not possible to wait for that long period, IVIG induction and/or LIT can be added to prevent AMR. Mycophenolate mofetil (MMF) is added pre LT as it removes plasma cells, which escape from rituximab action. With increasing success in preventing AMR with rituximab, most of the centers have stopped using LIT for desensitization.

5.2. Intraoperative measures

In order to prevent transfer of preformed antibodies in blood products the following principles are used according to blood group of donor and recipient (Table 2).

5.3. Post transplantation IA rebound control

To prevent rebound rise in IA levels regular monitoring of IA levels are done post transplantation and triple immunosuppression is used. If there is rebound rise in IA beyond 32, plasmapheresis is restarted with or without IVIG. At times, another dose of rituximab is used if CD19 titers go up in the posttransplant period.

6. ABO-I liver transplantation (LT) — different clinical scenarios

6.1. Pediatric liver transplantation (LT)

Children tolerate ABO-I graft very well as they lack preformed antibodies and their immune system is highly tolerant. Gurevich *et al.* examined

58 pediatric patients undergoing ABO-I LDLT with a preoperative isotitre of <16. No graft rejection or death was reported and 93% had a survival beyond 10 years [40]. Rejection rates were lower in cases of biliary atresia where mother was the donor [41–43]. The successful use of rituximab for desensitization in pediatric ABO-I LT was first described by Okada *et al.* from Japan in the year 2004 [44]. In the preoperative management of patients undergoing pediatric ABO-I LDLT, the administration of 200 mg/BSA rituximab three weeks prior to LDLT was safe and effective [44].

6.2. *Acute liver failure*

The use of ABO-I LDLT for acute liver failure is more common in Asia compared to Europe and the USA, where ABO-I LDLT is conducted only in absence of a compatible donor [45, 46]. Three-year survival rates in ABO compatible (ABO-C) vs. ABO-I LT were 83% vs. 86%, reported by Shen *et al.* [47]. They recommended simplified treatment consisting of single dose rituximab (375 mg/BSA) and IVIG for 10 days to prevent AMR for ABO-I LT patients. With this treatment, the patients did not need plasma exchange, splenectomy, and graft local infusion. This treatment was found to be safe and efficient for LT of the patients with ALF. Lee *et al.* reported that a MELD >30 puts patients at higher risk of mortality and ABO-I transplant should be avoided in these patients if titers are high [48]. However, there was no difference in outcome was found between ABO-C and ABO-I LDLT in a series reported by Shinoda *et al.* [49].

6.3. *Hepatocellular carcinoma (HCC)*

An alternative treatment option for patients with HCC in cirrhosis is living donor transplantation when no deceased donor organ is available because of low MELD scores or tumor burden beyond Milan criteria. However, Lee *et al.* recommended refrainment from transplantation of HCC patients after they experienced a recurrence of 57% in first year of ABO-I LDLT [50, 51]. HCC patients have very high anti-A/B titers and strong rebound due to altered expression of blood group antigens on their biliary tree in disease conditions. Antibody production is boosted by aberrant expression or neo-expression of A/B substances in malignant cells. In cases of HCC, the bulk of tumor defines antibody titer and recurrence. Matsuno *et al.* reported good long-term survival in their series of eight patients who underwent ABO-I LT [52]. Nakamura *et al.* reported 7-year recurrence-free survival after ABO-I

LT patient with HCC exceeding Milano criteria [53]. Rummler *et al.* studied plasma treatment procedure (PTP) related titer reduction rate and titer rebound after treatment. Based on the results of the study, they consider cancelling further scheduling for transplantation if titer reduction rate is below titer rebound in HCC patients after five PTPs. These patients are at high risk for arterial thrombosis and graft loss. Other transplant centers performed up to 12 PTPs before transplantation. No upper limit of PTP has been reported so far [54].

7. Predictors of survival in ABO-I liver transplantation (LT) and clinical significance

The survival outcomes of ABO-I LT essentially depend on the pre-transplant patient's severity of liver disease and age. The causes of graft failure in ABO-I LT are acute rejection, biliary complication, and infections [55]. In the early posttransplant period, formation of antibodies against the donor-blood group antigens bound to the graft vascular endothelium, induction of complement fixation, endothelial damage, and the formation of platelet thrombi followed by the clotting cascade, causing hemorrhagic necrosis, cause graft failure. This has significantly come down after the introduction of desensitization protocols especially rituximab and plasmapharesis.

Diffuse and multiple intrahepatic biliary strictures occurring several months after transplantation still remain a major challenge after ABO-I LT [56]. The overall prognosis is very poor because of refractory cholangitis leads to sepsis and graft failure and only option left is retransplantation in them.

Following factors have been identified as the predictors of survival:

1. Pretransplant patient condition:
   The survival outcomes of ABO-I LT largely depend on the patients' pre-transplant clinical condition and MELD score. A Japanese multicenter retrospective study reported that pretransplant intensive care unit stay and high MELD score were the most significant risk factors for patient survival. The most common cause of death in patients with high MELD score was infectious complications, which were attributed to potent immunosuppression with high-dose steroid, calcineurin inhibitor or a combination of cell-depleting agents, etc. Therefore, prudent patient selection and prevention of AMR are crucial factors for successful outcomes in ABO-I LT [9].

2. Patient age:

   Age is also a powerful indicator of survival outcomes. The immune system is usually immature in children, especially in infants. In the latter, the titer of IA is very low or zero, and B-cell responses to antigenic stimuli are very weak. Therefore, the incidence of AMR in infants was very low even before the era of rituximab. Survival after ABO-I LT was comparable with that after ABO-C LT, without any special measures to prevent AMR. However clinical outcomes deteriorate with increasing patient age, generally starting at age 8 [9, 40–44].

3. Pretransplant and posttransplant peak IA titers:

   High IA titers tends to be a significant risk factors for AMR. For the same reason, recipient blood type O has been considered a risk factor for AMR because IA titers are intrinsically higher in type O than in other blood types. However, a high pretransplant IA titer can be lowered by immunoadsorption or repetitive TPE, and the posttransplant rebound rise of IA can be efficiently suppressed by rituximab prophylaxis and posttransplant TPE. Thus, the impact of IA titer upon AMR has been diminished, and no relationship with patient survival has been found in recent studies, nor is the recipient's blood type or mismatch pattern related to AMR or patient survival [9, 50].

4. Use of rituximab:

   The epoch-making event in ABO-I LT was the introduction of rituximab for DSZ, so that the history of ABO-I LT can be divided into before, and after, rituximab. In post-rituximab era, 3-year survival has increased from 30% to 80% and on analysis of multicenter study from Japan desensitization protocol without rituximab was the only factor predictive of AMR [9, 11, 55]. In a single-center study cohort of 142 adult patients who underwent ABO-I LDLT, 3-year graft and patient survival rates of 90.9% and 96.3% was achieved. In a single-center comparative study of ABO-I and ABO-C LT recipients, there was no significant difference in 1-, 3-, and 5-year graft survival between the two groups. Patient selection and desensitization by rituximab are the most important factors in present era that determine the successful outcome in ABO-I LT [56].

8. Conclusion

The ABO-I transplant has now become an accepted method of LT worldwide. After the development of different desensitization protocols over a period of time the graft and overall survival rates have significantly improved. The introduction of rituximab and plasma exchange has revolutionized the management of these patients and has made ABO-I LT feasible and less complicated. The overall results in pediatric LT have shown a similar graft survival rates at 1, 3, 5, and 10 years between the ABO-C and ABO-I LT. However, in the adults the 1-, 3-, and 5-year graft survival rates in ABO-I LT are slightly inferior. With the evolution of LT and improved understanding of the liver immunology the future of ABO-I LT looks good.

References

1. Gordon RD, Iwatsuki S, Esquivel CO, Tzakis A, Todo S, and Starzl TE. Liver transplantation across ABO blood groups. *Surgery* 1986;100:342–8.
2. Wolfe RA, Roys EC, and Merion RM. Trends in organ donation and transplantation in the United States, 1999–2008. *Am J Transplant* 2010;10:961–72.
3. Petrowsky H and Busuttil RW. Evolving surgical approaches in liver transplantation. *Semin Liver Dis* 2009;29:121–33.
4. Stegall M. ABO-incompatible liver transplant: is it justifiable? *Liver Transpl* 2003;9:31.
5. Hunto DW, Fecteuu AH, Alonso MH, et al. ABO-incompatible liver transplantation with no immunological graft losses using total plasma exchange, splenectomy, and quadruple immunosuppression: evidence for accommodation. *Liver Transpl* 2003;9:22–30.
6. Sugawara Y and Makuuchi M. Adult liver transplantation using live ABO-incompatible grafts in Western countries. *Liver Transpl* 2006;12:1324–25.
7. Haga H, Egawa H, Fujimoto Y, et al. Acute humoral rejection and C4d immunostaining in ABO blood type-incompatible liver transplantation. *Liver Transpl* 2006;12:457–64.
8. Egawa H, Teramukai S, Haga H, et al. Present status of ABO incompatible living donor liver transplantation in Japan. *Hepatology* 2008;47:143–52.
9. Egawa H, Oike F, Buhler L, et al. Impact of recipient age on outcome of ABO-incompatible living-donor liver transplantation. *Transplantation* 2004;77:403–11.
10. Usuda M, Fujimori K, Koyamada N, et al. Successful use of anti-CD20 monoclonal antibody (rituximab) for ABO-incompatible living-related liver transplantation. *Transplantation* 2005;79:12–16.
11. Egawa H, Teramukai S, Haga H, et al. Impact of rituximab desensitization on blood-type-incompatible adult living donor liver transplantation: a Japanese multicenter study. *Am J Transplant* 2014;14:102–14.
12. Kozaki K, Egawa H, Kasahara M, et al. Therapeutic strategy and the role of apheresis therapy for ABO incompatible living donor liver transplantation. *Ther Apher Dial* 2005;9:285–91.

13. Troisi R, Noens L, Montalti R, *et al*. ABO-mismatch adult living donor liver transplantation using antigen-specific immunoadsorption and quadruple immunosuppression without splenectomy. *Liver Transpl* 2006;12:1412–17.
14. Alexandre GP, De Bruyere M, Squifflet JP, *et al*. Human ABO-incompatible living donor renal homografts. *Neth J Med* 1985;28:231–4.
15. Haga H, Egawa H, Fujimoto Y, *et al*. Acute humoral rejection and C4d immunostaining in ABO blood type-incompatible liver transplantation. *Liver Transpl* 2006;12:457–64.
16. Tanabe M, Kawachi S, Obara H, *et al*. Current progress in ABO-incompatible liver transplantation. *Eur J Clin Invest* 2010;40:943–9.
17. Tanabe M, Shimazu M, Wakabayashi G, *et al*. Intraportal infusion therapy as a novel approach to adult ABO-incompatible liver transplantation. *Transplantation* 2002;73:1959–61.
18. Nakamura Y, Matsuno N, Iwamoto H, *et al*. Successful case of adult ABO-incompatible liver transplantation: beneficial effects of intrahepatic artery infusion therapy: a case report. *Transplant Proc* 2004;36:2269–73.
19. Monteiro I, McLoughlin LM, Fisher A, de la Torre AN, and Koneru B. Rituximab with plasmapheresis and splenectomy in abo-incompatible liver transplantation. *Transplantation* 2003;76:1648–9.
20. Kawagishi N, Takeda I, Miyagi S, *et al*. Management of anti-allogeneic antibody elimination by apheresis in living donor liver transplantation. *Ther Apher Dial* 2007;11:319–24.
21. Mor E, Skerrett D, Manzarbeitia C, *et al*. Successful use of an enhanced immunosuppressive protocol with plasmapheresis for ABO-incompatible mismatched grafts in liver transplant recipients. *Transplantation* 1995;59:986–90.
22. Takahashi K. Accommodation in ABO-incompatible kidney transplantation. *Transplant Proc* 2004;36:193–6.
23. Egawa H, Ohmori K, Haga H, *et al*. B-cell surface marker analysis for improvement of rituximab prophylaxis in ABO-incompatible adult living donor liver transplantation. *Liver Transpl* 2007;13:579–88.
24. Morioka D, Togo S, Kumamoto T, *et al*. Six consecutive cases of successful adult ABO-incompatible living donor liver transplantation: a proposal for grading the severity of antibody-mediated rejection. *Transplantation* 2008;85:171–8.
25. Kim BW, Park YK, Kim YB, Wang HJ, and Kim MW. Effects and problems of adult ABO-incompatible living donor liver transplantation using protocol of plasma exchange, intra-arterial infusion therapy, and anti-CD20 monoclonal antibody without splenectomy: case reports of initial experiences and results in Korea. *Transplant Proc* 2008;40:3772–7.
26. Broelsch CE, Malagó M, Testa G, and Gamazo CV. Living donor liver transplantation in adults: outcome in Europe. *Liver Transpl* 2000;6:S64–5.
27. Raut V and Uemoto S. Management of ABO-incompatible living-donor liver transplantation: past and present trends. *Surg Today* 2011;41:317–22.
28. Urbani L, Mazzoni A, Bianco I, *et al*. The role of immunomodulation in ABO-incompatible adult liver transplant recipients. *J Clin Apher* 2008;23:55–62.

29. Morioka D, Togo S, Kumamoto T, *et al*. Six consecutive cases of successful adult ABO-incompatible living donor liver transplantation: a proposal for grading the severity of antibody-mediated rejection. *Transplantation* 2008;85:171–8.
30. Uchiyama H, Mano Y, Taketomi A, *et al*. Kinetics of anti-blood type isoagglutinin titers and B lymphocytes in ABO-incompatible living donor liver transplantation with rituximab and plasma exchange. *Transplantation* 2011;92:1134–9.
31. Lee SG. A complete treatment of adult living donor liver transplantation: a review of surgical technique and current challenges to expand indication of patients. *Am J Transplant* 2015;15:17–38.
32. Raut V, Mori A, Kaido T, *et al*. Splenectomy does not offer immunological benefits in ABO-incompatible liver transplantation with a preoperative rituximab. *Transplantation* 2012;93:99–105.
33. Thalgahagoda S, Webb NJ, Roberts D, *et al*. Successful ABO incompatible renal transplantation following rituximab and DFPP after failed immunoadsorption. *Pediatr Transplant* 2014;18:E74–6.
34. Schwartz J, Winters JL, Padmanabhan A, *et al*. Guidelines on the use of therapeutic apheresis in clinical practice-evidence-based approach from the Writing Committee of the American Society for Apheresis: the sixth special issue. *J Clin Apher* 2013;28:145–284.
35. Bensinger WI. Plasma exchange and immunoadsorption for removal of antibodies prior to ABO incompatible bone marrow transplant. *Artif Organs* 1981;5:254–8.
36. Tanabe M, Kawachi S, Obara H, *et al*. Current progress in ABO-incompatible liver transplantation. *Eur J Clin Invest* 2010;40:943–9.
37. Ikegami T, Taketomi A, Soejima Y, *et al*. Rituximab, IVIG, and plasma exchange without graft local infusion treatment: a new protocol in ABO incompatible living donor liver transplantation. *Transplantation* 2009;88(3):303–7.
38. Kim JD, Choi DL, and Han YS. Fourteen successful consecutive cases of ABO-incompatible living donor liver transplantation: new simplified intravenous immunoglobulin protocol without local infusion therapy. *Transplant Proc* 2014;46(3):754–7.
39. Song GW, Lee SG, Hwang S, Ahn CS, *et al*. A desensitizing protocol without local graft infusion therapy and splenectomy is a safe and effective method in ABO-incompatible adult LDLT. *Transplantation* 2014;97(Suppl 8): S59–66.
40. Gurevich M, Guy-Viterbo V, Janssen M, *et al*. Living donor liver transplantation in children: surgical and immunological results in 250 recipients at Université Catholique de Louvain. *Ann Surg* 2015;262(6):1141–9.
41. West LJ. Antibodies and ABO-incompatibility in pediatric transplantation. *Pediatr Transplant* 2011;15:778–83.
42. Sanada Y, Kawano Y, Miki A, *et al*. Maternal grafts protect daughter recipients from acute cellular rejection after pediatric living donor liver transplantation for biliary atresia. *Transpl Int* 2014;27:383–90.

43. Nijagal A, Fleck S, Hills NK, *et al.* Decreased risk of graft failure with maternal liver transplantation in patients with biliary atresia. *Am J Transplant* 2012;12:409–19.

44. Okada N, Sanada Y, Hirata Y, *et al.* The impact of rituximab in ABO-incompatible pediatric living donor liver transplantation: the experience of a single center. *Pediatr Transplant* 2015;19(3):279–86.

45. Mendes M, Ferreira AC, Ferreira A, *et al.* ABO incompatible liver transplantation in acute liver failure: a single Portuguese center study. *Transplant Proc* 2013;45:1110–5.

46. Maitta RW, Choate J, Emre SH, Luczycki SM, and Wu Y. Emergency ABO-incompatible liver transplant secondary to fulminant hepatic failure: outcome, role of TPE and review of the literature. *J Clin Apher* 2012;27:320–9.

47. Shen T, Lin BY, Jia JJ, *et al.* A modified protocol with rituximab and intravenous immunoglobulin in emergent ABO-incompatible liver transplantation for acute liver failure. *Hepatobiliary Pancreat Dis Int* 2014;13:395–401.

48. Lee SG. A complete treatment of adult living donor liver transplantation: a review of surgical technique and current challenges to expand indication of patients. *Am J Transplant* 2015;15:17–38.

49. Shinoda M, Obara H, Kitago M, *et al.* Emergency adult living donor liver transplantation using ABO incompatible donor for acute liver failure. *HPB* 2015;17:206.

50. Lee SD, Kim SH, Kong SY, Kim YK, and Park SJ. Kinetics of B, T, NK lymphocytes and isoagglutinin titers in ABO incompatible living donor liver transplantation using rituximab and basiliximab. *Transpl Immunol* 2015;32:29–34.

51. Lee J, Lee JG, Lee JJ, *et al.* Results of ABO-incompatible liver transplantation using a simplified protocol at a single institution. *Transplant Proc* 2015;47:723–6.

52. Matsuno N, Iwamoto H, Nakamura Y, *et al.* ABO-incompatible adult living donor liver transplantation for hepatocellular carcinoma. *Transplant Proc* 2008;40(8):2497–500.

53. Nakamura Y, Hama K, Iwamoto H, *et al.* Long-term recurrence-free survival after liver transplantation from an ABO-incompatible living donor for treatment of hepatocellular carcinoma exceeding Milano criteria in a patient with hepatitis B virus cirrhosis: a case report. *Transplant Proc* 2012;44:565–9.

54. Rummler S, Bauschke A, Baerthel E, *et al.* ABO-incompatible living donor liver transplantation in focus of antibody rebound. *Transfus Med Hemother* 2017;44(1):46–51.

55. Kawagishi N and Satomi S. ABO-incompatible living donor liver transplantation: new insights into clinical relevance. *Transplantation* 2008;85:1523–5.

56. Song GW, Lee SG, Hwang S, *et al.* Biliary stricture is the only concern in ABO-incompatible adult living donor liver transplantation in the rituximab era. *J Hepatol* 2014;61:575–82.

10. New Trends in Immunosuppression for Liver Transplantation: Minimization, Avoidance, and Withdrawal

Shoko Kimura, Fermin Fontan, and James F. Markmann

Massachusetts General Hospital Transplant Center, 55 Fruit Street, Boston, MA 02144, USA

1. Introduction

In 1967, Dr. Thomas E. Starzl and his team in Denver, Colorado performed the first liver transplant (LTx) with a documented 1-year survival [1, 2]. The immunosuppressive (IS) regimen included an antilymphocyte globulin (ALG), azathioprine (AZA) and prednisolone [2]. Despite his groundbreaking results, liver transplant(ation) (LT) remained experimental through the 1970s with a 1-year patient survival close to 25% (United Network for Organ Sharing (UNOS) data). From IS regimens mainly based on steroids and AZA in the 1970s to the inclusion of cyclosporine (CYA), and the discovery of University of Wisconsin (UW) preservation solution [3], the 1980s firmly established LT as the gold standard surgical treatment for patients with end-stage liver disease.

The field has come a long way with 1-year patient survival currently close to 90%. Adam *et al.* report of the European Liver Transplant Registry (ELTR), where 44,286 LTs were analyzed, showed an 83% 1-year patient survival (UNOS data). More currently, Schoening *et al.* single-center experience in the USA of 313 consecutive cases showed an 88% survival rate at the 1-year limit which is representative of the outcomes in most of the large transplant centers in the USA [4–6]. Since the 1980s, the number of LTs and specialized centers in the USA have grown from around 1,000 to well over 6,000 a year, and from a few dozens to over 100 respectively. In parallel to refinements in mortality risk scoring systems, organ procurement, allocation protocols, surgical technique and preservation modalities, the evolution of immunosuppression (IS) has shown to have a leading role in the field [7].

Defined as the level of drug therapy that achieves a stable allograft function with the least suppression of systemic immunity, the ideal transplant IS regimen remains the goal as other IS strategies continue to gain a solid identity. The art-science of IS represents a very challenging aspect of transplantation in that therapies are targeted to each patient, often requiring adjustments in the type and proportions of agents used. Denton *et al.* review of IS strategies in transplantation describes how overimmunosuppression and underimmunosuppression are common and almost inevitable [7]. Although the induction and maintenance-protocolled intervals commonly define more predictable stages in liver IS, salvage therapy for acute rejection represent a dynamic problem [8]. The poor correlation between rejection and liver test markers as well as drug levels reflect how liver biopsies remain as the gold standard in diagnosing rejection [9]. Individualized decisions based on the patient's immune sensitization status prior to transplantation, causal disease process, and the overall behavior after the graft is implanted are also fundamental to a successful IS regimen.

The long-term side effects of current IS drugs are the driving forces behind the development of less noxious regimens. A diverse pool of medications is available in the market and based on their pharmacokinetics and pharmacodynamics they can be conveniently selected for each patient and specific phase (Table 1). The concept "polypharmacy", which refers to the use of small doses of multiple drugs in order to avoid dose-dependent complications (Table 2), represents the historic therapeutic strategy to approach the different phases in IS after transplantation [10]. More dated IS streams show that there can be a benefit in decreasing the number of drugs utilized.

Three well-described phases in IS regimens, which will be discussed next, are induction and maintenance with the addition of a salvage phase in the case of acute rejection [8].

2. Induction therapy

The initial phase known as induction entails a 30-day period that occurs right after transplantation when alloreactivity is at its peak. This course of

Table 1. Classification of immunosuppression drugs

Biological agents	Mechanism of action
T-cell-depleting agents	
Anti-CD3: OKT3	Targets the CD3 molecule on T cells and causes depletion of lymphocytes with activation and T-cell lysis with cytokine release
Antithymocyte globulins (ATGs): horse and rabbit ATG and ALG	Rapid lymphocyte depletion due to complement-mediated cell lysis and uptake by the reticuloendothelial system (RES) of opsonized T cells, partial T-cell activation and blockade of T-cell proliferation
Anti-CD52: (Alemtuzumab)	Targets lymphocytes, monocytes, macrophages, natural killer cells and thymocytes but spares plasma cells and memory lymphocytes
Non-T-cell-depleting agents	
Anti-IL-2 receptors	
Basiliximab	Inhibition of T-cell proliferation and signal 3
Daclilumumab	
Belatacept	Binds CD80 and CD86 and inhibits T-cell activation by competition with CD28 for CD80/CD86 binding
Non-biological agents	
Corticosteroids	Effects on antigen presentation by dendritic cells and induction of a decrease in the number of circulating CD4 + T cells, IL-1 transcription and IL-1-dependent lymphocyte activation
Calcineurin inhibitors (CNIs)	
Cyclosporine (CYA)	Inhibition of T-cell activation inhibition of the calcium/calmodulin-dependent phosphatase
Tacrolimus (TAC)	
Antimetabolites	
Mycophenolic acid (MPA)	Inhibition of IMPDH, rate-limiting enzyme in purine and DNA synthesis and prevention of T-cell proliferation
Mycophenolate mofetil (MMF)	
Azathioprine (AZA)	Inhibition of purine and DNA synthesis and prevention of T-cell proliferation
mTOR inhibitors	
Sirolimus (SRL)	Inhibits IL-2 signaling to T cells, thus preventing T-cell proliferation
Everolimus (EVL)	

Table 2.   IS drugs and their most common adverse effects.

IS drug	Adverse effects
Corticosteroids	Cushingoid features, psychosis, poor wound healing, adrenal suppression, cataracts, diabetes, hypertension, obesity, osteoporosis, avascular necrosis, growth retardation
Cyclosporine	Nephrotoxicity, neurotoxicity, metabolic acidosis, gingival hyperplasia, hypertrichosis diabetes, hyperlipidemia, hypertension, hyperkalemia
TAC	Nephrotoxicity, neurotoxicity, hypertension, hyperlipidemia, diabetes, hyperkalemia, metabolic acidosis
MMF	Myelosuppression, gastrointestinal side effects (diarrhea, nausea, emesis), viral infections (cytomegalovirus (CMV), herpes simplex virus (HSV)), candida infections, miscarriages
Sirolimus	Hyperlipidemia, myelosuppression, poor wound healing, pneumonitis, skin rash proteinuria

IS has been defined as a prophylactic intensive regimen given to prevent acute rejection [11]. In contrast to other organs, the application of the induction therapy in LT was relatively infrequent, although throughout the last 15 years it has gained more ground as more benefits have been proven. In an era where patients with higher Model for End-Stage Liver Disease (MELD) scores and more prevalence of renal dysfunction represent the average recipients, attempts to reduce the need for early CNIs and steroids use have become the trend. One of the most current strategies is called "minimization" [12]. It defines an IS approach formulated to avert the infectious and metabolic complications of steroids and the renal toxicity, hepatitis C virus (HCV) reinfection, and tumor-promoting effects of CNIs.

Historically, the most common regimens included a triple-drug therapy with an antimetabolite, a CNI, and corticosteroids. In fact, data reported by the Scientific Registry of Transplant Recipients (SRTR), done in this decade, showed that almost 60% of patients in the USA receive initial IS with TAC and MMF plus steroids, with almost 13% of patients only receiving MMF and TAC without the steroids. MMFs have raised the possibility of withdrawing or avoiding steroids or CNIs altogether. As described by Samuel *et al.*, the cumulative dose of steroids administered during the first weeks has been drastically reduced. From faster taper strategies to steroid-free regimens, the use of this potent medication has significantly dropped with aims to fully avoid its use and so its deleterious side effects. Steroid avoidance strategies have been well described by multiple authors [12]. As Llado *et al.*

have shown, IS without steroids is safe and reduces metabolic and infectious complications [13]. Besides, in HCV-infected patients, IS without steroids does not increase the risk of rejection and can avoid HCV activation. Graft rejection responsiveness to steroids has been well studied showing that, although beneficial in early acute rejection, the use of glucocorticoids for late acute rejection and chronic rejection can negatively impact graft survival. These changes in practice have been associated with a drastic fall in the incidence of chronic rejection. The fine line between steroid-free therapies and the eventual need for steroid boluses in the case of acute rejection is one of the main reasons why multiple centers haven't adopted steroid-free regimens yet. Additionally, a steroid-free regimen usually balances its efficacy by incremental increases in CNI doses which puts renal function preservation at higher risk [14].

The high incidence of renal dysfunction, in LTx patients managed with CNIs, has been associated with a decrease in graft and patient survival, with even worse outcomes observed when hemodialysis is required. Surprisingly, the rate of severe renal failure is estimated at 20–25% at 5 years. In response to CNIs overuse, global awareness has led to the development of CNI reduction, delay and even CNI-free regimens [14]. A meta-analysis of 64 trials found that a lower trough concentrations of TAC showed superiority over standard regimens. Reduction or withdrawal of CNI along with the introduction of MMF has been shown to be safe and to improve renal function [15]. Conversion to everolimus (m-TOR) from CNIs has shown substantial renal benefits with similar incidence of rejection [16]. A randomized prospective multicenter study assessing reduced TAC doses benefits in addition to everolimus compared with standard TAC doses found similar rates of graft loss and better renal function in the everolimus group [16]. This topic will be further discussed under the section "CNI avoidance."

As shown by Cai *et al.* through his analysis of the United Network for Organ Sharing registry data, the use of antibody regimens, and more specifically anti-IL-2 receptors, has gained more popularity over the last 10 years [17]. Patients and grafts survival rates have displayed a significant improvement and up to 30% of USA centers currently implement this strategy.

3. Maintenance therapy

Maintenance is considered as the period that follows induction; it usually starts 30 days after transplantation and is generally used indefinitely thereafter.

After the first year, most patients are being treated with monotherapy having a CNI drug as the most common agent [7, 8].

Even though IS minimization strategies have shown to reduce the complications of chronic IS, the amount of LT recipients able to achieve complete withdrawal still represent a small percentage [12]. Approximately 20% of patients will develop spontaneous operational tolerance, defined as long-term allograft survival without the need for maintenance IS while maintaining immunity to pathogens [18–20]. Different studies aiming to reproduce these phenomena have shown great results. Prospective protocols carried out on pediatric and adult patients showed feasibility and promising outcomes. A pediatric prospective multicenter trial of children receiving a living-related parental split graft found that 60% (12/20) of these patients remained off IS therapy at 1 year with normal histology about any form of rejection [21]. In the adult series, which was a prospective multicenter trial including 98 patients, IS was successfully withdrawn in 41% of the participants. Despite these IS withdrawal outcomes, almost 60% of these patients showed rejection evidence which catalogued them as operationally nontolerant [22]. Importantly, these rejection episodes were readily treated and graft loss and significant compromise of organ function was not observed.

4. Acute rejection

The incidence of clinically significant acute liver rejection is 10–40% in most series and is commonly seen between 5 and 30 days after transplantation [23–25]. The final diagnosis is confirmed by histopathological findings such as (1) portal inflammation, containing blastic or activated lymphocytes, neutrophils and eosinophils; (2) bile duct inflammatory changes and signs of damage; and (3) sub-endothelial inflammation of portal and/or terminal hepatic veins. Recent international consensus stablished that at least two of these findings are necessary for final diagnosis. In further detail, the Banff Schema is used for grading of rejection severity [26, 27]. The management of acute liver rejection refers to the addition of IS therapy which complexity requires a multidisciplinary approach. Steroids can be used as a first line antirejection medication, but in the case of steroid-resistant rejection the patient usually receives an antilymphocyte antibody. A difficult situation arises in patients with active HCV infection; in this circumstance increases in CNI and antimetabolite doses might be tried before bolus steroids, which could potentially enhance HCV infectivity leading to graft fibrosis and eventual failure [28]. Fortunately, the unprecedented efficiency of new classes of antivirals such as direct acting antivirals (DAAs) may effectively address this concern by eliminating the virus in most patients.

5. Steroid minimization

Steroid withdrawal has become a popular current trend implemented to minimize IS after LT. Two large meta-analysis reports found that steroid withdrawal regimens had significant advantages over standard steroid-based regimens, by showing a significant lower rate of side effects [29, 30]. On Shin EJ *et al.* metaanalysis on steroid avoidance, the steroid-free group appeared to benefit in terms of *de novo* diabetes mellitus development, CMV infection, cholesterol levels, severe acute rejection, and overall acute rejection. Additionally, the HCV+ group demonstrated a significant advantage when undergoing treatment with steroid-free protocols considering the HCV recurrence rate, acute graft hepatitis, and treatment failure. Interestingly, no unfavorable effects were observed after steroid withdrawal during short-term follow-up [30]. Fouzas I, *et al.* analysis showed similar benefits such as reduced hypertension, cholesterol levels and CMV infection incidences. This cohort also showed a lower risk of diabetes and overall rejection [29]. On the other hand, a prospective study on the influence of steroids on HCV recurrence after LT published by La Barba *et al.* found the beneficial effects of low-dose steroids indefinite maintainence over the course of recurrent hepatitis C although their outcomes were critisized based on the small size of their patient population [31]. In 2010, a long-term study with a mean follow-up period of 89.3 ± 21 months was published, showing that a steroid-free IS regimen did not increase the risk of graft fibrosis [32]. They concluded that long-term graft survival with steroid withdrawal protocols is still unclear but given the benefit of a substantial decrease in side effects, including lower *de novo* diabetes, CMV infection, and HCV recurrence, the trend of reducing steroid use after LT will continue to be explored. At MGH Transplant Center, for our HCV+ recipients, we quickly taper steroids and subsequently discontinue their use 5 days post transplantation and have not observed increased rates of acute rejection.

6. Calcineurin inhibitor (CNI) reduction

For many years, CNIs have been considered an essential maintenance IS drug after LT; however, because of the known associated nephrotoxicity and other common adverse effects, multiple CNI-reduction trials have been conducted. There are two general types of CNI-reduction strategies. One is set to target the TAC concentration after LT, aiming to accomplish beneficial effects at the expense of lower levels. The other one, more aggressive, is set to avoid CNIs use altogether. As briefly discussed under the maintenance section, on a recently published large systematic review, the authors concluded that lower trough concentrations of TAC (6–10 ng/mL during the first month) could be more appropriate after LT. Compared to a higher TAC concentration group, the group with the lowest levels was not adversely affected in terms of acute rejection rate and clearly resulted in less renal impairment [15]. Another study published in 2013 by Cros *et al.* showed that the low-dose CNI group (TAC baseline levels <5 ng/mL or CYA levels <50 ng/mL at $t = 0$ or <100 ng/mL at $t = 2$ hours) had significant low rates of acute rejection episodes ($p = 0.028$), and generally better renal function markers ($p = 0.04$). They concluded that minimization, or even cessation of CNIs may be an achievable goal in the long term for most liver graft recipients [33]. Using MMF is one of the options available to be able to reduce CNIs after LTx. There's significant published data showing that reduction or withdrawal of TAC in conjunction with MMF therapies in fact decreases renal function impairment without increasing the occurrence of graft rejection [34–36]. Saliba *et al.*'s randomized control study revealed that a reduced TAC and MMF dose group had a statistically significant reduction in the incidence of acute graft rejection and renal dysfunction compared to the full dose TAC treatment group [34].

7. Calcineurin inhibitor (CNI) avoidance

Conversion to an mTOR inhibitor such as everolimus or sirolimus from CNIs is another strategy to avoid long term CNIs use. The first randomized control trial reported in 2007 in UK interrogated the idea of exchanging from a CNI-based IS to Sirolimus-based regimen [37]. Patients enrolled showed a significant improvement in glomerular filtration rate (GFR) following conversion to sirolimus at 3 months and 1 year, and the authors concluded that this modest improvement in renal function could be attributed to a sirolimus IS regimen. Side effects were common but tolerable in most patients and essentially controlled with dose-reduction measures. However, in 2012, a large prospective, open-label randomized trial concluded that LTx patients showed no demonstrable benefit 1 year after conversion from a CNI-based IS to a sirolimus-based IS. In this trial, they found no renal function benefits in the sirolimus-treated arm, and in fact they found correlation with higher rates of biopsy-confirmed acute rejection ($p = 0.02$)

and drug discontinuation ($p < 0.001$), primarily due to adverse events [38]. The "spare-the-nephron trial" is another large randomized trial comparing CNI-free MMF/sirolimus maintenance that was recently published. This paper concluded that treatment with MMF/sirolimus is associated with a significantly better renal function but with an increased risk of rejection (but not enough to develop into graft loss) [39]. Everolius, the other approved mTOR inhibitor has also been tested during the maintenance phase in LTx. In 2009, a European group commenced the first prospective, randomized, multicenter, 6-month study and evaluated whether everolimus with CNI reduction or discontinuation would improve renal function when used as maintenance therapy in LT recipients experiencing CNI-related renal impairment [16]. They concluded that everolimus allows for discontinuation or major reduction of CNI exposure in liver allograft recipients suffering from CNI-related renal dysfunction without a loss of efficacy. Recently another prospective, multicenter, randomized control study was published by De Carlis *et al.* in which patients were randomized to three groups: (1) everolimus initiation with TAC elimination (2) everolimus initiation with reduced-exposure TAC and (3) standard-exposure to TAC. The TAC elimination group was terminated prematurely due to a higher rate of biopsy-proven acute rejection (BPAR). The everolimus plus reduced TAC group was noninferior to the control group and had a superior renal function compared to a standard TAC exposure regimen 12 months after LT [40]. A 3-year-long follow-up update was reported in 2015, after which it was concluded that there's a clinically meaningful outcome on renal function after using everolimus and reduced exposure to TAC after LT. Additionally they reported a comparable efficacy and no late safety concerns [41]. Furthermore, mTOR-inhibitor treatments have been known to possess anticancer benefits. It has been demonstrated in renal transplant recipients that maintenance IS with mTOR inhibitor drugs, such as sirolimus and everolimus, is associated with a significantly reduced risk of developing any posttransplant *de novo* malignancy and nonskin solid malignancy [42]. Additionally, everolimus has been reportedly effective in the management of patients with HCC recurrence after LTx [43]. Therefore, HCC patients with a high risk of tumor recurrence can have a valuable therapeutic benefit from regimens containing everolimus.

8. Operational tolerance (Immunosuppresive (IS) withdrawal)

The liver has long been known to be more tolerogenic when compared to other solid organ transplants. Multiple experimental animal allogeneic LT models have recorded spontaneous tolerance while other organs are simply rejected without immunosuppression [44–46]. There have also been multiple single reports of human LT recipients whose immunosuppression was discontinued for noncompliance or as a medical necessity for reasons such as PTLD [18, 47–53]. Sanchez-Fueyo *et al.* review concluded that after careful scrutiny of accumulated clinical experience, elective IS drug weaning is feasible in almost 20% of selected LT recipients [19]. This is associated with an incidence of 12–76% of acute cellular rejection (ACR), but these episodes are commonly mild and often show complete resolution with return to baseline IS, often without the need of steroid boluses. However, most of these reports were based on retrospective data analysis as well as single-center experiences, both limiting their conclusion power. More recent data derived from multicenter IS withdrawal trials have helped clarify the prevalence and natural history of spontaneous operational tolerance. As briefly mentioned under the maintenance section, a prospective multicenter clinical trial performed in Europe reported that IS withdrawal was indeed successful in a high proportion of carefully selected liver recipients when conducted at late time points after transplantation [22]. They enrolled 102 stable liver recipients at least 3 years after transplantation. Out of the 98 recipients evaluated, 57 rejected and 41 successfully discontinued all IS drugs. Of note, in nontolerant recipient rejection, episodes were mild and resolved over 5–6 months. In tolerant recipients, no progressive clinically significant histological damage was apparent in follow-up protocol biopsies performed up to 3 years following drug withdrawal. Tolerance was independently associated with time post transplant, recipient age, and male gender. They concluded that the proportion of adult liver recipients who can discontinue IS drugs is higher than previously estimated, particularly in selected non-HCV and non-autoimmune patients in whom drug withdrawal is performed at an adequate set time point away from the transplantation date. As previously introduced, reports on a prospective pilot trial of IS withdrawal for pediatric recipients of living-donor liver allografts, 60% (12 out of 20) of pediatric recipients remained off IS therapy for 1 year with normal graft function and stable allograft histology [21]. Longer follow-up results were published in 2016 reporting that operationally tolerant pediatric recipients maintained overall stable allograft histology despite apparently active humoral alloimmune responses. The absence of increased inflammation or progressive fibrosis suggests that a subset of liver allografts seem resistant to the chronic injury that is characteristic of antibody-mediated damage [54]. In summary, there's well-supported evidence that in a selected group of patients, IS withdrawal can be accomplished. Additional prospective randomized controlled studies will be needed to confirm the potential generalizability of this approach, to establish safety and efficacy compared to maintenance IS.

9. Tolerance induction

There have been multiple clinical trials to induce tolerance in LT recipients; however, most of the trials failed to succeed in most patients. The Miami group investigated the role of donor bone marrow cell infusions in IS withdrawal in adult LT, showing that this therapeutic approach did not increase the likelihood of being fully weaned from IS [53]. Another novel approach that has been investigated is to induce tolerance via aggressive lymphocyte depletion prior to transplantation [55–57]. Recent studies on this topic, attempting to minimize IS by ATG induction therapy, concluded that the use of ATG induction was in fact associated with a high rate of rejection and so failed to provide a clinical benefit.

Recently, one promising outcome pilot study to induce tolerance with regulatory T-cell-based cell therapy in living donor LTx was reported by a Japanese team [58]. The authors adoptively transferred an *ex vivo*-generated regulatory T-cell-enriched cell product in 10 consecutive adult patients during the early post-LT phase. Cells were generated using a 2-week coculture of recipient lymphocytes with irradiated donor cells in the presence of anti-CD80/86 monoclonal antibodies. IS agents were tapered beginning at about 6 months, and reduced every 3 months thereafter until completely discontinued by 18 months (Figure 1). Seven out of 10 patients had successfully completed weaning and cessation of IS agents and had been drug free for 16–33 months at the time of the report. The other three recipients with liver disease of autoimmune etiology developed mild rejection during weaning and then resumed conventional low-dose immunotherapy. Even though the size of this study was small and needed a longer observation period and there were several limitations (living-donor LTx and splenectomy for all recipients), this Treg-enriched cell therapy is so far the most promising modality to induce tolerance in the setting of transplantation.

10. Conclusion

IS drug regimens have evolved over the last two decades and their positive impact on extending the functional life of liver allografts is undeniable. We are now living in an era where IS drug complications have replaced rejection

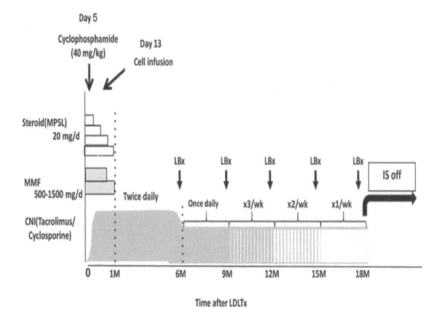

Figure 1. Postoperative immunosuppression and weaning protocol. Cyclophosphamide was administered on POD 5, and generated cells were infused on POD 13. Weaning was initiated at 6 months, repeated every 3 months, and terminated by 18 months. MPSL, methylprednisolone; CNI, calcineurin inhibitor; LBx, liver biopsy.

as the main therapeutic challenge. With the current therapies it is estimated that around 20% of transplanted patients will develop diabetes mellitus, 40% will experience a form of skin cancer (squamous cell and basal cell carcinoma), 50% hyperlipidemia, 75% hypertension and up to 80% will experience some form of renal dysfunction [59]. In general, the data reflects that LT patients are being overimmunosuppressed, and it is our responsibility as transplant physicians to improve patient quality of life while prolonging graft survival. Active attempts to reduce IS to the minimum tolerated level without rejection are well justified.

The current trend in IS therapy has evolved from polypharmacy approaches to minimizing the number and dossing of IS agents to avoid collateral damage. Studies continue to expand the knowledge in areas such as minimization, avoidance and withdrawal, and defining biomarkers predictive of which patients will tolerate withdrawal will be a major advance for the field. Equally important will be the exploration of approaches that engender a state of generational tolerance. The work detailed above using donor antigen specific TRegs may be the first glimpse of a new era in LT.

References

1. Starzl TE. The saga of liver replacement, with particular reference to the reciprocal influence of liver and kidney transplantation (1955–1967). *J Am Coll Surg* 2002;195:587–610.
2. Sass DA and Doyle AM. Liver and kidney transplantation: a half-century historical perspective. *Med Clin North Am* 2016;100:435–48.
3. Belzer FO and Southard JH. Principles of solid-organ preservation by cold storage. *Transplantation* 1988;45:673–6.
4. Schoening WN, Buescher N, Rademacher S, *et al.* Twenty-year longitudinal follow-up after orthotopic liver transplantation: a single-center experience of 313 consecutive cases. *Am J Transplant* 2013;13:2384–94.
5. Roberts MS, Angus DC, Bryce CL, Valenta Z, and Weissfeld L. Survival after liver transplantation in the United States: a disease-specific analysis of the UNOS database. *Liver Transpl* 2004;10:886–97.
6. Lodhi SA, Lamb KE, and Meier-Kriesche HU. Solid organ allograft survival improvement in the United States: the long-term does not mirror the dramatic short-term success. *Am J Transplant* 2011;11:1226–35.
7. Denton MD, Magee CC, and Sayegh MH. Immunosuppressive strategies in transplantation. *Lancet* 1999;353:1083–91.
8. Wiesner RH and Fung JJ. Present state of immunosuppressive therapy in liver transplant recipients. *Liver Transpl* 2011;17(Suppl 3):S1–9.
9. Snover DC, Freese DK, Sharp HL, Bloomer JR, Najarian JS, and Ascher NL. Liver allograft rejection. An analysis of the use of biopsy in determining outcome of rejection. *Am J Surg Pathol* 1987;11:1–10.
10. Starzl TE, Iwatsuki S, Shaw BW, Jr., Gordon RD, and Esquivel CO. Immunosuppression and other nonsurgical factors in the improved results of liver transplantation. *Semin Liver Dis* 1985;5:334–43.
11. Adams DH, Sanchez-Fueyo A, and Samuel D. From immunosuppression to tolerance. *J Hepatol* 2015;62:S170–85.
12. Humar A, Crotteau S, Gruessner A, *et al.* Steroid minimization in liver transplant recipients: impact on hepatitis C recurrence and post-transplant diabetes. *Clin Transplant* 2007;21:526–31.
13. Llado L, Xiol X, Figueras J, *et al.* Immunosuppression without steroids in liver transplantation is safe and reduces infection and metabolic complications: results from a prospective multicenter randomized study. *J Hepatol* 2006; 44:710–6.
14. Moini M, Schilsky ML, and Tichy EM. Review on immunosuppression in liver transplantation. *World J Hepatol* 2015;7:1355–68.
15. Rodriguez-Peralvarez M, Germani G, Darius T, Lerut J, Tsochatzis E, and Burroughs AK. Tacrolimus trough levels, rejection and renal impairment in liver transplantation: a systematic review and meta-analysis. *Am J Transplant* 2012;12:2797–814.

16. De Simone P, Metselaar HJ, Fischer L, *et al*. Conversion from a calcineurin inhibitor to everolimus therapy in maintenance liver transplant recipients: a prospective, randomized, multicenter trial. *Liver Transpl* 2009;15:1262–9.

17. Cai J and Terasaki PI. Induction immunosuppression improves long-term graft and patient outcome in organ transplantation: an analysis of United Network for Organ Sharing registry data. *Transplantation* 2010;90:1511–5.

18. Takatsuki M, Uemoto S, Inomata Y, *et al*. Weaning of immunosuppression in living donor liver transplant recipients. *Transplantation* 2001;72:449–54.

19. Lerut J and Sanchez-Fueyo A. An appraisal of tolerance in liver transplantation. *Am J Transplant* 2006;6:1774–80.

20. Orlando G, Soker S, and Wood K. Operational tolerance after liver transplantation. *J Hepatol* 2009;50:1247–57.

21. Feng S, Ekong UD, Lobritto SJ, *et al*. Complete immunosuppression withdrawal and subsequent allograft function among pediatric recipients of parental living donor liver transplants. *JAMA* 2012;307:283–93.

22. Benitez C, Londono MC, Miquel R, *et al*. Prospective multicenter clinical trial of immunosuppressive drug withdrawal in stable adult liver transplant recipients. *Hepatology* 2013;58:1824–35.

23. Wiesner RH, Demetris AJ, Belle SH, *et al*. Acute hepatic allograft rejection: incidence, risk factors, and impact on outcome. *Hepatology* 1998;28:638–45.

24. Regev A, Molina E, Moura R, *et al*. Reliability of histopathologic assessment for the differentiation of recurrent hepatitis C from acute rejection after liver transplantation. *Liver Transpl* 2004;10:1233–9.

25. Klintmalm GB, Nery JR, Husberg BS, Gonwa TA, and Tillery GW. Rejection in liver transplantation. *Hepatology* 1989;10:978–85.

26. Demetris A, Adams D, Bellamy C, *et al*. Update of the International Banff Schema for liver allograft rejection: working recommendations for the histopathologic staging and reporting of chronic rejection. An international panel. *Hepatology* 2000;31:792–9.

27. Banff schema for grading liver allograft rejection: an international consensus document. *Hepatology* 1997;25:658–63.

28. Chinnadurai R, Velazquez V, and Grakoui A. Hepatic transplant and HCV: a new playground for an old virus. *Am J Transplant* 2012;12:298–305.

29. Segev DL, Sozio SM, Shin EJ, *et al*. Steroid avoidance in liver transplantation: meta-analysis and meta-regression of randomized trials. *Liver Transpl* 2008;14:512–25.

30. Sgourakis G, Radtke A, Fouzas I, *et al*. Corticosteroid-free immunosuppression in liver transplantation: a meta-analysis and meta-regression of outcomes. *Transpl Int* 2009;22:892–905.

31. Vivarelli M, Burra P, La Barba G, *et al*. Influence of steroids on HCV recurrence after liver transplantation: a prospective study. *J Hepatol* 2007;47:793–8.

32. Manzia TM, Toti L, Angelico R, Di Cocco P, Orlando G, and Tisone G. Steroid-free immunosuppression after liver transplantation does not increase the risk of graft fibrosis. *Transplant Proc* 2010;42:1237–9.

33. Barbier L, Garcia S, Cros J, *et al*. Assessment of chronic rejection in liver graft recipients receiving immunosuppression with low-dose calcineurin inhibitors. *J Hepatol* 2013;59:1223–30.

34. Boudjema K, Camus C, Saliba F, *et al*. Reduced-dose tacrolimus with mycophenolate mofetil vs. standard-dose tacrolimus in liver transplantation: a randomized study. *Am J Transplant* 2011;11:965–76.

35. Creput C, Blandin F, Deroure B, *et al*. Long-term effects of calcineurin inhibitor conversion to mycophenolate mofetil on renal function after liver transplantation. *Liver Transpl* 2007;13:1004–10.

36. Orlando G, Baiocchi L, Cardillo A, *et al*. Switch to 1.5 grams MMF monotherapy for CNI-related toxicity in liver transplantation is safe and improves renal function, dyslipidemia, and hypertension. *Liver Transpl* 2007;13:46–54.

37. Watson CJ, Gimson AE, Alexander GJ, *et al*. A randomized controlled trial of late conversion from calcineurin inhibitor (CNI)-based to sirolimus-based immunosuppression in liver transplant recipients with impaired renal function. *Liver Transpl* 2007;13:1694–702.

38. Abdelmalek MF, Humar A, Stickel F, *et al*. Sirolimus conversion regimen versus continued calcineurin inhibitors in liver allograft recipients: a randomized trial. *Am J Transplant* 2012;12:694–705.

39. Teperman L, Moonka D, Sebastian A, *et al*. Calcineurin inhibitor-free mycophenolate mofetil/sirolimus maintenance in liver transplantation: the randomized spare-the-nephron trial. *Liver Transpl* 2013;19:675–89.

40. De Simone P, Nevens F, De Carlis L, *et al*. Everolimus with reduced tacrolimus improves renal function in de novo liver transplant recipients: a randomized controlled trial. *Am J Transplant* 2012;12:3008–20.

41. Fischer L, Saliba F, Kaiser GM, *et al*. Three-year outcomes in de novo liver transplant patients receiving everolimus with reduced tacrolimus: follow-up results from a randomized, multicenter study. *Transplantation* 2015;99: 1455–62.

42. Kauffman HM, Cherikh WS, Cheng Y, Hanto DW, and Kahan BD. Maintenance immunosuppression with target-of-rapamycin inhibitors is associated with a reduced incidence of de novo malignancies. *Transplantation* 2005;80: 883–9.

43. Saliba F, Dharancy S, Lorho R, *et al*. Conversion to everolimus in maintenance liver transplant patients: a multicenter, retrospective analysis. *Liver Transpl* 2011;17:905–13.

44. Calne RY, Sells RA, Pena JR, *et al*. Induction of immunological tolerance by porcine liver allografts. *Nature* 1969;223:472–6.

45. Kamada N, Brons G, and Davies HS. Fully allogeneic liver grafting in rats induces a state of systemic nonreactivity to donor transplantation antigens. *Transplantation* 1980;29:429–31.

46. Qian S, Demetris AJ, Murase N, Rao AS, Fung JJ, and Starzl TE. Murine liver allograft transplantation: tolerance and donor cell chimerism. *Hepatology* 1994;19:916–24.

47. Assy N, Adams PC, Myers P, *et al*. Randomized controlled trial of total immunosuppression withdrawal in liver transplant recipients: role of ursodeoxycholic acid. *Transplantation* 2007;83:1571–6.

48. Devlin J, Doherty D, Thomson L, *et al*. Defining the outcome of immunosuppression withdrawal after liver transplantation. *Hepatology* 1998;27:926–33.

49. Eason JD, Cohen AJ, Nair S, Alcantera T, and Loss GE. Tolerance: is it worth the risk? *Transplantation* 2005;79:1157–9.

50. Mazariegos GV, Reyes J, Marino IR, *et al*. Weaning of immunosuppression in liver transplant recipients. *Transplantation* 1997;63:243–9.

51. Pons JA, Yelamos J, Ramirez P, *et al*. Endothelial cell chimerism does not influence allograft tolerance in liver transplant patients after withdrawal of immunosuppression. *Transplantation* 2003;75:1045–7.

52. Starzl TE, Demetris AJ, Trucco M, *et al*. Cell migration and chimerism after whole-organ transplantation: the basis of graft acceptance. *Hepatology* 1993;17:1127–52.

53. Tryphonopoulos P, Tzakis AG, Weppler D, *et al*. The role of donor bone marrow infusions in withdrawal of immunosuppression in adult liver allotransplantation. *Am J Transplant* 2005;5:608–13.

54. Feng S, Demetris AJ, Spain KM, *et al*. Five-year histological and serological follow-up of operationally tolerant pediatric liver transplant recipients enrolled in WISP-R. *Hepatology* 2017;65(2):647–60.

55. Benitez CE, Puig-Pey I, Lopez M, *et al*. ATG-Fresenius treatment and low-dose tacrolimus: results of a randomized controlled trial in liver transplantation. *Am J Transplant* 2010;10:2296–304.

56. Donckier V, Craciun L, Lucidi V, *et al*. Acute liver transplant rejection upon immunosuppression withdrawal in a tolerance induction trial: potential role of IFN-gamma-secreting CD8+ T cells. *Transplantation* 2009;87:S91–5.

57. Donckier V, Craciun L, Miqueu P, *et al*. Expansion of memory-type CD8 + T cells correlates with the failure of early immunosuppression withdrawal after cadaver liver transplantation using high-dose ATG induction and rapamycin. *Transplantation* 2013;96:306–15.

58. Todo S, Yamashita K, Goto R, *et al*. A pilot study of operational tolerance with a regulatory T-cell-based cell therapy in living donor liver transplantation. *Hepatology* 2016;64:632–43.

59. Parekh J, Corley DA, and Feng S. Diabetes, hypertension and hyperlipidemia: prevalence over time and impact on long-term survival after liver transplantation. *Am J Transplant* 2012;12:2181–7.

11. Antibody-Mediated Rejection in Liver Transplantation

James F. Trotter

Baylor University Medical Center, 3410 Worth Street, #860, Dallas, TX 75246, USA

1. Introduction

Antibody-mediated rejection (AMR) has been identified from the earliest period of liver and kidney transplantation. The first identified form of AMR was from mismatched donor–recipient blood types and occurred after transplanting a donor organ into a recipient with an incompatible blood type (A donor to O recipient). However, there is evidence that early transplant physicians were uncertain whether transplanting incompatible blood types was clinically relevant. In an early paper from Thomas E. Starzl entitled "Renal homograft in patients with major donor-recipient blood group incompatibilities," the authors concluded that they had demonstrated "both immediate and prolonged renal function despite the presence of major blood group incompatibilities" [1]. However, an addendum was added to the paper while it was in press that further such cases fared quite poorly with diffuse small vessel and glomerular injury characteristic of hyperacute rejection. As a result, subsequent renal and liver transplant(ation)s (LTs) have largely been done only with identical or compatible blood types to avoid this problem. However, in desperate cases, ABO-incompatible (ABO-I) transplants were performed especially in younger patients, with clinicians discovering that while many such LTs failed, some patients experienced favorable long-term survival. The full impact of ABO-I LT was not apparent for a few decades. One reason for this was that the initial results of LT were so poor

223

(approximately 20% survival) that attributing risk to many factors was difficult to discern since so many patients died perioperatively due to technical complications. Over the decades, outcomes improved and the relevance of specific risk factors was then more apparent. In addition, the total number of LTs was so small that there was insufficient statistical "power" to discern the effects of many risk factors. Finally, some ABO-I patients survived, being less sensitive to this form of tissue incompatibility [2]. Younger patients who had yet to develop significant titers of anti-ABO antibodies were shown to fare particularly well. Starzl more definitively demonstrated the poor outcomes in ABO-I LT along with the pathologic findings in a large case series in the 1980s [3]. Specifically, ABO incompatibility caused sinusoidal congestion, coagulative necrosis and generalized hepatocyte cell death [4]. Many of these patients developed chronic, diffuse biliary strictures as a result of this vascular injury. In the past decade, protocols have been developed to allow successful LT in ABO-I patients using preconditioning regimens to remove the offending antibody with plasmapheresis and agents that inhibit antibody production, namely, rituxan and velcade [5, 6]. These cases have almost exclusively been performed in living-donor liver transplantation (LDLT) in Asia where there are effectively no other options for transplant for some patients. However, in general, in the western world transplantation using ABO-I donors is very rarely done and only in desperate cases especially in infants.

2. The four eras of antibody-mediated rejection (AMR)

There have been four eras of studying donor-specific antibodies (DSAs) in AMR. The first phase was their initial discovery in renal and then LT. Aside from antibodies to blood type antigens, preformed cytotoxic antibodies against human leukocyte antigen (HLA) epitopes were first postulated in the early 1960s [7]. The HLA system is a gene complex encoding cell surface proteins that are responsible for regulation of the immune system. Different classes have different functions. HLA class I are present on all nucleated cells and present antigens from inside the cell such as proteins from viruses that may have infected the cell. In this way, infected cells may be recognized by the immune system and destroyed. HLA class II antigens are found primarily in inflammatory cells such as macrophages, B-cells and activated T-cells and present antigens from outside of the cell to T-lymphocytes and, in part, are responsible for initiating antibody production from B-cells. The hepatic expression pattern of HLA class I and II antigens is that class I HLA is found on all cell types, but expression on hepatocytes is weaker [8–12]. HLA class II is largely restricted to dendritic cells, and Kupffer cells and there is weak expression on portal capillaries and sinusoidal and central vein endothelial cells. Increased expression of class I and II can occur after an inflammatory stimulus so that hepatic inflammatory pathology could alter the expression of these antigens. In a landmark study in 1969, Patel and Terasaki definitively demonstrated the importance of HLA matching in renal transplantation [13]. In a large cohort of kidney transplant recipients they found that 63/226 had preformed antibodies against lymphocytes of randomly selected people before transplant. In addition, they performed a crossmatch (testing the recipient's serum for cytotoxic antibody against donor lymphocytes). Of the 30 recipients with positive crossmatches, 25 (83%) of grafts failed within 120 days. In contrast, the recipients with a negative crossmatch had only four of 168 grafts (2.4%) fail. This study was the foundation for crossmatching recipient serum against donor lymphocytes as a standard means of matching specific kidney donors for recipients. The early poor experience in renal transplant in recipients with a positive crossmatch initially led to trepidation in LT. There was obvious concern that the same process would occur in the liver patients. The second phase was 1970s and early 1980s where DSA was identified, but the liver was considered "protected" from AMR due to its unique anatomy and physiology. Initial reports suggested that the liver was more resilient than the kidney. Starzl initially documented favorable long-term survival in a number of LT patients with positive crossmatches in the 1970s [14–15]. In 11 of 179 cases of orthotopic LT in Denver, patients received liver homografts from donors to whom the recipients' sera showed strong lymphocyte cytotoxic activity by standard cytotoxicity crossmatch tests. Two had early graft dysfunction, the remaining nine did not and the crossmatch appeared to be unimportant. Thus, from the earliest era of LT, the liver appeared to be more resistant to AMR compared to the kidney. As described above some of the more subtle effects of risk factors on patient survival were more difficult to discern in the early era of LT when the high mortality rates masked the contribution of other factors in patient survival. Over time with closer observation and improved survival rates, a more definitive description of the impact of the positive crossmatch was later reported by Starzl in 1992 with worse outcomes. This started the third phase in the 1990s and early 2000s where the negative effects of DSA and their participation in AMR were noted in the literature, but largely ignored due to their apparent minimal impact. In the report by Starzl, 25 patients whose crossmatch became negative in the first 2 months post transplant were compared to comprised 15 patients who had an increased or stable titer over the same time after transplant [16]. The graft survival rate of crossmatch positive patients was much lower with graft survival rates of 33% at 3 months vs. 88.0% in the negative group. At that same time, one of the first studies to link the role of alloantibodies and chronic rejection was published by Demetris *et al.* which showed seven of 22 patients with chronic rejection had high panel reactive antibodies (PRAs) peritransplant and the majority showed deposition of Ig or complement components in the rejected liver tissue [17]. Later, Piazza *et al.* showed that 65% of LT recipients had DSA after transplant and this was associated with rejection [18]. Kasahara *et al.* reported that all patients with DSA detected immediately after transplant developed rejection compared to only 17% without DSA [19]. Takaya reported a 29% 1-month graft loss rate in patients with a positive crossmatch vs. 16% with a negative crossmatch ($p < 0.05$) [20]. Similarly, Ogura *et al.* found a 47% vs. 12% 1-month graft loss in patients with vs. without a positive crossmatch, ($p = 0.001$) [21]. Despite the negative findings associated with DSA, the effects were deemed clinically irrelevant to the extent that clinicians did not measure DSA before or after transplant or seek to diagnose or treat AMR. There were several reasons for this. First, the impact of AMR on outcomes is relatively modest, with only a small, if any, decrement on survival, especially compared to ABO incompatibility. Next, DSA was identified in only 10–15% of recipients, so it might only impact a small fraction of patients. In addition, acute AMR occurring soon after the transplant operation is very rare (see below) and is often manifest along with classic T-cell rejection. The treatment of the T-cell rejection with corticosteroids was almost always effective, so there was no apparent penalty incurred by transplanting crossmatch positive patients. Finally, any long-term effects of AMR were not recognized because any decrement in outcome was difficult to discern over the years because of the multiple confounding effects of other problems on survival including recurrent hepatitis C, malignancy, and renal failure. Consequently, the importance of AMR was minimized in the LT literature and the liver was designated as uniquely resistant to AMR based on its unusual anatomic design compared to the kidney [22]. The porous hepatic sinusoidal microvascular bed which is lined with Kupffer cells allows phagocytosis of immune complexes mitigating their effect. The dual blood supply from the portal vein and hepatic artery helps to preserve blood flow to the graft even in the face of microscopic graft vasculitis caused by AMR. In addition, the liver secretes soluble HLA antigen which can bind and consume the offending antibody preventing it from causing graft damage.

Finally, the liver has the capacity to regenerate after injury to a far greater extent than other organs. Consequently, the LT community has, until recently, considered DSA to be clinically irrelevant in terms of outcomes.

The final and current era is the effective "rediscovery" of the potential clinical relevance of AMR and DSA which has been reported in a number of studies, most of which have shown DSA's negative effects on outcomes in LT recipients. Kozlowski *et al.* reported that preformed DSA was associated with early rejection [23]. Other groups have reported increased graft loss rates in orthotopic LT (OLT) patients with a positive crossmatch compared to OLT patients with a negative crossmatch. Castillo-Rama *et al.* reported outcomes in 896 liver recipients and found increased graft loss on patients with preformed DSA using a solid-phase assay and Luminex assay which showed an increased graft loss rate in patients with preformed DSA [24]. Fontana and colleagues, found post-OLT anti-HLA antibodies in 24% of liver recipients [25]. Of those, 75% had biliary complications when the allograft biopsy was analyzed, and 50% had biopsy-proven chronic rejection. Another report found that DSA-positive recipients with diffuse portal C4d deposition had significantly more acute cellular rejection ACR and steroid-resistant rejection compared to controls (88% vs. 50% and 41% vs. 19%, respectively), $p < 0.03$ [26]. Some centers have discounted the effect of DSA on outcomes in LT recipients. In 90 liver recipients, 22% had preformed DSA, but in all but three patients, the levels dropped substantially and there was no higher rate of ACR, liver function tests, or graft function in the patients with DSA [27].

3. The detection of donor-specific antibodies (DSA)

The manner in which DSAs are detected has evolved over the years [28–30]. In its earliest form, serum from the recipient, potentially containing cytotoxic antibody to donor-specific antigens, was assayed for lysis of donor lymphocytes. The presence of cytotoxic antibody is determined by the number or amount of lymphocyte death in the assay. This is a relatively crude test, requiring viable donor lymphocytes, subjective interpretation of the results and does not identify they type or concentration of the antibody responsible for the reaction. This technology has since been supplanted by more sophisticated measures including flow cytometry and solid-phase immunoassays (SPIs), immunoassays in which the antigen or serum is bound to a solid surface, such as a microplate wall with the other reactants (antibodies) being free in solution. SPI using purified class I and/or II HLA antigens as targets allows the detection of specific HLA antibodies with great specificity and sensitivity. The results of this antibody assay are reported in mean fluorescent intensity (MFI) which is an indirect measure of the antibody concentration. While SPI is clearly more efficient and precise compared to the cross-match test, it only measures the presence of the antibody and not its biologic activity. As such, there are some problems in the interpretation of its results as it relates to AMR. The precise level of MFI which reflects the presence of clinically significant cytotoxic antibody may vary from lab to lab based on the specific technical variations. These include the antigen source, its density and conformation on the solid phase as well as specific aspects of antibody–antigen binding including cross-reactivity and variations between different lots from the manufacturer. Therefore, it is not surprising that there is some divergence of views on the role of SPIs in kidney transplantation.

4. The histologic diagnosis of antibody-mediated rejection (AMR)

The outcomes attributed to the presence of DSA in the serum to clinically relevant outcomes from AMR are further complicated by a number of clinical factors. While there are strict criteria for the diagnosis of AMR, confirmation of the diagnosis is made with some degree of subjectivity. The criteria for AMR in LT are critical in attributing graft injury to the AMR [31]. The criteria include (1) presence of DSA in the serum, (2) positive C4d staining in the tissue, (3) histopathologic evidence of diffuse microvascular endothelial cell injury, and (4) exclusion of other causes. As noted above, the definition of "presence of DSA in the serum" depends on the assay and its specific technical aspects. The definition of positive C4d staining in the tissue is subjective and the exclusion of other causes of graft injury invokes of plethora of other causes (T-cell rejection, recurrent liver disease, vascular complications) whose diagnosis can be subjective as well. The utility of C4d as it relates to the diagnosis of AMR is important to understand. Essentially, C4d is a footprint for antibody-mediated tissue injury; its presence in a histologic specimen is evidence for antibody-mediated tissue injury. The classical pathway of complement is initiated by binding of its complement factor C1q to immune complex deposits. This activates C1q which, in turn, activates complement factor C4 creating its split product C4d which is without a biological function. Although C4d is mainly interpreted as evidence classical pathway activation, nonspecific production of C4d has been reported as derived from carbohydrate ligands on the surface of a wide variety of pathogens results in activation of the lectin pathway and cleavage of C4. Normal liver allograft biopsies are usually negative for endothelial cell C4d staining, but nonspecific C4d can be seen in portal and arterial elastic lamina, necrotic hepatocytes, and fibrotic areas. So, hepatic damage from viral hepatitis or recurrent liver disease could cause confounding results. However, C4d staining is more commonly seen in patients with a positive crossmatching or DSA (in portal venous, arterial, or capillary endothelial cells) compared to negative controls [32].

5. The three types of antibody-mediated rejection (AMR)

While many patients with DSA have no clinically relevant outcomes, there are three recognized broad types of AMR based on their temporal occurrence after transplant. Hyperacute AMR is caused by preformed cytotoxic DSAs which caused graft loss due to antibody-mediated microvascular injury to the hepatic endothelium within minutes to hours after its implantation. While it has been reported in LT, this type of rejection is extremely rare [33, 34]. Acute AMR typically occurs days to weeks after the transplant and is characterized clinically by allograft dysfunction in the presence of DSA along with markers of its clinical activity including hypocomplementemia and thrombocytopenia. The histologic appearance of acute AMR is similar to acute AMR in other organs: diffuse microvascular endothelial cell injury, C4d deposits, microvasculitis, centrilobular hepatocyte swelling, and cholestasis. Acute AMR is also uncommon. Only about 10–15% of liver recipients are DSA positive and only 5% of those develop acute AMR. Therefore, acute AMR occurs only in <1% of all liver recipients. Consequently, in the absence of testing and thoughtful consideration, it may not be considered or recognized as a specific entity and could otherwise be diagnosed and treated as severe classic T-cell rejection. A study evaluated 3,137 ABO-compatible liver-only transplants at Administrative Support + Knowledge (ASK) Center, University of Wisconsin, and evaluated DSA in 337 (10.7%) patients who experienced unexplained allograft loss within 90 days [35]. AMR was identified in 3/337 patients (1%) and 5% (3/60) of previously unexplained early graft loss. Furthermore, they found that graft loss from AMR occurred in 40% of patients with high-titer preformed DSA (bead saturation at ≥1:27 dilution). This suggests that there could be some value in pretransplant testing for DSA in all LT candidates and performing conducting protocol postreperfusion biopsies. This might identify which highly sensitized patients might be at risk for this phenomenon. Chronic AMR is more difficult to identify, because it is a much more indolent process occurring over many months to many years. However, it is the form of AMR that has recently been most associated with negative clinical outcomes. Strongly linked to serum class II DSA, chronic AMR is characterized histologically by low-grade lymphoplasmacytic portal and perivenular inflammation along with fibrosis patterns and variable microvascular C4d deposition.

6. Clinical studies of chronic antibody-mediated rejection (AMR)

Emerging data has shown that AMR may be a relevant cause of long-term graft loss or injury in LT. A study from our center demonstrated the risk of *de novo* DSA on long-term survival. This study of 749 patients found that 61 (8.1%) patients developed *de novo* DSA at 1 year post LT, 95% of which were against HLA class II antigens only [36]. The following risk factors for developing DSA were identified by multivariable logistic regression analysis: cyclosporine (vs. tacrolimus (TAC) at 1 year) (OR = 2.50, p = 0.004) and low calcineurin inhibitor (CNI) levels (TAC <3 ng/mL or cyclosporine <75 ng/mL) in the first year (OR = 2.66, p = 0.015). On the other hand, MELD score >15 (OR = 0.47, p = 0.021) at transplant and recipients >60 years old (OR = 0.26, p = 0.03) had a significantly lower likelihood of *de novo* DSA. More important, patients with *de novo* DSA had a significantly lower patient (p = 0.002) and graft survival (p = 0.005) than patients without *de novo* DSA. However, the effect on survival was relatively small, only 7% difference at 5 years for patient survival and 6% for graft survival). The role of *de novo* DSA in predicting patient and graft survival was analyzed using Cox proportional hazard analysis which showed that final multivariable model identified *de novo* DSA (hazard ratio (HR) = 1.99, p = 0.005), hepatitis C virus (HCV) viremia post transplant, donor age >50 years old, recipient age >60 years old, and African-American race as independent predictors of patient death. There are several instructive points from this study. The choice of immunosuppression may impact AMR. Since TAC has generally been shown to be a more efficacious agent compared to cyclosporine, AMR may be prevented by more effective immunosuppression. Similarly, low levels of any type of CNI were associated with AMR demonstrating the vendor in adequate immunosuppression in the potential prevention of AMR. This also suggests that nonadherence to treatment as evidenced by low levels of these drugs could play a role in AMR, as discussed below. The lower occurrence in older and less sick patients suggests that recipients who might be less able to mount an immune response may be less likely to develop AMR. Finally, it is known that there is a differential expression of class I and II

HLA antigens on the surface of liver cells, including endothelial cells, hepatocytes, and biliary epithelial cells and that this expression can be altered by different events, such as rejection, infection, and inflammation related to transplantation. Consequently, the higher rate of HLA antigen expression during any type of hepatic inflammation suggests that these processes could induce a more intense immune response including worse AMR. DSA has also been linked to chronic rejection. In a study from our center of 39 patients with chronic rejection, 92% had DSA vs. 61% in control patients, $p = 0.003$ [37]. Since induction with antilymphocyte antibodies is sometimes employed during the initiation of immunosuppressive therapy and might reduce DSA, recipients were compared who did or did not receive such induction. Graft survival was markedly improved when induction therapy with either daclizumab or OKT3 was used. In fact, five out of five class I preformed antibodies were eliminated in patients who received antibody induction therapy and had a follow-up sample for analysis. In fact, Moonka and colleagues in surveying the UNOS database found improved early graft survival in patients who received induction antibody therapy regardless of their HCV status [38]. Given these results, it is interesting to hypothesize that this may be the mechanism of improved graft survival. This possibly warrants further investigation given the small number of patients with preformed DSA who received induction therapy in our study. Another study in pediatric LT recipients found DSA in 68% of patients with chronic rejection compared to 33% in controls [39]. These antibodies were primarily HLA class II. AMR may also contribute to the progression of recurrent liver disease. A recent study evaluated the effect of DSA on fibrosis (with protocol liver biopsies) in 607 HCV-infected liver recipients [40]. Both preformed class I DSA (HR) = 1.44, $p = 0.04$ and class II DSA (HR = 1.86, $p < 0.001$) antibodies were independent predictors of progression to stage 2–4 fibrosis. *De novo* DSA (HR = 1.41, $p = 0.07$) had borderline significance. In addition, preformed class I DSAs (HR = 1.63, $p = 0.03$) and class II DSAs (HR = 1.72, $p = 0.03$) were statistically significantly associated with an increased risk of death.

7. Clinical management of AMR

One of the current difficulties in the diagnosis and management of AMR in LT is how to test and monitor patients after transplant, as well how to treat patients once AMR is potentially identified. Most patients who develop low levels of class I DSA have no long-term consequences relative to graft function. Therefore, one challenge is to identify patients who are presensitized before transplant and likely to experience graft injury as well as how to identify long-term survivors after transplant who might be experiencing chronic graft injury and benefit from a change or increase in immunosuppression.

While there is no known therapy demonstrating efficacy in the treatment of AMR in LT, interventions focused on both removal of antibody or pharmacologic suppression of its production have been employed. Plasmapheresis is the most direct means to remove antibody from the patient. However, it is very expensive and time consuming. While it has clear appeal in the short-term management of AMR, its role in the management of chronic AMR is less apparent. Intravenous immune globulin may also be beneficial for short-term management. Rituximab, a monoclonal antibody against CD20 which is found primarily on B-cells, targets these cells for destruction thereby eliminating the cellular source of the DSA. Since it is commonly used in the clinical treatment of lymphoma (including posttransplant lymphoproliferative disease (PTLD), rituximab has greater familiarity to transplant physicians. Eculizumab is a monoclonal antibody that inhibits complement activity and has been used for AMR. It has efficacy in atypical hemolytic uremic syndrome and is quite expensive. Bortezomib is a proteasome inhibitor with particular activity against plasma cells. It has been used to treat acute AMR in liver recipients [41]. Aside from the lack of proven efficacy in the treatment of AMR, many of these treatment strategies are expensive, short-lived (plasmapheresis, intravenous immunoglobulin (IVIg)) or further immunosuppressive (eculizumab, bortezomb, rituximab). Consequently, if these agents are used, their immunosuppressive effects have to be carefully considered as liver recipients who are considered for treatment for AMR have already been heavily treated for classic T-cell rejection. Because of the uncertainties related to the management of AMR, there is a clear need for prospective trials to provide guidance in patient management.

Chronic DSA is almost always directed against class II, but DSA should always be correlated with biopsy findings as other etiologies of graft damage must be considered and rule out. If histologic inflammation and fibrosis are present, there are several considerations to help in the management of the patient. First, adequate immunosuppression should be confirmed including adherence to treatment. Using TAC may have some benefit over cyclosporine (refer to the preceding discussion). Next, increasing immunosuppression levels may be beneficial balancing the negative effects of this approach. Finally, treating any concomitant disease that may be contributing to chronic allograft inflammation, such as chronic viral hepatitis B or C may reduce

HLA antigen expression and reduce associated immune reaction. However, it is important to remember that none of these treatment recommendations have demonstrated efficacy and the best approach is unknown.

8. Ongoing challenges in antibody-mediated rejection (AMR)

There are important challenges related to the routine integration of AMR into the practice of LT. First, there are many skeptics who seriously doubt the clinical utility of this proven biological phenomenon on LT patients. Most, but not all, of these skeptics are experienced clinicians who have raised the following questions. If AMR is so important in LT, then how can we have been missing the diagnosis for so long? If there is no therapy for this phenomenon, then why should we worry about its diagnosis? Many patients who have DSA experience no clinical problems; so how important can this be? While these are important questions, it is important to recognize what is known and what is not known about AMR. This was described in a recent consensus conference [42]. Despite its identification for decades in LT recipients, AMR was initially recognized as being clinically irrelevant to long-term outcomes, as described earlier in this chapter. However, there is clear evidence that AMR can have a statistically significant independent impact on patient survival. Different forms of AMR can occur including acute AMR (<1%) of patients and chronic AMR up to 8% of patients. Different classes of antibody are typically responsible for these different types of AMR: preformed class I for acute AMR and *de novo* class II for chronic AMR. The diagnosis of AMR requires the presence of the strict diagnostic criteria. Perhaps the most subjective and difficult is C4d staining which has to be on the vascular endothelium to be of the greatest clinical importance. Equally important, other causes of graft injury have to be ruled out. This is a very important point because AMR can at times be used as a "histologic excuse" for another serious and unrelated problem such as hepatic artery thrombosis or a drug interaction. The depth at which alternative causes of this injury are sought is associates with the strength of the AMR diagnosis. There is no known therapy for AMR which has clinical efficacy. Further studies to better characterize patients with AMR await agent which could provide clinically efficacious therapies.

Another important and potential existential question about AMR is fundamentally whether this is a predetermined immunologic phenotype or whether it is an epiphenomenon of another problem including nonadherence to immunosuppression. While adherence has been shown to be more common in renal transplant recipients with AMR such studies have not been performed in liver patients, although it is known that lower level of immunosuppression are associated with AMR [43, 44]. Therefore, the contribution of nonadherence to AMR is an important question to evaluate in LT. The recent "rediscovery" of the importance of AMR in LT should lead many clinical investigators to study this interesting phenomenon in the coming years.

References

1. Starzl TE, Marchioro TL, Herman G, Brittain RS, and Waddell WR. Renal homografts in patients with major donor-recipient blood group incompatibilities. *Surg Forum* 1963;14:214–6.
2. Starzl TE, Ishikawa M, Putnam CW, Porter KA, Picache R, Husberg BS, *et al*. Progress in and deterrents to orthotopic liver transplantation, with special reference to survival, resistance to hyperacute rejection, and biliary duct reconstruction. *Transplant Proc* 1974;6:129–39.
3. Gordon RD, Iwatsuki S, Esquivel CO, Tzakis A, Todo S, and Starzl TE. Liver transplantation across ABO blood groups. *Surgery* 1986;100:342–8.
4. Demetris AJ, Jaffe R, Tzakis A, Ramsey G, Todo S, Belle S, *et al*. Antibody-mediated rejection of human orthotopic liver allografts. A study of liver transplantation across ABO blood group barriers. *Am J Pathol* 1988;132: 489–502.
5. Egawa H, Teramukai S, Haga H, Tanabe M, Mori A, Ikegami T, *et al*. Impact of rituximab desensitization on blood-type-incompatible adult living donor liver transplantation: a Japanese multi center study. *Am J Transplant* 2014;14:102–14.
6. Egawa H, Teramukai S, Haga H, Tanabe M, Fukushima M, and Shimazu M. Present status of ABO-incompatible living donor liver transplantation in Japan. *Hepatology* 2008;47:143–52.
7. Terasaki PI, Mandell M, Vandewater J, and Edgington TS. Human blood lymphocyte cytotoxicity reactions with allogenic antisera. *Ann N Y Acad Sci* 1964;120:322–34.
8. Daar AS, Fuggle SV, Fabre JW, Ting A, and Morris PJ. The detailed distribution of MHC Class II antigens in normal human organs. *Transplantation* 1984;38:293–8.
9. Lautenschlager I, Taskinen E, Inkinen K, Lehto VP, Virtanen I, and Hayry P. Distribution of the major histocompatibility complex antigens on different cellular components of human liver. *Cell Immunol* 1984;85:191–200.
10. Demetris AJ, Lasky S, Thiel DHV, Starzl TE, and Whiteside T. Induction of DR/IA antigens in human liver allografts: an immunocytochemical and clinicopathologic analysis of twenty failed grafts. *Transplantation* 1985;40:504–9.

11. Ballardini G, Bianchi FB, Mirakian R, Fallani M, Pisi E, and Bottazzo GF. HLA-A,B,C, HLA-D/DR and HLA-D/DQ expression on unfixed liver biopsy sections from patients with chronic liver disease. *Clin Exp Immunol* 1987;70:35–46.

12. Steinhoff G, Wonigeit K, and Pichlmayr R. Analysis of sequential changes in major histocompatibility complex expression in human liver grafts after transplantation. *Transplantation* 1988;45:394–401.

13. Patel R, and Terasaki PI. Significance of the positive crossmatch test in kidney transplantation. *N Engl J Med* 1969;280:735–9.

14. Kashiwagi N, Corman J, Iwatsuki S, Ishikawa S, Fiala JM, Johanaen TS, *et al.* Mixed lymphocyte culture and graft rejection. *Surg Forum* 1973;24:345–8.

15. Iwatsuki S, Iwaki Y, Kano T, Klintmalm G, Koep LJ, Weil R, and Starzl TE. Successful liver transplantation from crossmatch-positive donors. *Transplant Proc* 1981;13:286–8.

16. Kobayashi M, Yagihashi A, Manez R, Takaya S, Noguchi K, Konno A, *et al.* Posttransplant donor-specific T-lymphocytotoxic antibody in liver transplant patients with a positive crossmatch. *Transplant Proc* 1992;24:2510–11.

17. Demetris AJ, Markus BH, Burnham J, Nalesnik M, Gordon RD, Makowka L, and Starzl TE. Antibody deposition in liver allografts with chronic rejection. *Transplant Proc* 1987;19D:121–5.

18. Piazza A, Adorno D, Torlone N, Valeri M, Poggi E, Monaco PI, *et al.* Flow cytometric analysis of antidonor-specific antibodies in liver transplant. *Transplant Proc* 1997;29:2975–6.

19. Kasahara M, Kiuchi T, Takakura K, Uryuhara K, Egawa H, Asonuma K, *et al.* Postoperative flow cytometry crossmatch in living donor liver transplantation: clinical significance of humoral immunity in acute rejection. *Transplantation* 1999;67:568–75.

20. Takaya S, Duquesnoy R, Iwaki Y, Demetris J, Yagihashi A, Bronsther O, *et al.* Positive crossmatch in primary human liver allografts under cyclosporine or FK 506 therapy. *Transplant Proc* 1991;23:396–9.

21. Ogura K, Terasaki PI, Koyama H, Chia J, Imagawa DK, and Busuttil RW. High one-month liver graft failure rates in flow cytometry crossmatch-positive recipients. *Clin Transplant* 1994;8:111–5.

22. Taner T, Stegall MD, and Heimbach JK. Antibody-mediated rejection in liver transplantation: current controversies and future directions. *Liver Transpl* 2014;20:514–27.

23. Kozlowski T, Rubinas T, Nickeleit V, Woosley J, Schmitz J, Collins D, *et al.* Liver allograft antibody-mediated rejection with demonstration of sinusoidal C4d staining and circulating donor-specific antibodies. *Liver Transpl* 2011;17:357–68.

24. Castillo-Rama M, Castro MJ, Bernardo I, Meneu-Diaz JC, Elola-Olaso AM, Calleja-Antolin SM, *et al.* Preformed antibodies detected by cytotoxic assay or multibead array decrease liver allograft survival: role of human leukocyte antigen compatibility. *Liver Transpl* 2008;14:554–62.

25. Fontana M, Moradpour D, Aubert V, Pantaleo G, Pascual M. Prevalence of anti-HLA antibodies after liver transplantation. *Transpl Int* 2010;23:858–9.

26. Musat AI, Agni RM, Wai PY, Pirsch JD, Lorentzen DF, Powell A, *et al*. The significance of donor-specific HLA antibodies in rejection and ductopenia development in ABO compatible liver transplantation. *Am J Transplant* 2011;11:500–10.

27. Taner T, Gandhi MJ, Sanderson SO, Poterucha CR, De Goey SR, Stegall MD, and Heimbach JK. Prevalence, course and impact of HLA donor-specific antibodies in liver transplantation in the first year. *Am J Transplant* 2012;12:1504–10.

28. Reed EF, Rao P, Zhang Z, Gebel H, Bray RA, Guleria I, *et al*. Comprehensive assessment and standardization of solid phase multiplex-bead arrays for the detection of antibodies to HLA. *Am J Transplant* 2013;13:1859–70.

29. Zachary AA, Vega RM, Lucas DP, and Leffell MS. HLA antibody detection and characterization by solid phase immunoassays: methods and pitfalls. *Methods Mol Biol* 2012;882:289–308.

30. Tait BD, Susal C, Gebel HM, Nickerson PW, Zachary AA, Claas FH, *et al*. Consensus guidelines on the testing and clinical management issues associated with HLA and non-HLA antibodies in transplantation. *Transplantation* 2013;95:19–47.

31. O'Leary JG, Cai J, Freeman R, Banuelos N, Hart B, Johnson M, *et al*. Proposed diagnostic criteria for chronic antibody-mediated rejection in liver allografts. *Am J Transplant* 2016;16:603–14.

32. Sakashita H, Haga H, Ashihara E, Wen MC, Tsuji H, Miyagawa-Hayashino A, *et al*. Significance of C4d staining in ABO-identical/compatible liver transplantation. *Mod Pathol* 2007;20:676–84.

33. Starzl TE, Demetris AJ, Todo S, Kang Y, Tzakis A, Duquesnoy R, *et al*. Evidence for hyperacute rejection of human liver grafts: the case of the canary kidneys. *Clin Transplant* 1989;3:37–45.

34. Knechtle SJ, Kolbeck PC, Tsuchimoto S, Coundouriotis A, Sanfilippo F, and Bollinger RR. Hepatic transplantation into sensitized recipients. Demonstration of hyperacute rejection. *Transplantation* 1987;43:8–12.

35. O'Leary JG, Kaneku H, Demetris AJ, Marr JD, Shiller SM, Susskind BM, *et al*. Antibody-mediated rejection as a contributor to previously unexplained early liver allograft loss. *Liver Transpl* 2014;20:218–227.

36. Kaneku H, O'Leary JG, Banuelos N, Jennings LW, Susskind BM, Klintmalm GB, and Terasaki PI. De novo donor-specific HLA antibodies decrease patient and graft survival in liver transplant recipients. *Am J Transplant* 2013;13:1541–48.

37. O'Leary JG, Kaneku H, Susskind BM, Jennings LW, Neri MA, Davis GL, *et al*. High mean fluorescence intensity donor-specific anti-HLA antibodies associated with chronic rejection postliver transplant. *Am J Transplant* 2011;11:1868–76.

38. Moonka DK, Kim D, Kapke A, Brown KA, and Yoshida A. The influence of induction therapy on graft and patient survival in patients with and without hepatitis C after liver transplantation. *Am J Transplant* 2010;10:590–601.
39. Grabhorn E, Binder TM, Obrecht D, Brinkert F, Lehnhardt A, Herden U, *et al*. Long-term clinical relevance of de novo donor-specific antibodies after pediatric liver transplantation. *Transplantation* 2015;99:1876–81.
40. O'Leary JG, Kaneku H, Jennings L, Susskind BM, Terasaki PI, and Klintmalm GB. Donor-specific alloantibodies are associated with fibrosis progression after liver transplantation in hepatitis C virus-infected patients. *Liver Transpl* 2014;20:655–63.
41. Paterno F, Shiller M, Tillery G, O'Leary JG, Susskind B, Trotter J, and Klintmalm GB. Bortezomib for acute antibody-mediated rejection in liver transplantation. *Am J Transplant* 2012;12:2525–31.
42. O'Leary JG, Demetris AJ, Friedman LS, Gebel HM, Halloran PF, Kirk AD, *et al*. The role of donor-specific HLA alloantibodies in liver transplantation. *Am J Transplant* 2014;14:779–87.
43. Dunn TB, Noreen H, Gillingham K, Maurer D, Ozturk OG, Pruett TL, *et al*. Revisiting traditional risk factors for rejection and graft loss after kidney transplantation. *Am J Transplant* 2011;11:2132–43.
44. Sellares J, de Freitas DG, Mengel M, Reeve J, Einecke G, Sis B, *et al*. Understanding the causes of kidney transplant failure: the dominant role of antibody-mediated rejection and nonadherence. *Am J Transplant* 2012;12:388–99.

12. Hepatitis C and Liver Transplantation in the Era of New Antiviral Treatments

Elizabeth C. Verna*,† and Robert S. Brown Jr.†,‡

*Department of Medicine, Columbia University College of
Physicians & Surgeons, New York, NY, USA
†Department of Medicine, Center for Liver Disease and
Transplantation, New York Presbyterian Hospital,
New York, NY, USA
‡Department of Medicine, Weill Cornell Medical College,
New York, NY, USA

1. Introduction

The availability of safe and effective direct acting antiviral (DAA) therapy for hepatitis C virus (HCV) infection has changed the landscape of liver transplant(ation) (LT). While HCV remains the leading indication for transplant in the United States, there is already evidence that this may soon change, with nonalcoholic fatty liver disease poised to soon surpass HCV as the indication for transplant listing among patients with decompensated cirrhosis [1]. In addition, while the accelerated progression of recurrent disease in the allograft previously led to diminished posttransplant survival among LT recipients with HCV [2], antiviral therapy has become sufficiently safe and effective that it is no longer debated whether patients can be cured, but rather the timing of therapy to maximize the overall survival of the patient [3].

Despite these remarkable advances, several important questions remain unanswered. There are small subgroups, especially those with advanced renal insufficiency, who still have limited treatment options and suboptimal outcomes. There is a great need for better safety and efficacy data on patients with high MELD scores on the waiting list, and a better understanding of the natural history of patients with decompensated cirrhosis following treatment with sustained virologic response (SVR) including the issues regarding "MELD purgatory" and the "point of no return" where decompensation will not reverse with virologic cure. In addition, trials are still ongoing for pre- and posttransplant treatment with the newest generation, pangenotypic regimens. Despite these questions, it is clear that for most LT candidates and recipients with HCV, the availability of DAAs has dramatically changed the field.

2. Natural history of posttransplant recurrent hepatitis C virus (HCV)

HCV remains the leading indication for LT in most of the world. Unfortunately, for patients with HCV viremia at the time of LT, recurrent disease in the allograft is universal. The natural history of untreated HCV post LT is accelerated compared to the pre-LT setting, with 10–20% of patients developing cirrhosis by 5 years post LT [4]. In addition, severe and often fatal forms of HCV including "cholestatic", or "fibrosing cholestatic" HCV occur almost exclusively in immunocompromised hosts such as transplant recipients [5].

Predictors of severe recurrence in untreated patients include donor factors such as older donor age [6], overall donor quality as represented by donor risk index [7], and donor HCV seropositivity [8], recipient factors such as female gender [9], and IL28B genotype [10], and immunosuppression type and intensity. As a result, overall survival among LT recipients with HCV has been lower than HCV negative recipients (Figure 1) [11, 12]. In addition, examination of the Scientific Registry of Transplant Recipients data in the United States has shown that there has been a significant improvement in post-LT survival throughout the last two decades in HCV-negative but not HCV-positive LT recipients [6].

Even in the pre-DAA era, it was clear that HCV treatment with SVR could improve posttransplant survival even once histologic recurrence was established [13]. Unfortunately, due to the poor tolerability and minimal

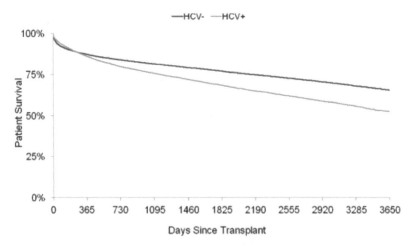

Figure 1. Reduction in LT wait-listing in the era of direct-acting antiviral therapy [1].`

efficacy of interferon and ribavirin in the pre- and posttransplant setting, many patients were left without hope for cure to slowing of disease progression. When pooled in a systematic review, post-LT SVR rates among all studies with pegylated interferon with ribavirin were 27% overall (95% confidence interval 23–31%), with only 21% tolerating full dose treatment and 66% tolerating the full duration [14]. These SVR rates were significantly augmented with the addition of the first-generation protease inhibitors (telaprevir and boceprevir) to interferon and ribavirin [15–18], though with the trade-off of additional toxicities. However, given the safety and efficacy of the interferon-free DAA regimens available, interferon-based regimens are no longer recommended [19].

As detailed below, safe and effective DAA treatment has revolutionized that care of these patients, as virtually all patients are now curable in the pre- or post-LT setting. The question is not whether they will be cured but when and with what regimen [3, 20]. While it is widely anticipated that this success in HCV treatment will translate into both improved posttransplant survival and decreased need for LT among patients with HCV (due to prevention of hepatic decompensation and hepatocellular carcinoma (HCC)), these improvements have yet to be clearly demonstrated. Recent reports have suggested that even in the few short years since interferon-free regimens have been available there may already be an impact in terms of a decline in wait-listing for HCV-related decompensated liver disease (Figure 2) [1]. Interestingly, wait-listing of patients

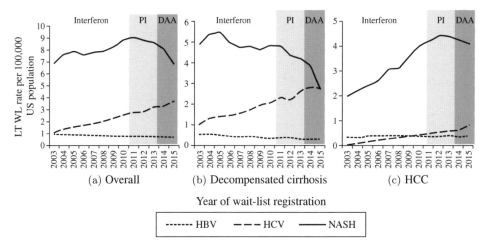

Figure 2. Posttransplant patients survival in HCV-positive patients compared to HCV negative patients [6].

with HCV and HCC has not yet significantly declined, highlighting the need for ongoing monitoring of patients even after SVR. Ongoing investigation will be needed in the years to come to both characterize this potential impact of DAAs on pre- and post-LT outcomes, as well as to identify new predictors of treatment failure and severe disease recurrence in this setting.

3. Pretransplant HCV treatment

The current revolution in HCV treatment is perhaps most remarkable for the incredible safety and efficacy that has been demonstrated even among the traditionally most difficult to treat populations. The management of patients with chronic HCV infection on the LT waiting list is thus evolving rapidly. Interferon-based treatment, especially among patients with decompensated cirrhosis, has generally been ineffective and associated with unacceptable risks, including up to 10% treatment-related mortality [21]. Given the significantly improved safety and efficacy of interferon-free DAA regimens, interferon is no longer recommended in pretransplant patients. There are now several prospective clinical trials as well as growing real-world datasets on the use of DAAs combinations in patients with compensated cirrhosis (Child–Turcotte–Pugh (CTP) class A), as well as more limited data on decompensated disease with moderate or severe hepatic impairment (CTP classes B and C).

4. Compensated cirrhosis

The current recommendations for patients on the LT wait list with compensated (CTP class A) cirrhosis but indications for LT such as HCC and are the same as for all patients with cirrhosis (Table 2) [19]. Table 1 describes the current first line and alternative DAA regimens by genotype, emphasizing the impact of cirrhosis on treatment recommendations. While overall it is still possible to achieve excellent SVR rates in patients with cirrhosis, for several regimens and/or genotypes, extension of therapy to 16 or 24 weeks, with or without the addition of ribavirin is required to achieve equivalent response rates.

Table 1. Characteristics of currently approved directly acting antiviral medications (Adapted with modifications from Ref. [53])

	NS3/4A protease inhibitors	Nucleos(t)ide NS5B polymerase inhibitors	Nonnucleoside NS5B polymerase inhibitors	NS5A replication complex inhibitors
Approved drugs in the class	Telaprevir, boceprevir, simeprevir, paritaprevir, grazoprevir	Sofosbuvir	Dasabuvir	Ledipasvir, daclatasvir, ombitasvir, elbasvir, velpatasvir
Potency	High (varies by HCV genotype)	Moderate to high (consistent across HCV genotypes)	Variable (by HCV genotypes)	High (multiple HCV genotypes)
Barrier to resistance	Low (1a < 1b)	High (1a = 1b)	Very low (1a < 1b)	Low (1a < 1b)
Potential for drug interactions	High	Low	Variable	Low to moderate
Toxicity	Rash, anemia, ↑ bilirubin, liver injury	Mitochondrial, NRTI interactions	Variable	Variable
Metabolism	Predominantly hepatic	Predominantly renal	Predominantly hepatic	Predominantly hepatic

Table 2.   Current recommendations for adjustment in antiviral regimen in patients with compensated cirrhosis [19].

HCV genotype	Regimen	Treatment-naïve	Treatment-experienced[#]
1	Sofosbuvir + ledipasvir for 12 weeks	No change	Extend to 24 weeks or + ribavirin (RBV)
	Sofosbuvir + velpatasvir for 12 weeks	No change	No change
	Elbasvir + grazoprevir* for 12 weeks	No change	No change
	Paritaprevir/r + dasabuvir + ombitasvir (Riba for 1a) for 12 weeks**	1a: Extend to 24 weeks 1b: no change	1a: Extend to 24 weeks 1b: no change
	Simeprevir + sofosbuvir ± Riba***	Extend to 24 weeks	Extend to 24 weeks
	Daclatasvir + sofosbuvir***	Extend to 16–24 weeks ± RBV	Extend to 16–24 weeks ± RBV
2	Sofosbuvir + velpatasvir for 12 weeks	No change	No change
	Daclatasvir + sofosbuvir***	Extend to 24 weeks ± RBV	Extend to 24 weeks ± RBV
3	Sofosbuvir + velpatasvir for 12 weeks	No change	No change
	Daclatasvir + sofosbuvir ± Riba	Extend to 24 weeks ± RBV	Extend to 24 weeks ± RBV
4	Sofosbuvir + ledipasvir for 12 weeks	No change	Extend to 24 weeks or ± RBV
	Sofosbuvir + velpatasvir for 12 weeks	No change	No change
	Elbasvir + grazoprevir for 12 weeks	No change	No change
	Paritaprevir/r + dasabuvir + ombitasvir for 12 weeks	No change	No change

Note: *For patients with genotype 1a, 12 weeks if no baseline resistance associated variants (RAVs), extend to 16 weeks if baseline RAVs.

**PrOD for 12 weeks is a recommended regimen for patients with HCV genotype 1b, and is an alternative regimen with ribavirin for HCV genotype 1a.

***These regimens are recommended as alternatives.

[#]Treatment-experienced indicates prior interferon-based treatment. Prior DAA exposure may require additional adjustments in the regimen.

5. Decompensated cirrhosis

In the first large clinical trials of patients with decompensated cirrhosis (the SOLAR-1 and SOLAR-2 trials), patients with CTP B and C cirrhosis were randomized to 12 or 24 weeks of the fixed dose combination of ledipasvir/ sofosbuvir with ribavirin [22, 23]. These complex trials included a "cohort A" of pre-LT patients with CTP B and C cirrhosis, and a "cohort B" of post-LT patients described in more detail below. Between the two studies, a total of 215 patients with HCV genotype 1 or 4 and decompensated cirrhosis were enrolled and overall SVR12 rates ranged from 78–96% (Table 3). SVR rates were numerically lower in the CTP C patients, but there was no difference between patients treated for 12 or 24 weeks in any arm. The treatment was well tolerated, with no deaths attributed to treatment. However, it is notable that all of these patients received ribavirin, and that the minority (27% overall) had a MELD score over 15. Thus additional data on the safety and efficacy of treatment among patients with decompensated cirrhosis with MELD over 15 and indications for transplant are urgently needed.

In the phase 3, open-label ALLY-1 study, patients with HCV genotypes 1–4 and advanced liver disease including 48 with CTP B or C cirrhosis were treated with daclatasvir, sofosbuvir, and ribavirin for 12 weeks [24]. The SVR12 rate was lower among the CTP C patients (56%) compared to CTP B (94%), though the cohort included 42% of patients with a MELD score greater than 15, perhaps indicative of a sicker underlying population. Again, treatment was well tolerated overall with no treatment-related serious adverse events of deaths and all patients received ribavirin, limiting our ability to determine whether this is necessary in all cases.

More recently, the phase 3 ASTRAL-4 trial enrolled the largest number of patients with decompensated cirrhosis to date [25]. A total of 267 patients with HCV genotypes 1–6 and CTP class B disease were randomized 1:1:1 to sofosbuvir/velpatasvir for 12 weeks, sofosbuvir/velpatasvir with ribavirin for 12 weeks, or sofosbuvir/velpatasvir for 24 weeks. Overall SVR12 rates were 83%, 94%, and 86% among these three groups, respectively. While this is a pangenotypic regimen, the vast majority of patients enrolled were genotype 1 (78%) or 3 (15%). In addition, this trial was limited to CTP class B patients, and only 5% had a MELD score greater than 15, perhaps limiting the applicability of these data to many patients on the transplant wait list.

Due to hepatic metabolism and reports of hepatotoxicity, the currently available NS3/4A protease inhibitors are not recommended for patients with moderate to severe hepatic impairment. The approved fixed-dose

Table 3. Directly acting antiviral clinical trials in patients with decompensated cirrhosis (CTP class B or C).

Trial	Treatment regimen	Patients	SVR12	Impact on liver function
SOLAR-1 [22].	Sofosbuvir/ ledipasvir + Riba × 12 or 24 weeks	N = 108 CTP B or C GT 1 or 4	86–89%	63/94 (67%) with improvement in MELD by posttreatment week 4 15/94 (16%) no change 16/94 (17%) worsening in MELD
SOLAR-2 [23]	Sofosbuvir/ ledipasvir + Riba × 12 or 24 weeks	N = 107 CTP B or C GT 1 or 4	78–96%	59/81 (73%) with improvement in MELD by posttreatment week 4 9/81 (11%) no change 13/81 (16%) worsening in MELD
ALLY-1 [24]	Sofosbuvir + daclatasvir + Riba × 12 weeks	N = 48 CTP B or C GT1, 2, 3, or 4	CTP B = 94% CTP C = 56%	20/43 (47%) with improvement in MELD by last posttreatment visit 7/43 (16%) no change 16/43 (37%) worsening in MELD
ASTRAL-4 [25]	Sofosbuvir/ velpatasvir ± Riba × 12 weeks or 24 weeks	N = 267 CTP B GT 1, 2, 3, 4, 5, or 6	83–94%	136/250 (54%) with improvement in MELD by posttreatment week 12 52/250 (21%) had no change 62/250 (25%) worsening in MELD
C-SALT [26]	Grazoprevir (50 mg daily) + elbasvir (50 mg daily)	N = 30 CTP B GT 1	90%	11/28 (39%) with improvement in MELD by posttreatment week 12 11/28 (39%) had no change 6/28 (21%) worsening in MELD

Note: CTP = Child–Turcotte–Pugh; SVR = sustained virologic response 12 weeks after stopping treatment; RCT = randomized controlled trial; GT = genotype.

combination of elbasvir/grazoprevir has not been studied in patients with decompensated cirrhosis. In a small phase 2 open-label study of 30 patients with HCV genotype 1 and CTP B cirrhosis, patients were given reduced dose grazoprevir (50 mg daily) and elbasvir (50 mg daily) [26]. The SVR12 rate was 90% and one patient died at week 4 post treatment. However, there are no data on the currently approved dosage and the safety of this regimen has not been established. Similarly, the mean steady state area under the curve (AUC) of simeprevir is 2.4-fold higher in patients with moderate hepatic impairment (CTP B) and 5.3-fold higher with severe hepatic impairment (CTP C) [27], and reports of cholestasis and hepatotoxicity [28, 29] with this regimen have prevented formal trials of simeprevir in these patients.

The PrOD regimen (paritaprevir/ritonavir with ombitasvir and dasabuvir) is also contraindicated in patients with CTP class B and C cirrhosis. Due to the predominantly hepatic elimination, the AUC of paritaprevir increases by 62% in subjects with moderate hepatic impairment and 94.5% in patients with severe hepatic impairment [30]. While PrOD has been used with high response rates in a small number of patients with CTP B cirrhosis reported in real-world efficacy reports, cases of hepatotoxicity have limited its use in this setting. In a multicenter European cohort of 209 patients treated with this regimen, the SVR12 rate was 100% among the 14 patients with CTP B disease. However, seven patients with cirrhosis experienced hepatic decompensation, two of which were possibly related to treatment. While pretreatment measures of liver function including CTP score and MELD were predictive of decompensation, not all of these patients were decompensated at baseline and there are now additional reports of hepatic decompensation in patients with CTP A disease at the start of therapy. These reports include an FDA Drug Safety Communication reporting 26 cases of liver injury considered possibly or probably due to medications [31] and a multicenter cohort from Israel reported seven patients who received PrOD and were decompensated [32]. These decompensation events appear to have occurred between 1 and 8 weeks of treatment initiation. Thus, PrOD remains contraindicated in patients with CTP B or C cirrhosis.

As a result of these data, the current multisociety guidelines [19] for the treatment of patients with decompensated cirrhosis and HCV genotype 1 or 4 recommend treatment with sofosbuvir/ledipasvir with initial low-dose ribavirin (600 mg divided daily and increased as tolerated) for 12 weeks, sofosbuvir/velpatasvir with weight-based ribavirin for 12 weeks, or sofosbuvir with daclatasvir and initial low-dose ribavirin for 12 weeks. For patients who are intolerant of ribavirin, extended duration of treatment is often utilized. For HCV genotype 2 or 3, sofosbuvir/velpatasvir with weight-based ribavirin for 12 weeks, or sofosbuvir with daclatasvir and initial low-dose ribavirin for 12 weeks are recommended.

6. Immediate pretransplant therapy

Due to the limited efficacy and significant safety concerns regarding interferon-based treatment in patients with decompensated cirrhosis, strategies specific to wait-listed patients such as the low accelerating dose regimen (LADR) were developed. With this approach, patients were started at low doses of pegylated-interferon and ribavirin, which were then titrated up to a maximally tolerated dose with the goal of undergoing LT on a truncate course of treatment with an undetectable viral load [33, 34]. While this approach did achieve intent-to-treat posttransplant virologic response (pTVR) of 28%, and up to 80% among patients with undetectable HCV RNA for over 16 weeks prior to LT, the overall safety and efficacy of this approach are poor.

In the first interferon-free trial in this immediate pre-LT setting, Curry and colleagues enrolled an open-label phase 2 study of sofosbuvir and ribavirin for up to 48 weeks in patients with CPT score ≤7 and HCC with exception points on the LT waiting list. A total of 46 patients underwent LT, 43 of whom had undetectable HCV RNA at the time of LT. Among these 43 patients, 70% achieved SVR12, 23% relapsed, and 7% died. Thus the overall SVR12 rate for the cohort was 49%. Among the patients with undetectable HCV RNA for at least 30 days prior to LT, the SVR12 rate was 96%.

It is clear that we now have more potent and effective DAA combinations available, though formal studies of these combinations with the specific intention of LT while on therapy have not been reported. In addition, it is not known how long pre-LT viral negativity is needed with these newer combinations, whether treatment can be safely continued in the immediate post-LT setting, and what the optimal total treatment duration is. It is likely that additional data from real-world cohorts will help to shed light on some of these important questions.

7. Impact of SVR on liver function

Now that SVR is achievable even in patients with decompensated liver disease, there is great interest in the potential for improvement in liver function and perhaps even complete "recompensation" of liver disease such that LT is no longer needed for long-term survival. In all of the clinical trials detailed above, all measures of liver function including MELD and CTP class or score were compared for available patients between baseline and the end-of-study follow-up (usually 4–12 weeks after starting treatment, Table 3). When data from all of the prospective and retrospective literature was recently pooled, 60% of treated patients experienced an improvement in MELD score of at least 1 point [3]. In addition, among the pre- and post-LT patients with decompensated liver disease in the SOLAR studies, 61% of patients with a baseline MELD >15 had an improvement in MELD to below the MELD of 15 threshold often utilized as minimal LT listing criteria [22, 23]. However, in the overall pooled analysis, 17% experienced no change in MELD and 23% experienced worsening of MELD score despite SVR in many of these patients, and clinical predictors of treatment response are currently lacking [7]. Data from real-world cohorts suggest that younger age and albumin >3.5 g/dL may predict improvement in liver function [35]. Others have suggested improvement in liver function may only occur in patients with a baseline MELD score <20, perhaps implicating a point of no return after which improvement is unlikely [36].

It is important to note that the follow up available for all of these studies is currently very short term, and whether prolonged transplant-free survival can be achieved in patients with small or moderate improvements in MELD or CTP scores is unknown. In addition, very few patients with a MELD above 15 and almost no patients with a MELD above 20 were included in any of the formal clinical trials. Thus, the impact on liver function in patients more likely to be actually prioritized or able to obtain an organ for LT is unknown. As discussed below, treatment in high MELD or CTP C patients needs to be individualized based upon treatment goals for the particular patient.

8. Posttransplant treatment

For patients who remain with HCV viremia at the time of LT, recurrent HCV-associated liver disease is universal. Recurrent HCV has traditionally been associated with an accelerated course post LT, leading to excess graft loss and mortality among LT recipients with HCV [4, 11]. As a result, transplant recipients are among the highest priority for treatment [19]. Fortunately, SVR rates among LT recipients with early-stage liver disease or compensated cirrhosis are comparable to those in the nontransplant setting (Table 4). An increasing proportion of post-LT treatment is being performed among patients with early-stage recurrent liver disease when liver function remains normal and even before significant histologic recurrence of fibrosis has occurred.

Table 4.   Directly acting antiviral clinical trials in LT recipients

Trial	Treatment regimen	Patients	Fibrosis stage	SVR12
SOLAR-1 [22]	Sofosbuvir/ledipasvir + Riba for 12 or 24 weeks	N = 310 post-LT GT 1 or 4	Stage F0–3 (n = 111) CTP A (n = 51) CTP B (n = 52) CTP C (n = 9) FCH (n = 6)	Stage 0–3 97% CTP A 96% CTP B 87% CTP C 67% FCH 100%
SOLAR-2 [23]	Sofosbuvir/Ledipasvir + Riba for 12 or 24 weeks	N = 226 post-LT GT 1 or 4	Stage 0–3 (n = 101) CTP A (n = 67) CTP B (n = 45) CTP C (n = 8) FCH (n = 5)	Stage 0–3 97% CTP A 97% CTP B 98% CTP C 63% FCH 100%
ALLY-1 [24]	Sofosbuvir + Daclatasvir + Riba for 12 weeks	N = 53 post-LT GT 1, 2, 3, 4, 5 or 6	F0 (n = 6) F1 (n = 10) F2 (n = 7) F3 (n = 13) F4 (n = 16)	94%
GALAXY [40]	Sofosbuvir + Simeprevir ± Riba for 12 or 24 weeks	N = 46 GT 1	F0–1 (n = 9) F2 (n = 23) F3 (n = 9) F4 (n = 1)	94%
CORAL-1 [43]	Paritaprevir/r + Dasabuvir + Ombitasvir for 24 weeks	N = 34 GT 1 No cirrhosis	F0 (n = 6) F1 (n = 13) F2 (n = 15)	97%

Note: SVR = sustained virologic response 12 weeks after stopping treatment; RCT = randomized controlled trial; GT = genotype.

9. Drug–drug interactions

The additional important consideration for HCV treatment in post-LT patients is the potential for significant drug–drug interactions, most prominently with the calcineurin inhibitors (CNIs) cyclosporine and tacrolimus (TAC). The impact of each DAA on the AUC for cyclosporine and TAC is summarized in Table 5. While there are several DAA regimens that do not require significant *a priori* CNI dose adjustment, there are agents including the NS3/4A protease inhibitors (especially those which are coformulated with ritonavir), which require both dose adjustment and intensive monitoring.

Table 5. Drug–drug interactions between antiviral therapy and CNIs.

	Cyclosporine		TAC	
	Healthy volunteers	*A priori* dose adjustment	Healthy volunteers	*A priori* dose adjustment
Sofosbuvir	No change	None	No change	None
Simeprevir*	AUC ↑19%	None	AUC ↓17%	None
Daclatasvir	No change	None	No change	None
Ledipasvir	No data	None	No data	None
PrOD	AUC ↑5.8-fold	↓5-fold	AUC ↑57-fold	↓100-fold
PrO	AUC ↑4.3-fold	↓5-fold	AUC ↑86-fold	↓100-fold
Elbasvir/grazoprevir**	No change	None	AUC ↑43%	None
Grazoprevir	No change	None	No change	None
Valpatasvir	No change	None	No change	None

Note: *Cyclosporine coadministration results in AUC ↑5.8-fold of simeprevir, and this combination is not recommended.

**Cyclosporine coadministration results in AUC ↑15-fold of grazoprevir and AUC ↑2-fold of elbasvir, and this combination is not recommended.

Unfortunately, data on drug–drug interactions are generally not available for other important classes of immunosuppressive drugs, including the mammalian target of rapamycin (mTOR) inhibitors, everolimus, and sirolimus [37].

9.1. *Sofosbuvir-based regimens*

Sofosbuvir is an important agent for the treatment of LT recipients as there are no cytochrome p450 interaction; thus no definite dose adjustment in immunosuppression is needed and it provides and a potent pangenotypic backbone to any chosen regimen. The largest trials of LT recipients to date were the SOLAR-1 and SOLAR-2 trials, in which the "cohort B" arms included LT recipients with HCV genotype 1 or 4 and early-stage disease as well as recurrent compensated or decompensated cirrhosis [22, 23]. As in the pretransplant setting, patients were randomized to 12 or 24 weeks of ledipasvir/sofosbuvir and ribavirin. Overall, the SVR12 rates were remarkable, including 97% in patients with early-stage recurrence, 96–97% among patients with recurrent compensated cirrhosis, and even 87–98% among patients with recurrent CTP B disease. As in the pretransplant setting, all patients received ribavirin, limiting our ability to determine whether it is necessary, especially in the early-stage patients. Importantly, no significant dose adjustments in immunosuppression were required.

Real-world data regarding ledipasvir/sofosbuvir post transplant has revealed similarly high response rates. In the largest series to date of 204 LT recipients, the overall SVR12 rate was 96% [38]. In addition, in this study the use of ribavirin did not significantly impact response rates. However, as this was a nonrandomized study, whether ribavirin is of benefit to select patients cannot be sufficiently answered in this type of analysis.

Additional sofosbuvir-based regimens have also been studied. The ALLY-1 study included 53 post-LT patients with HCV genotypes 1–6 who received sofosbuvir and daclatasvir with ribavirin for 12 weeks. None of these patients had recurrent decompensated cirrhosis, though 30% had recurrent cirrhosis. The overall SVR12 rate was 94%, treatment was well tolerated and *a priori* dose adjustments in immunosuppression were not needed. Real-world cohort data on the use of daclatasvir and sofosbuvir even in patients with more advanced or severe recurrent disease has also confirmed the excellent safety and efficacy of this regimen [39].

In addition, as sofosbuvir and simeprevir were the first two DAAs available, many post-LT patients have been treated with this combination. In the recently published GALAXY trial, 33 patients with GT 1 HCV without cirrhosis were randomized to sofosbuvir and simeprevir for 12 weeks, sofosbuvir and simeprevir with ribavirin for 12 weeks, or sofosbuvir and simeprevir for 24 weeks [40]. An additional group of 13 patients were entered into the third 24-week arm. The overall SVR12 rate was 94% (82%, 100%, and 94% in the three arms, respectively). Treatment was well tolerated with no serious adverse events attributable to study drug. Simeprevir exposure was increased compared to the nontransplant setting, but not to a degree that was thought to be clinical relevant. Importantly, although a variety of immunosuppressive regimens were included, no patients were on cyclosporine due to the known increase in simeprevir AUC in with coadministration of cyclosporine (Table 5). Larger real-world datasets on the use of simeprevir in LT recipients are also available, including a recent meta-analysis of nine studies [41]. The pooled SVR12 rate was 88%. In a larger more recent cohort of 151 patients treated with simeprevir and sofosbuvir with or without ribavirin for 12 or 24 weeks, the overall SVR12 rate was also 88% [42].

The use of sofosbuvir/velpatasvir in LT recipients is currently being studied, and no data are currently available on the use of this combination in the post-LT setting. It is likely that as with the regimens above, there with not be a clinically significant interaction with CNIs.

9.2. *Protease inhibitor-based regimens*

The PrOD regimen, has been tested in small clinical trials in transplant recipients, though with very few patients reported to date. In the initial trial, 34 LT recipients with early-stage fibrosis (stage F0–F2) and HCV genotype 1 were treated with PrOD and weight-based ribavirin for 24 weeks [43]. The overall SVR12 rate was 97%. There were no episodes of acute rejection, though significant adjustments in CNI dose were required due to the drug–drug interactions with ritonavir and paretaprevir. For most patients, 0.5-mg and 0.2-mg doses of TAC were given with a median frequency of 10 days and 5 days, respectively. A larger trial of the PrOD regimen among liver and kidney transplant recipients is ongoing.

Real-world data on the use of PrOD in transplant recipients are also available. In a multicenter European series of the use of PrOD with or without ribavirin for HCV genotype 1 or 4, 21 patients included were LT recipients, and SVR12 was 100% in this subgroup [44]. While the report notes that changes in immunosuppression were required, additional details were not provided. Three of the patients with recurrent cirrhosis experienced decompensation of liver function on treatment and further data on the use of this regimen in patients with recurrent cirrhosis are needed.

Clinical trials of the fixed-dose combination of elbasvir/grazoprevir have not yet been reported in solid organ transplant recipients. There is a small pilot study planned among LT recipients, as well as a trial of the use of HCV seropositive grafts in HCV negative kidney transplant recipients. From preliminary pharmacokinetic studies, there is likely no need for *a priori* dose adjustment in TAC, coadministration with cyclosporine is not recommended due to a significant increase in the AUC for elbasvir and grazoprevir. These trials along with real-world effectiveness studies will provide essential information about the safety and immunosuppressive and DAA pharmacokinetics needed to treat transplant recipients, especially for those with advanced renal insufficiency which is unfortunately common in this population.

Finally, a trial of the next generation pangenotypic glecaprevir/pibrentasvir combination in liver and kidney transplant recipients is also now ongoing. Glecaprevir (which does not require ritonavir boosting) is expected to have fewer interactions with TAC and less interaction with cyclosporine than other PI-based regimens.

9.3. *Current recommendations for posttransplant treatment*

The recommended first line regimens in these patients include fixed dose sofosbuvir/ledipasvir with weight-based ribavirin for 12 weeks or sofosbuvir and daclatasvir with low-dose ribavirin (600 mg daily initially and increased as tolerated) for 12 weeks genotype 1 or 4, with alternative regimens including extension of these therapies to 24 weeks for ribavirin intolerant patients [19]. Additional alternatives for genotype 1 include sofosbuvir and simeprevir with weight-based ribavirin for 12 weeks, or PrOD and weight-based ribavirin for 24 weeks. For genotypes 2 and 3, sofosbuvir and daclatasvir with low-dose ribavirin (600 mg daily initially and increased as tolerated) for 12 weeks is the current first line regimen due to a lack of data with sofosbuvir and velpatasvir, though many experts believe this is a reasonable treatment choice as well.

10. Fibrosing cholestatic hepatitis C virus (HCV)

Fibrosing cholestatic HCV (FCH) is a severe forms of HCV recurrence with a predominantly cholestatic presentation and unique pathological features [5]. Although it is relatively rare, impacting <10% of patients in the pre-DAA era, the severity of this type of recurrence and its profound impact on post-LT survival led FCH to be among the most feared complications in these patients. While the numbers of patients with FCH included in formal clinical trials of DAA therapy post LT have been small, the efficacy for the patients with FCH in the SOLAR-1 and SOLAR 2 trials was 100% [22, 23]. Similar results have been seen in real-world cohort, including with sofosbuvir and daclatasvir [39, 45]. In one report of 23 patients with FCH and severely decompensated liver disease treated with sofosbuvir and daclatasvir-based regimens, the SVR12 rate was 96% [45]. Perhaps more importantly, 96% of patients experienced "complete clinical response" with normalization of bilirubin and resolution of symptoms by the end of follow-up. This, the new DAA therapies have very dramatically changed the natural history for patients with FCH, and this entity may become rarer and patients are being treated pre-LT or in the early post-LT setting.

11. Novel approaches to perioperative therapy

The remarkable safety and efficacy of ledipasvir/sofosbuvir in transplant recipients has led to additional investigation of novel approaches including a pilot study of a shortened duration of treatment in the perioperative or pre-emptive setting. Pre-emptive therapy with interferon-based treatment had never before been shown to have a benefit in terms of prevention of disease progression [46]. Thus, treatment previously had been reserved for patients with established histological recurrence. However, in this DAA study, ledipasvir/sofosbuvir was given to 16 patients with genotype 1 HCV, with the first dose prior to the transplant, and then for a total of only 4 weeks of treatment [47]. The concept behind shortened duration of treatment in this setting is that perhaps removal of the hepatic reservoir will diminish the chance of relapse in this setting, even on the high-dose immunosuppression given in this setting. Among these 16 patients, there was one treatment failure due to early discontinuation of therapy in the setting of prolonged kidney injury (and thus contraindication to ongoing sofosbuvir use), and one on-treatment breakthrough for an overall SVR12 rate of 88%. Importantly, both of these patients were successfully retreated with ledipasvir/sofosbuvir for 12 weeks. While this is just a pilot trial, it highlights the ongoing work needed to determine the optimal timing of treatment in this population.

Finally, there has been considerable interest in the development of a perioperative immunoglobulin infusion analogous to the hepatitis B virus (HBV) immunoglobulin used for LT recipients with HBV. Previous attempts at this formulation had failed to reveal benefit from administration. However, a more recent trial studied the use of a human hepatitis C antibody enriched immune globulin product in the setting of viral suppression prior to transplant with DAAs. Although the final results are pending in terms of both prevention of posttransplant recurrence and safety, preliminary results support of the safety of this approach in transplant recipients [48]. This could be perhaps of particular interest in patients with confirmed or suspected drug resistance going into LT [49]. However, how best to utilize HCV immunoglobulin in the current DAA era is not yet well understood.

12. Timing of treatment

There is significant interest in determining the optimal timing of treatment (i.e., pre or post LT), in terms of patient outcomes and cost effectiveness [50–52]. Treatment prior to LT is desirable given the potential benefit of improvement in liver function with SVR, clinical stabilization prior to LT, and prevention of post-LT recurrent disease. However, there is concern that pre-LT treatment may inadvertently diminish access to transplant due to a decline in MELD score without complete resolution of transplant indications. Successfully treated patients and their providers may also be reluctant to accept an HCV seropositive graft, further diminishing access. Finally, overall SVR rates may be higher in the early post-LT period compared to in patients with severe hepatic impairment and in the case of patients with a high MELD on the waiting list, it is not clear that there will be significant clinical benefit from treatment just prior to LT rather than in the early postoperative period.

Modeling to inform an approach to treatment timing for a population is complex, and requires taking into account multiple variables specific to a patient's circumstance. Important factors include the patient's prognosis on the list with and without treatment, as well as the dynamics of allograft allocation including the availability of HCV-positive donors. This was recently simulated using a Markov-based microsimulation model that incorporated information from HCV treatment trials pre and post LT, as well as UNOS data on waiting-list activity [52]. The authors conclude that the optimal MELD threshold below which patients awaiting LT should receive HCV treatment may be between 23 and 27, depending on the UNOS region. However, given the limited data upon which many essential assumptions are made in modeling analyses, and the virtual absence of patients with MELD >20 in the current treatment literature, treatment decisions must remain individualized.

One proposed strategy for timing of HCV treatment in LT candidates is presented in Figure 3. Treatment is clearly indicated in patients on the waiting list with compensated cirrhosis and/or low MELD candidates who have access to transplant through MELD exception points or living donation. Patients with low MELD may also benefit from treatment to improve liver function and avoid transplant, though how to predict who will achieve prolonged transplant-free survival is unknown. There are also patients with MELD scores above which treatment is detrimental and/or not possible, especially those with concomitant renal dysfunction. However, for patients with moderate MELD scores, the best approach is difficult to generalize. The lack of data on safety and efficacy in these patients and the variability in access to transplant by MELD render treatment recommendations in this scenario highly individualized.

13. Conclusions

The availability of safe and effective anti-HCV therapy has undoubtedly changed the field of HCV in LT. The ability to cure these traditionally and

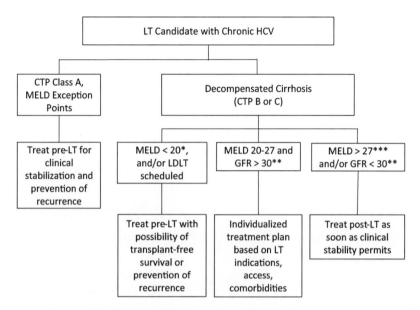

Figure 3. Proposed algorithm for HCV treatment in LT candidates with chronic HCV [54].

*MELD <20 is based upon the limited data on safety and efficacy of treatment in patients with MELD >20, however treatment above this MELD may be beneficial in some patients.

**GFR >30 mL/min/1.73 m^2 is based upon the need for use of sofobuvir in all currently recommended treatment regimens for patients with decompensated cirrhosis, and the contraindication to use of sofosbuvir in patients with severe renal impairment.

***MELD >27 is based upon the LT-SIM model presented in this issue [52], which found that even if treatment is assumed to be safe and effective above this MELD, there may be a survival benefit by delaying therapy to the posttransplant setting.

CTP = Child–Turcotte–Pugh, MELD = model for end stage liver disease, LT = liver transplant, LDLT = living donor liver transplant, GFR = glomerular filtration rate, expressed as ml/min/1.73 m^2.

the difficulty in treating patients before and after LT will surely lead to both a decline in the need for LT among patients with HCV, as well as improved post-LT survival. However, significant questions remain. The optimal regimen and timing of therapy is yet to be clarified, and more work is needed to identify clinical predictors of improvement in liver function among patients with decompensated cirrhosis on the waiting list. In addition, there remain small groups of patients that are underserved by our current treatment options. These include those with highly resistant variants (either *de novo* or the result of prior DAA failure), as well as those with both decompensated cirrhosis and advanced renal insufficiency (and therefore contraindications to both protease-inhibitor and sofosbuvir-based therapy). Finally, for these improvements in outcomes to be realized, expanded access to treatment will be essential. However, despite these important questions, it is remarkable that these patients who are at highest risk of HCV-related complications now have life-saving therapy.

References

1. Flemming JA, Kim WR, Brosgart CL, and Terrault NA. Reduction in liver transplant wait-listing in the era of direct-acting antiviral therapy. *Hepatology* 2017;65(3):804–12.
2. Verna EC and Brown RS, Jr. Hepatitis C and liver transplantation: enhancing outcomes and should patients be retransplanted. *Clin Liver Dis* 2008;12(3): 637–59, ix–x.
3. Bunchorntavakul C and Reddy KR. Treat chronic hepatitis C virus infection in decompensated cirrhosis — pre- or post-liver transplantation? the ironic conundrum in the era of effective and well-tolerated therapy. *J Viral Hepat* 2016;23(6):408–18.
4. Berenguer M. Natural history of recurrent hepatitis C. *Liver Transpl* 2002;8 (10 Suppl 1):S14–8.
5. Verna EC, Abdelmessih R, Salomao MA, Lefkowitch J, Moreira RK, and Brown RS, Jr. Cholestatic hepatitis C following liver transplantation: an outcome-based histological definition, clinical predictors, and prognosis. *Liver Transpl* 2013;19(1):78–88.
6. Thuluvath PJ, Guidinger MK, Fung JJ, Johnson LB, Rayhill SC, and Pelletier SJ. Liver transplantation in the United States, 1999-2008. *Am J Transplant* 2010;10(4 Pt 2):1003–19.
7. Maluf DG, Edwards EB, Stravitz RT, and Kauffman HM. Impact of the donor risk index on the outcome of hepatitis C virus-positive liver transplant recipients. *Liver Transpl* 2009;15(6):592–9.
8. Lai JC, O'Leary JG, Trotter JF, Verna EC, Brown RS, Jr., Stravitz RT, *et al.* Risk of advanced fibrosis with grafts from hepatitis C antibody-positive donors: a multicenter cohort study. *Liver Transpl* 2012;18(5):532–8.
9. Lai JC, Verna EC, Brown RS, Jr., O'Leary JG, Trotter JF, Forman LM, *et al.* Hepatitis C virus–infected women have a higher risk of advanced fibrosis and graft loss after liver transplantation than men. *Hepatology* 2011;54(2):418–24.
10. Charlton MR, Thompson A, Veldt BJ, Watt K, Tillmann H, Poterucha JJ, *et al.* Interleukin-28B polymorphisms are associated with histological recurrence and treatment response following liver transplantation in patients with hepatitis C virus infection. *Hepatology* 2011;53(1):317–24.
11. Forman LM, Lewis JD, Berlin JA, Feldman HI, and Lucey MR. The association between hepatitis C infection and survival after orthotopic liver transplantation. *Gastroenterology* 2002;122(4):889–96.

12. Charlton M, Ruppert K, Belle SH, Bass N, Schafer D, Wiesner RH, *et al.* Long-term results and modeling to predict outcomes in recipients with HCV infection: results of the NIDDK liver transplantation database. *Liver Transpl* 2004;10(9):1120–30.
13. Crespo G, Carrion JA, Coto-Llerena M, Marino Z, Lens S, Perez-Del-Pulgar S, *et al.* Combinations of simple baseline variables accurately predict sustained virological response in patients with recurrent hepatitis C after liver transplantation. *J Gastroenterol* 2013;48(6):762–9.
14. Wang CS, Ko HH, Yoshida EM, Marra CA, and Richardson K. Interferon-based combination anti-viral therapy for hepatitis C virus after liver transplantation: a review and quantitative analysis. *Am J Transplant* 2006;6(7):1586–99.
15. Forns X, Didier S, Mutimer D, Fagiuoli S, Navasa M, Agarwal K, *et al.* Efficacy of telaprevir-based therapy in stable liver transplant patients with chronic genotype 1 hepatitis C. *Ann Hepatol* 2016;15(4):512–23.
16. Coilly A, Roche B, Dumortier J, Leroy V, Botta-Fridlund D, Radenne S, *et al.* Safety and efficacy of protease inhibitors to treat hepatitis C after liver transplantation: a multicenter experience. *J Hepatol* 2014;60(1):78–86.
17. Burton JR, Jr., O'Leary JG, Verna EC, Saxena V, Dodge JL, Stravitz RT, *et al.* A US multicenter study of hepatitis C treatment of liver transplant recipients with protease-inhibitor triple therapy. *J Hepatol* 2014;61(3):508–14.
18. Verna EC, Saxena V, Burton JR, Jr., O'Leary JG, Dodge JL, Stravitz RT, *et al.* Telaprevir- and boceprevir-based triple therapy for hepatitis C in liver transplant recipients with advanced recurrent disease: a multicenter study. *Transplantation* 2015;99(8):1644–51.
19. HCV Guidance: Recommendations for Testing, Managing, and Treating Hepatitis C, http://hcvguidelines.org/. Accessed 1 October 2017.
20. Verna EC. We can cure hepatitis C virus after transplant, but what is the best regimen? *Liver Transpl* 2016;22(11):1463–5.
21. Verna EC and O'Leary JG. Hepatitis C treatment in patients on the liver transplant waiting list. *Curr Opin Organ Transplant* 2015;20(3):242–50.
22. Charlton M, Everson GT, Flamm SL, Kumar P, Landis C, Brown RS, Jr., *et al.* Ledipasvir and sofosbuvir plus ribavirin for treatment of HCV infection in patients with advanced liver disease. *Gastroenterology* 2015;149(3):649–59.
23. Manns M, Samuel D, Gane EJ, Mutimer D, McCaughan G, Buti M, *et al.* Ledipasvir and sofosbuvir plus ribavirin in patients with genotype 1 or 4 hepatitis C virus infection and advanced liver disease: a multicentre, open-label, randomised, phase 2 trial. *Lancet Infect Dis* 2016;16(6):685–97.
24. Poordad F, Schiff ER, Vierling JM, Landis C, Fontana RJ, Yang R, *et al.* Daclatasvir with sofosbuvir and ribavirin for hepatitis C virus infection with advanced cirrhosis or post-liver transplantation recurrence. *Hepatology* 2016;63(5):1493–505.
25. Curry MP, O'Leary JG, Bzowej N, Muir AJ, Korenblat KM, Fenkel JM, *et al.* Sofosbuvir and velpatasvir for HCV in patients with decompensated cirrhosis. *N Engl J Med* 2015;373(27):2618–28.

26. Jacobson IJ, Poordad F, Pirpi-Morrell R, Everson GT, Verna EC, Bhanja S, *et al*. Efficacy and safety of grazoprevir and elbasvir in hepatitis C genotype 1-infected patients with Child–Pugh class B cirrhosis. *J Hepatol* 2015;62:S193.

27. Simeprevir US prescribing information. (http://www.accessdata.fda.gov/drugsatfda_docs/label/2013/205123s001lbl.pdf) (Accessed December 2016).

28. Stine JG, Intagliata N, Shah NL, Argo CK, Caldwell SH, Lewis JH, *et al*. Hepatic decompensation likely attributable to simeprevir in patients with advanced cirrhosis. *Dig Dis Sci* 2015;60(4):1031–5.

29. Igawa T, Fushimi S, Matsuo R, Ikeda F, Nouso K, Yoshino T, *et al*. Severe liver injury associated with simeprevir plus pegylated interferon/ribavirin therapy in a patient with treatment-naive genotype 1b hepatitis C virus: a case report. *Clin J Gastroenterol* 2014;7(5):465–70.

30. Viekira Pak US prescribing information (http://www.accessdata.fda.gov/drugsatfda_docs/label/2014/206619lbl.pdf) (Accessed November 2016).

31. FDA Drug Safety Communication: FDA warns of serious liver injury risk with hepatitis C treatments Viekira Pak and Technivie, http://www.fda.gov/Drugs/DrugSafety/ucm468634.htm. Accessed 1 October 2017.

32. Zuckerman E, Ashkenasi E, Kovaleve Y, *et al*. The real world Israeli experience of treating chronic hepatitis C genotype 1 patients with advanced fibrosis with parataprevir/ritonavir/ombitasvir, dasabuvir with or without ribavirin: a large, multi-center cohort. *J Hepatol* 2016;64:PS004.

33. Everson GT, Trotter J, Forman L, Kugelmas M, Halprin A, Fey B, *et al*. Treatment of advanced hepatitis C with a low accelerating dosage regimen of antiviral therapy. *Hepatology* 2005;42(2):255–62.

34. Everson GT, Terrault NA, Lok AS, Rodrigo del R, Brown RS, Jr., Saab S, *et al*. A randomized controlled trial of pretransplant antiviral therapy to prevent recurrence of hepatitis C after liver transplantation. *Hepatology* 2013;57(5):1752–62.

35. Foster GR, Irving WL, Cheung MC, Walker AJ, Hudson BE, Verma S, *et al*. Impact of direct acting antiviral therapy in patients with chronic hepatitis C and decompensated cirrhosis. *J Hepatol* 2016;64(6):1224–31.

36. McCaughan G, Roberts SK, Strasser SI, *et al*. The TOSCAR study: sofosbuvir and daclatasvir therapy for decompensated HCV cirrhosis with MELD scores >/=15: what is the point of no return? *Hepatology* 2015;62(Suppl 1):738A.

37. Kwo PY and Badshah MB. New hepatitis C virus therapies: drug classes and metabolism, drug interactions relevant in the transplant settings, drug options in decompensated cirrhosis, and drug options in end-stage renal disease. *Curr Opin Organ Transplant* 2015;20(3):235–41.

38. Kwok RM, Ahn J, Schiano TD, Te HS, Potosky DR, Tierney A, *et al*. Sofosbuvir plus ledispasvir for recurrent hepatitis C in liver transplant recipients. *Liver Transpl* 2016;22(11):1536–43.

39. Fontana RJ, Brown RS, Jr., Moreno-Zamora A, Prieto M, Joshi S, Londono MC, *et al*. Daclatasvir combined with sofosbuvir or simeprevir in liver

transplant recipients with severe recurrent hepatitis C infection. *Liver Transpl* 2016;22(4):446–58.

40. O'Leary JG, Fontana RJ, Brown K, Burton JR, Jr., Firpi-Morell R, Muir A, *et al.* Efficacy and safety of simeprevir and sofosbuvir with and without ribavirin in subjects with recurrent genotype 1 hepatitis C post-orthotopic liver transplant: the randomized GALAXY study. *Transpl Int* 2017;30(2):196–208.

41. Nguyen NH, Yee BE, Chang C, Jin M, Lutchman G, Lim JK, *et al.* Tolerability and effectiveness of sofosbuvir and simeprevir in the post-transplant setting: systematic review and meta-analysis. *BMJ Open Gastroenterol* 2016; 3(1):e000066.

42. Brown RS, Jr., O'Leary JG, Reddy KR, Kuo A, Morelli GJ, Burton JR, Jr., *et al.* Interferon-free therapy for genotype 1 hepatitis C in liver transplant recipients: real-world experience from the hepatitis C therapeutic registry and research network. *Liver Transpl* 2016;22(1):24–33.

43. Kwo PY, Mantry PS, Coakley E, Te HS, Vargas HE, Brown R, Jr., *et al.* An interferon-free antiviral regimen for HCV after liver transplantation. *N Engl J Med* 2014;371(25):2375–82.

44. Flisiak R, Janczewska E, Wawrzynowicz-Syczewska M, Jaroszewicz J, Zarebska-Michaluk D, Nazzal K, *et al.* Real-world effectiveness and safety of ombitasvir/paritaprevir/ritonavir ± dasabuvir ± ribavirin in hepatitis C: AMBER study. *Aliment Pharmacol Ther* 2016;44(9):946–56.

45. Leroy V, Dumortier J, Coilly A, Sebagh M, Fougerou-Leurent C, Radenne S, *et al.* Efficacy of sofosbuvir and daclatasvir in patients with fibrosing cholestatic hepatitis C after liver transplantation. *Clin Gastroenterol Hepatol* 2015;13(11):1993–2001 e1–2.

46. Bzowej N, Nelson DR, Terrault NA, Everson GT, Teng LL, Prabhakar A, *et al.* PHOENIX: a randomized controlled trial of peginterferon alfa-2a plus ribavirin as a prophylactic treatment after liver transplantation for hepatitis C virus. *Liver Transpl* 2011;17(5):528–38.

47. Levitsky JL, Verna EC, O'Leary JG, *et al.* Perioperative ledipasvir–sofosbuvir for HCV in liver-transplant recipients. *N Engl J Med* 2016;375:2106–8.

48. Terrault NA, Shrestha R, Satapathy SK, Linda S, Rosenau J, O'Leary JG, *et al.* Prevention of recurrent hepatitis C in liver transplant (LT) recipients with Civacir®: preliminary results on safety and efficacy, including patients with renal/liver dysfunction. *Hepatology* 2015;62(Suppl 1):310A.

49. Tawar RG, Heydmann L, Bach C, Schuttrumpf J, Chavan S, King BJ, *et al.* Broad neutralization of hepatitis C virus-resistant variants by Civacir hepatitis C immunoglobulin. *Hepatology* 2016;64(5):1495–506.

50. Tapper EB, Hughes MS, Buti M, Dufour JF, Flamm S, Firdoos S, *et al.* The optimal timing of hepatitis C therapy in transplant eligible patients with Child B and C cirrhosis: a cost-effectiveness analysis. *Transplantation* 2017; 101(5):987–95.

51. Njei B, McCarty TR, Fortune BE, and Lim JK. Optimal timing for hepatitis C therapy in US patients eligible for liver transplantation: a cost-effectiveness analysis. *Aliment Pharmacol Ther* 2016;44(10):1090–101.

52. Chhatwal J, Samur S, Kues B, Ayer T, Roberts MS, Kanwal F, *et al.* Optimal timing of hepatitis C treatment for patients on the liver transplant waiting list. *Hepatology* 2017;65(3):777–88.

53. Schaefer EA and Chung RT. Anti-hepatitis C virus drugs in development. *Gastroenterology* 2012;142(6):1340–50 e1.

54. Verna EC. The dynamic landscape of liver transplant in the era of effective HCV therapy. *Hepatology* 2017;65(3):763–6.

13. Obesity in Liver Transplantation

Michele Molinari* and Subhashini Ayloo[†]

*Department of Surgery, Thomas Starzl Transplant Institute,
University of Pittsburgh, Pittsburgh, PA, USA
[†]Department of Surgery, Rutgers New Jersey Medical School,
Newark, NJ, USA

1. Introduction

Over the last few decades, the incidence and prevalence of obesity, nonalcoholic fatty liver disease (NAFLD) and nonalcoholic steatohepatitis (NASH) have increased worldwide [1]. Recent epidemiological studies have shown that 35.7% of the adults currently living in the USA are obese, 30% have NAFLD, and 12% are affected by NASH [2, 3]. As a consequence, the indication for liver transplant(ation) (LT) for NASH has risen from 1.2% to 9.7% and is currently the third most common cause of liver failure with the prediction to become the leading indication by 2025 [4]. These statistics [5] deserve particular attention since the number of individuals affected by liver failure and obesity has increased at a higher pace than the rate of available organs. The discrepancy between demand and offer of liver grafts has risen some concerns that patients in need of a LT for NAFLD and NASH might, one day, exhaust the pool of grafts available for other recipients [5]. There are also concerns about the rise incidence of steatosis in deceased donors and the overall declining quality of liver grafts. Since a large number of transplant programs are facing the epidemics of obesity, the primary aim of this chapter is to review the most current literature on the short- and long-term effects of obesity in LT, and the possible strategies that might enhance the quality of steatotic grafts from obese patients and improve patients' outcomes.

2. Definition of obesity

Obesity is defined by the World Health Organization [6] as the presence of excessive body fat that poses health risks. Although it has many limitations, body mass index (BMI) is the most common metric used to stratify patients in different categories by normalizing their weight to their height. Individuals with a BMI $\geq$30 kg/m^2 are defined as obese and individuals with a BMI $\geq$40 kg/m^2 are categorized as morbidly obese.

3. The effects of obesity on the liver

Among many of the metabolic abnormalities associated with obesity, dysregulation of insulin [7] is responsible for the abnormal deposition of fat in the liver with subsequent chronic inflammation and fibrosis [7, 8]. Major predisposing factors for the dysregulation of insulin are sedentary lifestyle, modern western nutrition, and genetic predisposition [9]. In a study of adults selected from the general population in Northern Italy, abdominal ultrasounds (US) showed fatty livers in 10–15% of individuals with normal BMI and 76% of obese participants [10] corroborating the hypothesis that excessive visceral and upper body fat plays a primary role in the pathogenesis of NAFLD [11]. In the adipose tissue, insulin resistance prevents the suppression of lipolysis with an increase in the production of free fatty acids [12–14]. When free fatty acids are not sufficiently oxidized, and accumulate in the body, they form intracytoplasmic lipid droplets containing diacylglycerols (DAGs) causing mitochondrial dysfunction [15]. Using stable isotope techniques, Donnelly *et al.* [16] have shown that, 59% of triglycerides found in steatotic livers originated from patients' own adipose tissue, 26% were formed *de novo* by lipogenesis, and 15% originated from dietary intake [14, 17, 18]. Liver injury occurs when the process of oxidant stress and lipotoxicity are long enough to activate intracellular stress kinases, apoptosis, and fibrogenesis [9].

The liver is not the only organ affected by chronic inflammation from excessive fat. Patients with NASH have also inflammatory changes in their peripheral adipose tissues where macrophages are upregulated by adipokines and cytokines that are downregulated by physical exercise and weight loss [9].

In 2–3% of patients, NASH leads to hepatic fibrosis that can progress to cirrhosis, liver failure, and hepatocellular carcinoma (HCC) [9]. Genetic factors seem to play a role since NASH is more common in patients who are Hispanic, females and with a positive family history for NASH [19–21]. Other factors that might contribute to the disease remain poorly understood [9]. In a meta-analysis [22] of 10 studies including a total of 221 patients, the strongest predictor of disease progression was the degree of necrosis and inflammation identified at the initial liver biopsy [19–21].

Besides NASH, obesity is a risk modifier in other liver diseases [23]. For example, obese patients have a lower response rate to interferon therapy for the treatment of HCV [24] and higher recurrence rates after initial response [25–27]. In comparison to normal weight patients, overweight and obese individuals produce higher levels of circulating C-reactive protein and IL-6 that are responsible for a systemic inflammatory status [28] that predisposes HCV patients to develop hepatic fibrosis [28]. Similar profibrotic effects might also occur in patients with nonviral hepatic diseases such as familial hemochromatosis or alcohol-induced liver disease [29].

4. Obesity-induced comorbidities

Several pathologies are associated with the presence of extra fat in obese patients (Table 1). Approximately 30% of people affected by morbid obesity develop structural and functional changes that lead to cardiomyopathy [30, 31]. In a recent meta-analysis, Mottillo *et al.* [32] have found that individuals with metabolic syndrome have a two-fold risk for cardiovascular and cerebral diseases compared to the rest of the population. The risk is even higher when obese patients have hypertension or decreased renal function [33–35].

5. Preoperative cardiac assessment

For LT recipients, cardiovascular complications represent the leading cause of nongraft-related mortality [36]. A key aspect of preventing poor outcomes for obese candidates is to identify those who are at a prohibitive cardiovascular risk. Coronary artery screening is performed, and patients undergo an extensive clinical history in addition to a standard 12-lead EKG and a transthoracic or transesophageal echocardiogram [37]. For the majority of nonobese patients, coronary angiograms are obtained only when patients have symptoms or findings suggestive of coronary artery insufficiency. Since most of the

Table 1. Common comorbidities observed in obese patients.

System	Comorbidity
Cardiovascular	Coronary artery disease
	Arterial hypertension
	Hypercoagulable state
	Cor pulmonale
	Cardiomyopathy
Pulmonary	Obstructive sleep apnea
	Restrictive lung disease
	Pulmonary embolism
Renal	Acute renal insufficiency
	Chronic renal dysfunction/insufficiency
	Urinary tract infections
Musculoskeletal	Arthrosis
	Osteoarthritis
	Osteoporosis
	Compression vertebral fractures
	Chronic back pain
Nervous	Sympathetic hyperactivity
	Increased risk for stroke
	Peripheral neuropathy
Metabolic	Diabetes
	Hypercholesterolemia
	Hypertriglyceridemia

obese patients have multiple risk factors for cardiovascular complications and very few can exercise to develop symptoms of coronary insufficiency during moderate to vigorous physical activity, obese patients require coronary angiograms to rule out critical stenosis or occlusions of the coronary arteries, presence of pulmonary hypertension, or abnormal contractility if considered otherwise suitable for LT [38].

6. Intraoperative and perioperative risks for obese recipients

Obesity represents a challenge not only for the surgical team but also for the anesthesiologists. Obese patients often have short and thick necks and require special skills and anesthesia techniques such as the use of fiberoptic bronchoscopy to guide the correct placement of endotracheal tubes [39]. Also, placement of arterial and venous access catheters for intraoperative monitoring is quite challenging as obesity makes identification of vascular structures difficult and more susceptible to iatrogenic injuries [39]. Also, obesity alters the distribution and response to anesthetic drugs particularly for lipophilic medications and gasses that face a large volume of distribution and unpredictable clearance [34, 40–42]. During surgery, and in the postoperative period, obese patients are at an increased risk for deep venous thrombosis [43], thromboembolic events [40], and pulmonary complications [40, 44]. Fat accumulation of the upper body reduces their chest wall and lung compliance in addition to the fact that the diaphragm is pressed upward by intra-abdominal adipose tissue and ascites. All these changes produce a restrictive pattern with patients becoming less tolerant of positional changes with frequent hypoxic spells commonly seen at the time of induction of general anesthesia and at the time of endotracheal extubation [45]. Often, obese patients have other pulmonary comorbidities, including airway hyperreactivity, sleep apnea, hypoventilation syndrome, and pulmonary hypertension that contribute to the challenges faced by the anesthesiology team during the operation and by the intensivists in the early perioperative period [46]. Postoperatively, the primary respiratory concerns for obese patients are related to their increased risk of hypoxemia and respiratory failure related to opioid-enhanced central respiratory depression, upper airway obstruction, and hypoventilation atelectasis [46]. Other common, but not life-threatening surgical complications seen in obese patients include poor wound healing and impaired drug clearance. The increased risk of wound infections is multifactorial [47]. In comparison to normal weight individuals, obese patients have lower levels of tissue oxygenation, insulin resistance with reduced immune function that play an important role for the normal wound healing [48]. Recent studies have shown that severely obese patients undergoing LT suffer from a significant increase in early postoperative wound infections (20% vs. 4%; $p = 0.0001$) and wound dehiscence (40% vs. 1.2%; $p = 0.0001$) in comparison to normal-weight recipients [49]. In addition, during the first year after LT, obese patients have an increased risk of hernias when compared to nonobese recipients (30% vs. 2.8%; $p = 0.0001$) [49]. Other minor wound problems such as superficial wound infections, seromas, hematomas, and fat necrosis are frequently observed in obese patients due to the thickness of the subcuticular adipose tissue that is inadequately vascularized and at an increased risk of mechanical trauma, dehydration, and exposure to airborne bacteria due to longer operative times [39].

7. Outcomes of obese patients undergoing liver transplantation (LT)

The effect of obesity on outcomes of patients undergoing LT remains a very controversial topic. All available studies are retrospective, with various quality of reporting and statistical methodology, and with heterogeneous populations since immunosuppression protocols and perioperative care have changed over the years. Dick *et al.* [50] found that the perioperative mortality for obese patients was extremely high (>30%) in the first era of LT (1987–1992) in comparison to 15% in most recent years (2002–2007); however it continued to be higher than in nonobese recipients [50].

Intuitively, obese patients should have inferior outcomes in comparison to nonobese recipients since obesity is associated with many comorbidities including diabetes, cardiovascular and pulmonary dysfunction that have been linked to higher risks of perioperative morbidity and overall mortality [51–57]. There are an increasing number of studies that have contradicted these assumptions (Table 2).

Due to the lack of randomized trials, the results of available studies are difficult to interpret as obese recipients who underwent LT are a very selected group of patients, and each study reports the experience of single centers or data from registries where selection and reporting bias certainly played an important role. Therefore, in the absence of well-designed randomized controlled trials, determining if obesity is indeed an independent factor for increased perioperative mortality and inferior long-term survival after LT is very challenging and there is no consensus among transplant specialists [58].

Historically, Keeffe *et al.* [59] were one of the first transplant groups reporting the outcomes of 276 LT recipients stratified by their BMI who were operated between 1988 and 1992 at California Pacific Medical Centre. The authors found that in 18 obese patients (BMI >30), LT was feasible and relatively safe with no increased perioperative mortality. Two years later, in 1996, Braunfeld *et al.* [60] compared the outcomes of obese patients (n. 40) undergoing LT at UCLA vs. nonobese recipients (n. 61) and found that there were no differences in reoperations, need for retransplantation, ICU and overall hospital stay, 30-day survival and 1-year survival between the two groups. The authors concluded that morbid obesity alone was not a predisposing factor for increased complications or decreased survival after LT.

During the following years, several other studies were published on the outcomes of obese recipients of LTs.

One of the first large studies that raised concerns about the outcomes of obese LT recipients was published in 2002 by Nair *et al.* [61]. The authors

Table 2. Summary of the risk ratio reported by recent studies that compared survival of obese *vs.* nonobese patients who underwent LT over two decades (1994–2013). Risk ratios between the two groups were not statistically significant.

Author	Medical center	Year	Number of patients	Study design	Risk ratio (95% confidence interval)	p value
Keeffe *et al.*	California Pacific Medical Center, California, USA	1994	276	Retrospective single center	7.08 (0.46, 108.6)	n.s.
Braunfeld *et al.*	University of California, Los Angeles, USA	1996	101	Retrospective single center	0.72 (0.47, 1.09)	n.s.
Sawyer *et al.*	University of Virginia, Virginia, USA	1999	277	Retrospective single center	0.76 (0.45, 1.29)	n.s.
Nair *et al.*	The Johns Hopkins University, Baltimore, Maryland, USA	2001	121	Retrospective cohort UNOS database	0.63 (0.31, 1.29)	n.s.
Hillingso *et al.*	Department of Surgical Gastroenterology and Liver Transplantation, Center of Abdominal Disease, Copenhagen	2005	40	Retrospective single center	0.38 (0.17, 0.88)	n.s.
Fujikawa *et al.*	University of Florida, Florida, USA	2006	700	Retrospective single center	1.18 (0.95, 1.48)	n.s.
Boin *et al.*	Faculty of Medical Science Campus, Brazil	2007	244	Retrospective single center	1.07 (0.76, 1.50)	n.s.
Leonard *et al.*	Mayo Clinic, Rochester, Minnesota, USA	2008	1,313	Retrospective cohort NIDDK LT database	1.13 (0.75, 1.69)	n.s.
Dick *et al.*	University of Washington, Seattle, Washington, USA	2009	71,446	Retrospective cohort UNOS database	1.23 (1.15, 1.30)	n.s.
Werneck *et al.*	Hospital Israelita Albert Einstein, San Paolo, Brazil	2011	136	Retrospective single center	0.84 (0.35, 2.04)	n.s.
La Mattina *et al.*	University of Wisconsin, Ann Arbor, Wisconsin, USA	2012	788	Retrospective single center	0.81 (0.59, 1.10)	n.s.
Perez-Protto *et al.*	Cleveland Clinic, Cleveland, USA	2013	230	Retrospective single center	0.91 (0.51, 1.64)	n.s.
Hakeem *et al.*	St James's University, Leeds, UK	2013	908	Retrospective single center	1.08 (0.75, 1.57)	n.s.

Note: n.s. nonsignificant.

analyzed a total of 18,172 LT patients transplanted in the USA between 1988 and 1996. Morbidly obese recipients had higher primary graft dysfunction and perioperative mortality at 1, 2, and 5 years in comparison to nonobese recipients due to cardiovascular events.

Another group led by LaMattina *et al.* [62] reported the perioperative morbidity of 813 LT patients transplanted at the University of Wisconsin in the period between 1997 and 2008, and found that obese patients had prolonged mean operative time (class I obesity: 7.7 hours, p = 0.009; class II obesity: 7.9 hours, p = 0.008; class III obesity: 8.2 h, p = 0.003 vs. normal weight: 7.2 hours), ICU stay (class II obesity: 4.1 days vs. 2.6 days; p = 0.04), higher number of blood transfusions (class I obesity: 15 units, p = 0.005; class II obesity: 16 units, p = 0.005; class III obesity: 15 units, p = 0.08 vs. normal weight: 11 units), higher incidence of infections (HR 7.21, CI: 1.6–32.4, p = 0.01), biliary complications requiring intervention (class II obesity: HR 2.04, CI: 1.27–3.3, p = 0.003) and, more importantly, decreased patient (class II obesity: HR 1.82, CI: 1.09–3.01, p = 0.02) and graft survivals (class II obesity: HR 1.62, CI: 1.02–2.65, p = 0.04).

Similar outcomes were observed in 1,325 obese LT recipients [63] in the United Kingdom where increased infectious complications, and longer ICU and hospital stay were observed in obese recipients when compared to normal weight patients. In another study of 73,538 LT recipients, the overall survival was significantly lower in patients with BMI higher than 40 and lower than 18.5, compared to the control group [50].

More recently, because of the increasing attention to optimizing patient outcome, Bambha *et al.* [64] addressed the question whether individuals with elevated BMI and high Model for End-Stage Liver Disease (MELD) have inferior outcomes in comparison to recipients with lower BMI (Table 3). Using UNOS data of all adult recipients of primary LT from March 2002 to September 2011, they identified 45,551 recipients. They stratified patients by BMI, gender, age, MELD, donor risk index and found that after adjustments at multivariable analysis, elevated BMI was not associated with increased risk of death or graft loss. The authors concluded that overweight and obese LT recipients do not have an increased risk of perioperative mortality or graft loss regardless of their MELD score at the time of transplantation [64].

Another group led by Perez-Protto *et al.* [65] compared graft and patient survival after LT of 47 obese patients and 183 normal-weight patients operated at the Cleveland Clinic between April 2005 and June 2011. After

Table 3. Summary of outcomes of the most recent observational studies comparing obese vs. nonobese patients undergoing LT (2013–2016).

Author	Medical center	Year	Number of patients	Study design	Outcomes	Findings	Authors' conclusions
Ayloo *et al.*	Dalhousie University, Halifax, Nova Scotia, Canada	2016	48,281	Retrospective cohort UNOS database	Impact of BMI on short- and long-term outcome of adult LT recipients	BMI <18.5 (no. of patients = 914) Median survival 11.5 years (95% CI 10.4–12.7) BMI 18.5–24.9 (no. of patients = 14,529) Median survival 13.1 years (95% CI 12.6–13.6) BMI 25–29.9 (no. of patients = 16,724) Median survival 12.8 years (95% CI 12.5–13.2) BMI 30–34.9 (no. of patients = 9,944) Median survival 12.4 years (95% CI 11.9–12.8)	After adjustment, BMI category remained a predictor for in hospital, 90-day and 1-year mortality. After adjustment for recipients' and donors' characteristics, cold- and warm-ischemia time, year of transplantation, underweight status and class III obesity remained significant predictors for lower survival in comparison to normal weight recipients.

(Continued)

Table 3. (*Continued*)

Author	Medical center	Year	Number of patients	Study design	Outcomes	Findings		Authors' conclusions
Terjimanian et al.	University of Michigan, Ann Arbor, Michigan, USA	2016	348	Retrospective single center	The relationship between body composition and survival after LT	BMI 35–39.9 (no. of patients = 4,438)	Median survival 12.2 years (95% CI 11.6–12.9)	Abdominal adiposity is associated with survival after LT, especially in patients with small trunk muscle size.
						BMI ≥40 (no. of patients = 1,732)	Median survival 11.3 years (95% CI 10.3–12.3)	
						High fat low muscle ratio (no. of patients = 85)	1-year survival 71.8%; 5-year survival 36.9%	
						Low fat small muscle ratio (no. of patients = 88)	1-year survival 81.8%; 5-year survival 58.2%	
						High fat large muscle ratio (no. of patients = 90)	1-year survival 91.1%; 5-year survival 68.4%	
						Low fat large muscle ratio (no. of patients = 85)	1-year survival 95.3%; 5-year survival 76.0%	

Andert et al.	Uniklinik RWTH Aachen, Germany	2016	163	Retrospective single center	Comparison of early allograft dysfunction and primary nonfunction of LT recipients receiving organs from donors with different BMI	Donor BMI <30 (no. of patients = 111)	Median hospital stay 30 days, early allograft dysfunction 33.3%; primary graft nonfunction 3.6%; 30-day patient survival 96.4%; 1-year patient survival 90.1%.	Significant difference among the donor BMI groups occurred only during the first three postoperative days. Optimal patient management intraoperatively and in the ICU can compensate these differences without causing permanent adverse outcomes for the recipients. Grafts from obese donors can safely be transplanted.
						Donor BMI 30–39 (no. of patients = 31)	Median hospital stay 33 days, early allograft dysfunction 64.5%; primary graft nonfunction 0%; 30-day patient survival 96.8%; 1-year patient survival 87.1%	
						Donor BMI >40 (no. of patients = 15)	Median hospital stay 25 days, early allograft dysfunction 26.7%; primary graft nonfunction 0%; 30-day patient survival 100%; 1-year patient survival 100%	

(Continued)

Table 3. (*Continued*)

Author	Medical center	Year	Number of patients	Study design	Outcomes		Findings	Authors' conclusions
Triguero *et al.*	Virgen de las Nieves University Hospital, Granada, Spain	2016	180	Retrospective single center	Short- and long-term survival and morbidity in obese patients compared to normal-weight LT recipients	BMI 20–25 (no. of patients = 36)	Portal vein thrombosis 13.9%; overall mortality 38.9%	There was a significant increase in mortality and portal vein thrombosis in obese patients undergoing LT. There were no significant differences of complications, length of stay in ICU, overall hospital stay between obese and nonobese recipients.
						BMI >35 (no. of patients = 11)	Portal vein thrombosis 36.5%; overall mortality 72.7%	
Febrero *et al.*	Regional Transplant Centre, Murcia, Spain	2015	343 (total number of patients in this study), 74 (total number of obese patients)	Retrospective single center	Postoperative respiratory complications	Patients with BMI 30–35 (no. of patients = 59)	5% had respiratory complications with 33% mortality rate	There were no significant differences in short-term respiratory complications between obese LT recipients and recipients with BMI <30.
						BMI >35 (no. of patients = 15)	20% had respiratory complications with 33% mortality rate	
						Control group BMI <30	17% had respiratory complications with 20% mortality rate	

	Year	N					
Wong *et al.*	2015	57,255	Alameda Health System, Oakland, California, USA	Retrospective cohort UNOS database	Survival of patients undergoing LT stratified by BMI and presence or absence of diabetes mellitus at the time of transplantation	BMI 18–24.9	5-year survival 72.5 (95% CI 71.7–73.3)	There was no significant difference in 5-year survival post LT among overweight, class II obese or class III obese patients when compared to patients with normal BMI at the time of transplantation. Presence of diabetes contributed significantly to lower posttransplant survival among patients with class I and II obesity.
						BMI 25–29.3	5-year survival 73.4 (95% CI 72.7–74.2)	
						BMI 30–34.9	5-year survival 74.1 (95% CI 73.1–75)	
						BMI 35–39.9	5-year survival 73.1% (95% CI 71.5–74.6)	
						BMI >40	5-yeear survival 71.4% (95% CI 68.7–74)	
Singhal *et al.*	2015	12,445	University of Cincinnati, Cincinnati, USA	Retrospective cohort SRTR database	Resource utilization and survival outcomes	Patients with BMI <40	Total length of stay 9 days; ICU length of stay 3; mortality 4.1%; readmissions in 30 days 37.8%; direct cost $100,469. With a median follow-up of 2 years, there was no statistically significant difference for overall patient and graft survival between the two groups	Morbid obesity patients have similar survival outcomes to patients with lower BMI. However, they require more healthcare resources and their MELD score at the time of transplantation is higher than patients with lower BMI.
						Patients with BMI ≥40	Total length of stay 11 days; ICU length of stay 3; mortality 4.8%; readmissions in 30 days 39.4%; direct cost $98,541	

(Continued)

Table 3.   (*Continued*)

Author	Medical center	Year	Number of patients	Study design	Outcomes	Findings		Authors' conclusions
Conzen et al.	Washington University, St. Louis, Missouri, USA	2015	758	Retrospective single center	Long-term graft and overall survival stratified by BMI	BMI <18 (no. of patients = 9)	ICU length of stay 6; hospital length of stay 12; re-exploration for bleeding 0%; acute rejection 33.3%	1-year overall survival is 91% for the entire cohort vs. 84.6% for patients with BMI >40 (*p* = n.s). Mean 5-year overall survival for patients with BMI >40 was significantly lower than the rest of the cohort (51.3% vs. 78.8%). Mean 7-year overall survival of patients with BMI >40 was significantly lower than the rest of the cohort (38.5% vs. 71.5%) (*p* = 0.009). Graft survival at 5 and 7 years was significantly decreased for recipients with BMI >40 in comparison to the rest of the cohort (49% vs. 75.8%, and 36.7% vs. 68.4%, respectively; *p* < 0.02).
						BMI 18–24.9 (no. of patients = 210)	ICU length of stay 2; hospital length of stay 7; re-exploration for bleeding 7.1%; acute rejection 24.3%	
						BMI 25–29.9 (no. of patients = 294)	ICU length of stay 2; hospital length of stay 7; re-exploration for bleeding 6.8%; acute rejection 24.8%	
						BMI 30–35 (no. of patients = 169)	ICU length of stay 2; hospital length of stay 7; re-exploration for bleeding 8.9%; acute rejection 16.6%	
						BMI 35.1–40 (no. of patients = 77)	ICU length of stay 3; hospital length of stay 9; re-exploration for bleeding 13%; acute rejection 27.3%	

Bambha *et al.*	University of Colorado, Denver, Colorado, USA and University of California, San Francisco, California, USA	2015	45,551	Retrospective cohort UNOS database	Early outcomes at 3 months and 1 year after LT	BMI <18.5 (no. of patients = 863)	Patient death 3 months post LT 7%; graft loss 3 months post LT 10%; patient death 1 year after LT 16%; graft loss 1 year after LT 19%	Very selected obese patients, even with high MELD scores, do well with LT. Underweight LT recipients with low MELD scores have increased risk for death and graft loss.
						BMI 18.5–24.9 (no. of patients = 13,262)	Patient death 3 months post LT 5%; graft loss 3 months post LT 7%; patient death 1 year after LT 12%; graft loss 1 year after LT 15%	
						BMI 25–29.9 (no. of patients = 16,329)	Patient death 3 months post LT 5%; graft loss 3 months post LT 8%; patient death 1 year after LT 11%; graft loss 1 year after LT 15%	
						BMI 30–34.9 (no. of patients = 9,639)	Patient death 3 months post LT 5%; graft loss 3 months post LT 8%; patient death 1 year after LT 11%; graft loss 1 year after LT 15%	
						BMI >40 (no. of patients = 26)	ICU length of stay 3; hospital length of stay 9; re-exploration for bleeding 7.7%; acute rejection 26.9%	

(Continued)

Table 3. (*Continued*)

Author	Medical center	Year	Number of patients	Study design	Outcomes	Findings	Authors' conclusions
						BMI 35–39.9 (no. of patients = 4,062)	Patient death 3 months post LT 6%; graft loss 3 months post LT 9%; patient death 1 year after LT 12%; graft loss 1 year after LT 16%	
						BMI ≥40 (no. of patients = 1,396)	Patient death 3 months post LT 7%; graft loss 3 months post LT 9%; patient death 1 year after LT 12%; graft loss 1 year after LT 17%	
Younossi et al.	Inova Health System, Falls Church, Virginia, USA	2014	85,194	Retrospective cohort SRTR database	Impact of type 2 diabetes and obesity on the long-term outcomes of LT recipients	Adjusted hazard ratio and 95% confidence intervals calculated for 35,870 adult LT recipients	Pretransplant diabetes was associated with increased mortality HR 1.21 (95% CI 1.12–1.30). Posttransplant diabetes was associated with increased mortality HR 1.06 (95% CI 1.02–1.11). Higher BMI, after adjustment for hypertension and donors' factors, was not associated with posttransplant mortality HR 0.99 (95% CI 0.99–1.00)	Major predictors for patient survival after LT are African American heritage, history of cardiovascular disease, history of type 2 diabetes, history of previous nonhepatic transplantation, hepatitis C, noncompliance. After adjustment, obesity was not associated with increased patients' mortality or risk of graft failure.

Dare *et al.*	Auckland City Hospital, Auckland, New Zealand	2014	202	Retrospective single center	Postoperative complications, length of hospital and ICU stay, patient survival	Obesity CR 1.03; 95% CI 1.01–1.04), diabetes mellitus (CR 1.4; 95% CI 1.16–1.69) and MELD score (CR 1.02; 95% CI 1.00–1.03) were each predictive of a higher postoperative complication rate. Obese patients with concomitant diabetes had hospital stay that was in average 5.8 days longer than nonobese patients. Duration of posttransplant ICU stay was not different in obese vs. nonobese patients. There was no significant survival difference between obese and nonobese patients. Early postoperative morbidity is highest for patients with concomitant obesity and diabetes mellitus. Metabolic risk factors had no effect on 30-day, 1-year, and 5-year patient survival.
Tanaka *et al.*	University of Toronto, Toronto, Ontario, Canada	2013	507	Retrospective single center	Retransplantation and mortality of adult LT recipients	BMI <18.5 (no. of patients = 11) BMI 18.5–25 (no. of patients = 162) ICU stay 2 days; hospital stay 21 days; vascular complications 9% ICU stay 3 days; hospital stay 14 days; vascular complications 5% Patient and graft survival showed that they were statistically significant lower for recipients with BMI >40 or <18.5 when compared to other BMI groups (*p* = 0.038 and *p* = 0.010 respectively).

(Continued)

Table 3. (*Continued*)

Author	Medical center	Year	Number of patients	Study design	Outcomes	Findings	Authors' conclusions
						BMI 25–30 (no. of patients = 185)	ICU stay 2 days; hospital stay 15.5 days; vascular complications 12%	
						BMI 30–35 (no. patients = 105)	ICU stay 2 days; hospital stay 15 days; vascular complications 10%	
						BMI 35–40 (no. patients = 30)	ICU stay 2 days; hospital stay 14.5 days; vascular complications 7%	
						BMI >40 (no. patients = 14)	ICU stay 3 days; hospital stay 26.5 days; vascular complications 8%	
Perez-Protto	Cleveland Clinic, Cleveland Ohio, USA	2013	230	Retrospective cohort UNOS database and perioperative health documentation system at Cleveland Clinics	Patient and graft survival	Obese patients (no. of patients = 47) and nonobese patients (no. of patients = 183)	The estimated hazard ratio for obese patients to experience graft failure or mortality in comparison with patients with normal BMI after transplantation was 1.19 (95% CI 0.85–1.67; p = n.s.). Patient survival at 1 year: 94% obese vs. 78% nonobese patients. At 3 years: 85% obese vs. 76% nonobese patients. At 4 years: 73% obese vs. 73% nonobese patients. Median ICU stay: 4 for obese vs. 3 for	Outcomes were comparable in lean and obese patients undergoing LT. Obesity per se should not exclude patients from consideration for LT. Efforts should be focused on posttransplant behavioral changes to decrease the incidence of metabolic syndrome.

nonobese patients ($p = 0.29$). Median hospital stay: 10 for obese vs. 10 for nonobese patients. Duration of surgery: 9.7 hours for obese vs. 9.3 for nonobese patients ($p = 0.58$). Intraoperative estimated blood loss: 6.2 L for obese vs. 5.0 L for nonobese patients ($p = 0.07$). Cardiovascular adverse events: 15% for obese vs. 6% for nonobese patients ($p = 0.047$). Posttransplantation metabolic syndrome: 46% for obese vs. 21% for nonobese patients ($p < 0.001$)

(*Continued*)

Table 3. *(Continued)*

Author	Medical center	Year	Number of patients	Study design	Outcomes		Findings	Authors' conclusions
Mathur et al.	University of South Florida, Florida, USA	2013	159	Retrospective single center	Survival and complications of patients transplanted for HCC	Patients with BMI <25 (no. of patients = 47)	90-day mortality rate was 3% in nonobese patients, 5% in overweight patients, 4% in obese patients	There was increased incidence of life-threatening complications in overweight (58%) and obese (70%) patients compared to nonobese patients (41%) ($p < 0.05$). The recurrence rate of HCC was doubled in the presence of overweight (15%) and obesity (15%) compared to nonobese patients (7%) ($p < 0.05$).
						Patients with BMI 25–29 (no. of patients = 112)	Primary graft nonfunction was 2% in nonobese patients, 4% in overweight patients, 3% in obese patients	
						Patients with BMI ≥30 (no. of patients = 58)	Mean survival for nonobese patients was 58 months, for overweight patients was 45 months and for obese patients was 41 months	

adjusting for several confounders, the authors did not find any significant differences in graft and patient survival between the two groups. A more recent study by Ayloo *et al.* [66] using UNOS data of adult recipients of cadaveric grafts transplanted for non-HCC liver failure, found that underweight and morbid obese LT recipients had lower survival when compared to the control groups, but these differences were clinically insignificant. Kaplan–Meier curves showed early separation in the first months after LT, resuming a parallel slope after the first year post LT. At 1-year after surgery, 13.6% of class II and 12.4% of class III obese recipients were dead in comparison to 10.6% for normal-weight recipients. Since obesity was associated with an increased mortality in the first year after surgery, Ayloo *et al.* performed an impact analysis of the hypothetical number of lives that could have been saved by allocating grafts only to low perioperative risk groups (normal weight, overweight, and obese class I patients). Using data from 48,281 patients transplanted in the USA between January 1994 until June 2013, the authors found that even in the best hypothetical scenario where all the grafts were allocated to patients with the longest median survival (normal weight recipients), the expected net survival gain for the entire cohort was only 2.7%. The authors concluded that this very limited improvement was due to two main reasons: the first one was that obese and underweight recipients represented only a small proportion of patients, the second one was that the median overall survival of underweight (11.5 years), class II obese (12.2 years), class III obese (11.3 years) was not far from the median overall survival of normal weight recipients (13.1 years) [66].

A recent review of the literature and meta-analysis by Saab *et al.* [58] using data of 2,275 obese patients and 77,212 nonobese recipients from 13 studies showed no significant differences in mortality between the two groups (RR = 0.97; 95% CI 0.82–1.13; $p = 0.66$). However, when survival was compared between obese patients and nonobese recipients with the same cause of liver disease, obesity resulted as a significant risk factor for inferior patient overall survival (RR = 0.69; 95% CI 0.52–0.92; $p = 0.01$).

8. New morphometric instruments

Current measures of obesity are unable to distinguish between lean body mass and adipose tissue. In humans, obesity is not monogenic [67] and current metrics used to stratify patients by using their overall body weight normalized by their height seem inadequate because they do not account for the presence of ascites or decline of muscle mass that is frequently observed in patients with liver disease. Therefore, better morphometric instruments are necessary to better predict the outcomes of obese patients in need of LT.

Terjimanian *et al.* [68] studied the content of adipose tissue in the abdominal cavity of 348 adult LT recipients at the University of Michigan between 2000 and 2011 (Table 3). Visceral fat area was calculated using T12 and L4 as bone landmarks in addition to the psoas area measured at the level of L4. Five-year survival of patients with high fat and small muscle mass was 37%, in comparison to 76% for patients with low fat and large muscle mass (p = 0.023). A similar correlation was noted after 1-year, as patients' survival was lower for the group of patients who had more visceral fat, particularly among those who had smaller trunk musculature. Regression analysis showed that visceral fat area was a significant independent predictor of mortality. This study and other studies suggest that the distribution of body fat and changes in body composition predict more accurately high-risk patients than BMI.

Changes in body composition due to age and liver failure result in a shift toward decreased muscle mass and increased fat [69], a process called sarcopenia [70]. Rubenoff hypothesized that both sarcopenia and obesity have similar biological behavior [71] that can be closely associated with the overall frailty status or LT recipients and their risk of postoperative morbidity and mortality [72].

9. Steatotic liver grafts

9.1. *Rationale for the use of steatotic liver grafts*

Since the rise in demand for LT has is not matched by the increase in the supply of deceased organs, the median pretransplant waiting time among adult patients in the USA has progressively increased from 12.9 months in 2009 to 18.5 months in 2011 [73]. The insufficient number of grafts is responsible for the rate of deaths on the waiting list. One of the strategies to expand the pool of potential donors is the acceptance of organs from individuals who, in the past, were considered unsuitable because of their advanced age, comorbidities, cause of death or suboptimal quality of their organs. The use of livers form extended criteria donors is associated with a higher risk of primary nonfunctioning grafts (PNF), early allograft dysfunction and inferior long-term survival [74]. However, with the experience accumulated over the last decades, most transplant centers are currently using steatotic livers with outcomes comparable to more ideal donors [75] (Table 4).

Table 4. Summary of published studies reporting primary graft nonfunction and 1-year graft survival after liver transplantation using steatotic grafts.

Author	Year	Institution	Macrosteatosis	No. of grafts transplanted	Primary nonfunction (%)	1-year graft survival
Adam et al.	1991	Paul Brousse Hospital, Vellejuif, France	30–60	31	13	—
Ploeg et al.	1993	University of Wisconsin Hospital and Clinics, Madison, USA	30–60	10	0	—
Ploeg et al.	1993	University of Wisconsin Hospital and Clinics, Madison, USA	>60	5	80	—
Urena et al.	1998	University Hospital 12 de Octubre, Madrid, Spain	30–60	27	0	—
Urena et al.	1998	University Hospital 12 de Octubre, Madrid, Spain	>60	4	50	—
De Carlis et al.	1999	Ospedale Niguarda, Milano, Italy	>60	21	66	—
Canelo et al.	1999	Georg-August-Universitat, Gottingen, Germany	30–60	14	14	—
Canelo et al.	1999	Georg-August-Universitat, Gottingen, Germany	>60	10	10	—
Busquets et al.	2001	Ciutat Sanitaria I Universitaria de Bellvitge, University of Barcelona, Spain	30–60	10	0	—
Zamboni et al.	2001	Molinette Hospital, Turin, Italy	>25	8	75	—
Verran et al.	2003	Royal Prince Alfred Hospital, Sydney, Australia	30–60	25	0	60
Alfonso et al.	2004	German Hospital, San Paulo, Brazil	>60	3	0	—
Briceno et al.	2005	Hospital Reina Sofia, Cordoba, Spain	30–60	67	1.5	—
McCormack et al.	2007	HPB Centre, Zurich, Switzerland	30–60	6	0	100
McCormack et al.	2007	HPB Centre, Zurich, Switzerland	>60	20	5	95
Nickeghbalian et al.	2007	Nemazee Hospital Shiraz, Iran	30–60	34	18	73
Reddy et al.	2008	Freeman Hospital, Newcastle upon Tyne, United Kingdom	30–60	10	10	—

(Continued)

Table 4. (Continued)

Author	Year	Institution	Macrosteatosis	No. of grafts transplanted	Primary nonfunction (%)	1-year graft survival
Angele et al.	2008	Klinikum Gosshader, Munich, Germany	30–60	36	4	77
Noujaim et al.	2009	Hospital Beneficencia Portuguesa, San Paolo, Brazil	30–60	6	0	53
Noujaim et al.	2009	Hospital Beneficencia Portuguesa, San Paolo, Brazil	>60	5	20	—
Burra et al.	2009	University of Padova, Padova, Italy	30–60	11	0	—
Li et al.	2009	West China Hospital Chengdu, China	20–40	18	5.6	90
Frongillo et al.	2009	Gemelli Hospital, Rome, Italy	30–60	3	33	3
Noujaim et al.	2009	Hospital Beneficencia Portuguesa, San Paolo, Brazil	30–60	6	0	50
Gao et al.	2009	Zhejiang University School of Medicine, Hangzhou, China	30–60	24	0	92
Doyle et al.	2010	Washington University, St. Louis, USA	30–60	22	0	81
Deroose et al.	2011	Erasmus Medical Center, Rotterdam, The Netherlands	30–60	19	0	95
Deroose et al.	2011	Erasmus Medical Center, Rotterdam, The Netherlands	>60	15	13	94
Gabrielli et al.	2012	Pontificia Universidad Catolica de Chile, Santiago, Chile	30–60	6	9	—
Gabrielli et al.	2012	Pontificia Universidad Catolica de Chile, Santiago, Chile	>60	2	20	—
Teng et al.	2012	Tianjin Medical University, Tianjin, China	30–60	6	0	—
de Graaf et al.	2012	University of Groningen Medical School, Groningen, The Netherlands	30–60	7	0	100
de Graaf et al.	2012	University of Groningen Medical School, Groningen, The Netherlands	>60	2	50	25
Chavin et al.	2013	Medical University of South Carolina, Charleston, USA	30–60	27	0	81
Chavin et al.	2013	Medical University of South Carolina, Charleston, USA	>60	11	0	82
Wong et al.	2016	University of Hong Kong, Pokfulam, Hong Kong	>60	19	0	100

9.2. *Characteristics of steatosis*

Histologically, hepatic steatosis is classified as macrovescicular or microvescicular depending on the visual appearance of the hepatic biopsies [76]. Macrovescicular steatosis has large fat droplets occupying more than half of the hepatocyte, usually causing displacement of the nucleus that is pushed to the edges of the cell [75]. Microvescicular steatosis, instead, presents an accumulation of less than $1 \mu m$ fat droplets with foamy appearance without nuclear displacement [75, 76].

The degree of steatosis is quantitatively classified into mild (<30%), moderate (30–60%) or severe (>60%) [77] and it is calculated by the percentage of hepatocytes that contain droplets. This is often reported using an objective histological scoring system that has been validated by Kleiner *et al.* in 2005 [78]. Steatosis increases the sensitivity to cold ischemia and ischemia/reperfusion injury of the grafts [79] because of the increased lipid peroxidation and enhanced proinflammatory response [80, 81].

9.3. *Macroscopic assessment of liver grafts*

The assessment of the quality of steatotic liver grafts can be challenging for the retrieving transplant team. The visual inspection is able to provide information on the color of the liver and the acuity or bluntness of the edges of the liver. However, these characteristics are very subjective and unreliable as shown by a recent study by Rey *et al.* [82] Radiological characteristics of CT scans or MRI are more objective but these imaging modalities are not routinely available before the organs are procured or allocated [83].

Histological analysis by a pathologist remains the gold standard to assess the quality and quantity of steatosis in liver grafts [84, 85]. Nevertheless, fat in the liver is heterogeneously distributed and there is interobserver variability among pathologists [76, 85]. Therefore, when a liver biopsy is performed before the decision to use a steatotic graft, it is recommended that two biopsies are obtained from both lobes to increase the accuracy of the pathological reading [86].

9.4. *Outcomes of steatotic liver grafts*

Data to guide the decision whether to use or discard a steatotic graft is quite limited. Early studies by Ploeg *et al.* [77] and De Carlis *et al.* [87] reported primary graft nonfunction (PGNF) in 80% and 66% of recipients of livers with severe (>60%) steatosis. Because of the concerns of PGNF and inferior graft survival, a survey study by Imber *et al.* in 2002 has shown that the majority of transplant surgeons in the USA would hesitate to use a liver graft with severe steatosis [88]. Among some of the characteristics associated with poor 1-year graft survival, there was the presence of ≥30% macrovescicular steatosis on postperfusion liver biopsy [89].

In recent years, however, several groups have reported acceptable patients' and grafts' outcomes after the use of liver grafts characterized by moderate or severe steatosis [75, 90–93] (Table 4). Wong *et al.* [75] from the University of Hong Kong analyzed the data of all patients who underwent brain-dead donor LT in their institution from 1991 to 2013. Among 373 adult LT recipients, 19 (5%) received liver grafts with macrovescicular steatosis present in ≥60% of hepatocytes. Among the control group, 155 patients received grafts with no macrovescicular steatosis, 167 had ≤30% steatosis and 32 patients had moderate (30–60%) steatosis. The authors found that there were no differences in 30-day and in-hospital mortality between the group of patients who received a ≥60% steatotic liver and the comparison group (0% for steatotic grafts vs. 3.1% for nonsteatotic grafts). Also, there were no significant differences between the two groups regarding hepatic artery thrombosis, perioperative bleeding, biliary anastomotic complications, and renal dysfunction or postreperfusion syndrome. Overall patients' survival at 1 year and 3 years for patients who received steatotic grafts was similar to the control group (95% vs. 92% at 1 year and 95% vs. 86% at 3 years). Grafts and patients' survivals were also comparable between the two groups regardless of the MELD scores at the time of transplantation. The authors concluded that despite the severity of steatosis present in liver grafts, they observed excellent perioperative and long-term outcomes. Therefore, they suggested that grafts with ≥60% macrovescicular steatosis should not routinely be discarded and should be considered, on an individual basis, for patients who can be transplanted with short cold ischemia time (ideally less than 7 hours). One of the limitations of this study is the small number of patients who received severe steatotic livers, in addition to the fact that most of the donors with severe macrovescicular steatosis were relatively young (median age 42 years) and with low BMI (24.2). These characteristics are not frequently observed in Western transplant centers and the results of this study might not be generalizable to western centers. In pediatric LT recipients, Perito *et al.* [126] reported that children receiving adult donor livers with BMI >35 had increased risk of graft loss and death. On the other hand, pediatric recipients receiving a liver from an overweight or obese pediatric donor did not show the same increase in graft loss or mortality [127]. Yoo *et al.* [128] reported on the effect of donor obesity on recipients' outcome in the adult population. They determined that severe donor obesity or moderate steatosis did not influence short- or long-term outcomes [128]. Beal *et al.* [129] analyzed the United Network of Organ Sharing (UNOS) database to assess the impact of donors' BMI on the outcome of LT recipients stratified by BMI. A total of 51,556 patients were included with a total of 5,044 obese recipients (9.7%) transplanted with a liver graft from an obese donor. The author found that mortality at 30 days was significantly higher in the obese recipients who received a graft from obese donors in comparison to the other group or patients ($p < 0.001$). However, the survival crossed over at the 3-month mark, with no statistical significant differences in survival at 30 days and 1 year after LT ($p = 0.08$). A multivariable Cox proportional hazards model showed that the lowest mortality hazards were found among obese recipients who received a nonobese donor's liver grafts.

The authors concluded that obesity represented a disadvantage in the very early period after LT but that the disadvantage disappeared and became a relative survival advantage 3 months post LT.

Chu and colleagues [94] performed a systematic review of all available studies reporting the outcomes of LT recipients of steatotic grafts. All the 34 included were retrospective, single-center studies published between 1991 and 2013. The incidence of primary nonfunction graft and 1-year graft and patient survival were comparable between the groups of patients who received steatotic livers vs. recipients who received nonsteatotic grafts [94]. However, there appeared to be a trend towards higher rates of primary nonfunctioning grafts and lower graft survival rates in the moderately and severe steatotic liver graft recipients [94].

As the current evidence is limited, the degree of acceptable hepatic steatosis varies among transplant centers and depends on many variables including the clinical experience of health-care providers, the rate of organ donation and the mortality rate of patients on the waiting list, the ability to accept low but still real risks of suboptimal outcomes, and the clinical conditions of potential recipients. Generally, ≤30% steatotic livers are not associated with poor graft outcome [76]. Steatotic livers with ≥60% steatosis are generally discarded while grafts with 30–60% steatosis might be used for recipients who have reasonable performance status, low MELD scores and who can be transplanted with short ischemia times (ideally less than <7 hours). In addition, it is important to keep in mind that posttransplant outcomes are determined not only by the percentage of steatotic hepatocytes, but more importantly by the quality of steatosis, with the macrovescicular feature being the one associated with the highest risk of PGNF and periop-erative morbidity.

10. Future directions

The epidemic of obesity has forced transplant programs to gain a significant experience in how to manage the medical and surgical needs of obese recip-ients with end-stage organ failure. However, there is consensus that despite the important advances that occurred in the recent decades, there is room for new strategies that could improve the overall health of obese patients on the waiting list and the quality of liver grafts with moderate to severe stea-tosis. Among these strategies, bariatric surgery (BS) and *ex vivo* perfusion machines are the ones that have shown promising results and are predicted to play a clinical role in the near future.

10.1. *Weight-loss strategies for obese transplant candidates*

Obese patients with ESLD should benefit from losing weight as it reduces their risk for cardiovascular diseases, type 2 diabetes mellitus, dyslipidemia, obstructive sleep apnea, wound infections and many other comorbidities. In addition, weight loss might improve their chance of being transplanted. A recent analysis of the United Network for Organ Sharing (UNOS) data [102] has shown that the likelihood of obese patients being transplanted was lower in comparison to normal weight individuals. This finding was also confirmed by another study where patients with NASH cirrhosis referred for LT were more commonly denied for comorbid conditions than their HCV counterparts [103].

There are some legitimate concerns about transplanting obese patients because of their higher risk for perioperative complications [61] and because there is some evidence that they have lower survival rates in comparison to normal-weight patients [4, 104]. However, declining LT to obese patients is against the principle of fairness as LT provides a better survival in compari-son to supportive therapies [65]. Nevertheless, since the number of available grafts is insufficient to the actual needs, transplant programs continue to face the dilemma of choosing between offering transplant surgery to all candidates who are in need or being selective and allocate organs only to candidates who have the best likelihood of short- and long-term survival [64, 66, 105, 106].

10.2. *Behavioral and medical therapy*

Over the last few decades, there have been significant advances in the medical and surgical management of obese patients. The only intervention that has proven to be effective in reducing the extra weight in obese patients is BS. Dieting, physical activity, behavioral therapy, and pharmacotherapy are acceptable but poorly effective options for the treatment of obese patients. The Food and Drug Administration (FDA) has approved orlistat, lorcaserin, and phentermine–topiramate for weight loss but not for cirrhotic patients [95]. Orlistat (Xenical®) acts by blocking gastric and pancreatic lipases and inhibits triglycerides absorption. Lorcaserin HCl (Belviq®) suppresses the appetite and promotes satiety by acting as an agonist for serotonin receptors in the hypothalamus. Finally, phentermine–topiramate (Qsymia®) decreases appetite by a catecholamine effect in the central nervous system [96].

Medically supervised weight loss (MSWL) has a low success rate [96–99] as patients fail to maintain their desired weight [100]. Additionally, possible interactions between immunosuppressive medications and drugs used to reduce BMI are unknown [101] and further research is needed before weight-loss medications can be recommended either before or after LT.

10.3. *Bariatric surgery for liver transplant (LT) candidates*

Theoretically, weight-loss interventions would reduce their risk of suboptimal outcomes and may prevent the development of MS and recurrent NASH after LT. On the other hand, perioperative morbidity and mortality risks might be too high to justify any surgery to reduce their BMI. The potential benefits of BS for patients in need of a LT have not been studied in randomized trials and the only available evidence is based on retrospective observational studies.

Adjustable gastric banding (AGB) is a relatively simple procedure that does not require the rerouting of the gastrointestinal tract and maintains the endoluminal access to the biliary system for endoscopic treatment of biliary complications. AGB has no risks of anastomotic dehiscence and it is reversible. The main drawback of AGB is the presence of a foreign body that could become infected and cause long-term complications from slippage, prolapse, port-site infection and erosion into the stomach with potential serious consequences especially in immunocompromised patients. Other potential issues with AGB are that the band is positioned near the gastroesophageal junction where varices from chronic portal hypertension usually develop, and the band could prevent access to the supraceliac aorta for arterial reconstructions if necessary.

Roux-en-Y gastric bypass (RYGB) and duodenal switch (DS) are more effective than AGB, but have significantly higher perioperative risks of anastomotic leaks, obstructions, marginal ulcers, malabsorption of immunosuppression medications, loss of endoscopic access to the biliary system and are contraindicated for patients who need a Roux limb for their biliary reconstruction.

In recent years, sleeve gastrectomy has been viewed as a good compromise as it has lower perioperative risks in comparison to RYGB or DS [109], maintains direct access to the biliary system, it is unlikely to cause malabsorption of immunosuppression medications [110] and provides a gradual and sustained weight loss [99, 111, 112].

10.4. *Timing for bariatric surgery*

10.4.1. *Before transplant*

The rationale for performing bariatric surgery prior to LT would be the intention of optimizing patients' medical conditions before surgery or to bring patients' BMI within the range considered acceptable by some transplant centers.

However, BS performed before LT might delay transplant surgery due to the time necessary to achieve the desired BMI or to the development of perioperative complications. Another drawback of BS before LT is that recipients undergo two separate operations and two hospitalizations with associated increased financial costs, stress, and pain.

Although no randomized controlled trials have ever been conducted to test whether BS is beneficial for obese patient requiring LT, case reports and observational studies have described the feasibility of BS either pre, during, or post LT. Lin *et al.* [113] published a retrospective review of all SGs performed in liver (20 patients) and kidney transplant candidates (six patients) between 2006 and 2012. The mean excess weight loss (EWL) at 1 month, 3 months, and 12 months was 17%, 26%, and 50% respectively without any perioperative death. Six cases (16%) experienced postoperative complications, including superficial wound infections, staple line leak, bleeding requiring transfusion, transient encephalopathy and renal insufficiency. All these patients became transplantable candidates by meeting institutional BMI requirements at 12 months and the authors concluded that SG is relatively safe and effective.

Similar conclusions were drawn by Takata *et al.* [114] who evaluated the effect of BS in end-stage liver, kidney, and lung disease in 15 obese patients who were considered unsuitable for transplantation. Mean EWL at or after 9 months was 61%, 33%, and 61% respectively. Obesity-associated comorbidities improved in all patients and, except for two individuals (13%) who suffered from perioperative complications, no deaths occurred after surgery. More importantly, 93% of patients became transplant candidates by meeting the institutional requirements on BMI. These authors concluded that laparoscopic RYGB and SG is safe and improves the candidacy for transplantation. With gain in experience in cadaveric LT and BS, feasibility is being evaluated also in living donor LT. Taneja *et al.* [115] published a successful outcome of SG in a patient with BMI of 55.6 and NASH undergoing living-donor LT.

10.4.2. *After transplant*

The main rationale for performing BS after LT would be to prevent the recurrence of NASH and improve survival by reducing obesity-related comorbidities [116]. In a recent publication, Duchini *et al.* [117] described two patients who were successfully treated by RYGB for severe graft dysfunction due to recurrent NASH.

However, BS after LT comes with the risk of dealing with severe adhesions, wound complications and anastomotic or staple lines dehiscences due to the use of steroids and/or m-TOR inhibitors. Despite these potential drawbacks, Lin *et al.* [118] published a pilot study on the safety and feasibility of SG in nine obese LT recipients with the intent to improve steroid-induced diabetes, steatohepatitis, and MS. Postoperative complications occurred in three patients (33%) who developed mesh infection in a concurrent ventral hernia repair, bile leak requiring drainage and one patient who underwent reoperation for dysphagia. At 6 months, 55% EWL was achieved without graft rejection and the authors concluded that SG does not adversely affect LT function. On the other hand, some technical challenges associated with BS after LT were reported by Tichansky *et al.* [119] who described major adhesions with complete obliteration of the gastrohepatic space during a successful laparoscopic RYGB after LT for a patient with a BMI of 54 kg/m^2.

10.4.3. *During liver transplantation (LT)*

Combining BS and LT could theoretically minimize delays, hospital stay and reduce patients' overall pain as the same incision can be used for both operations. However, one of the biggest trade-offs is that the operation for LT will take longer and that patients might suffer from more severe complications due to the increased complexity of the procedure.

Campsen *et al.* [120] performed a successful simultaneous LT and AGB and reported that at 6 months, patients' BMI went from 42 kg/m^2 to 34 kg/m^2 with 45% EWL and resolution of T2DM, hypertension, and osteoarthritis. In 2013, Heimbach *et al.* [121] published their experience of BS in obese patients (BMI ≥35) undergoing LT. Obese patients with a BMI ≥35 were divided into two groups. Patients who successfully completed MSWL underwent LT ($n = 37$) alone. Seven patients who failed MSWL underwent simultaneous LT and SG ($n = 7$). In patients who underwent LT alone, weight regain (BMI >35) was noted in 21 of 34 patients (61%), posttransplant diabetes in 12 patients (35%), steatosis in seven (20%), graft losses and deaths in three (8%). In the group of patients who underwent simultaneous LT and SG ($n = 7$), all maintained their weight loss, one had a gastrointestinal leak from the staple line (14%) and one had excessive weight loss. Although the majority of patients who did not undergo BS achieved some weight loss with a nonsurgical approach, most regained weight within a mean follow-up of 33 months. On the other hand, patients treated with combination of SG and LT achieved effective and sustained weight loss and fewer metabolic complications over a mean follow-up of 17 months.

10.5. *Optimization of steatotic liver grafts*

Given that obesity in the USA and in many other Western countries has increased up to 30% of the general population [3], it is expected that the proportion of steatotic liver grafts will continue to increase causing a decline in the number of eligible grafts [79].

The extent of preservation injury in steatotic livers is mediated by the reduced levels of adenosine triphosphate (ATP) and by the elevated reactive oxygen species (ROS)-related stress that is correlated to the content of intrahepatic triglycerides and the number of macrosteatotic lipid droplets [80, 122, 123].

To improve the quality of fatty grafts, experimental animal models have been developed to study pathways that might optimize their function by minimizing the risk of ischemia/reperfusion stress [79]. Current models have studied new molecules, heat shock preconditioning, ischemic preconditioning, and *ex vivo* perfusion machines [79].

Normothermic *ex vivo* perfusion machines might provide a potential solution for borderline or severely steatotic livers. With normothermic perfusion, organs are maintained in a physiological state without depletion of cellular energy and without accumulation of waste products. This new approach has the potential to enable the assessment of the viability of organs prior to transplantation and reduce the risk of transplanting dysfunctional organs that should be discarded.

Because of the intracytoplasmatic accumulation of lipids, macrosteatotic hepatocytes increase in size causing the narrowing of the sinusoidal space with exacerbation of ischemia reperfusion injury [123]. Animal studies have shown that when steatotic livers have cleared excessive intracellular lipids, they recover the normal response to ischemia/reperfusion stress [80, 90] and that defatting hepatocytes is possible within a few hours using *ex vivo* normothermic perfusion of livers from Zucker rats [124].

The use of perfusion machines is still in the initial phases and has not reached universal acceptance in LT because there are several technical challenges including their weight, costs and above all the risk of failure.

Malfunctions of normothermic perfusion systems with flow interruption come with the risk of graft loss. This is not the case for hypothermic perfusion machines since such systems have a backup static hypothermic mode that replicates simple cold storage [125].

On the other hand, one of the most attractive features of normothermic perfusion machines is their ability to provide the liver graft an environment that promotes a metabolically active state of the organ, giving the transplant team the opportunity of evaluating its function and suitability for transplantation. This is not possible when livers are stored in cold perfusion solutions. Another important advantage for both the cold and normothermic perfusion systems is their ability of prolonging the time between retrieval and transplantation. During this period, the transplant team can modulate and optimize the liver grafts by using new pharmaceutical molecules or other interventions that decrease the percentage of steatosis and improve the quality and function of suboptimal organs.

11. Ethics

Transplantation in obese patients is technically more challenging and requires more resources in comparison to recipients with lower BMI [61, 63] and in the most recent guidelines of the American Association for the Study of Liver Disease [107], class III obesity (BMI ≥ 40 kg/m^2) remains a relative contraindication for LT [64, 66, 106, 108]. Since transplant centers have insufficient number of grafts for all their patients, and they are under an intense scrutiny of their outcomes by several regulatory bodies that demand excellent results, it seems logical to think that avoidance of high-risk groups is a rational response based on the principle of maximizing a very limited resource such as cadaveric liver grafts. However, this position creates an ethical dilemma because even for class III obese recipients undergoing LT, 5-year survival was 71.5% vs. 73.9% for normal weight recipients [66]. Although statistically significant the absolute difference is clinically irrelevant and the exclusion of patients based only on their BMI might be unethical since 5-year survival of obese and underweight LT recipients is higher than 50% that is conventionally considered the minimum survival benefit to justify the allocation of liver grafts to patients with end-stage liver disease [130].

12. Conclusions

The obesity epidemic has a significant impact on the field of transplantation. Over time, the number of obese patients who are in need of an LT has grown with a rate that has mirrored the increasing prevalence of obesity in the general population. Obesity is associated with many comorbidities including cardiopulmonary diseases that are the main causes of perioperative morbidity and mortality in patients undergoing major abdominal surgeries. However, several studies have shown that the outcomes of obese patients who undergo LT are comparable to the outcomes of nonobese recipients with the exception of morbidly obese patients (BMI $\geq$40). There is still controversy regarding the interpretation of these results since they are retrospective and selection bias might have played a significant role. The experience accumulated over the last decades has made LT safer and has improved patients' outcomes; nevertheless, LT in obese patients remains technically challenging not only for the surgeons, but also for anesthesiologists, intensivists, nursing staff, physiotherapists, and many other health-care providers. Therefore, strategies to induce weight loss in obese patients prior to their transplantation are desirable, although hardly applicable.

Obesity not only affects recipients, but it also has an impact on the quality of liver grafts since obesity correlates with the presence of hepatic steatosis. The preoperative use of *ex vivo* perfusion machines, with or without pharmacological or biological compounds, has shown to reduce the percentage of fat in the liver and improve the overall function of borderline grafts. Therefore, we anticipate that the use of pretransplant conditioning using perfusion machines and new medications or biologic molecules will increase the pool of available grafts by rescuing a significant proportion of borderline grafts.

References

1. Agopian VG, Kaldas FM, Hong JC, *et al.* Liver transplantation for nonalcoholic steatohepatitis: the new epidemic. *Ann Surg* 2012;256:624–33.
2. Phongsamran PV, Kim JW, Abbbott JC, and Rosenblatt A. Pharmacotherapy for hepatic encephalopathy. *Drugs* 2010;70:1131–48.
3. Ogden CL, Carroll MD, Kit BK, and Flegal KM. Prevalence of obesity among adults: United States, 2011–2012. NCHS Data Brief 2013:1–8.
4. Charlton MR, Burns JM, Pedersen RA, Watt KD, Heimbach JK, and Dierkhising RA. Frequency and outcomes of liver transplantation for nonalcoholic steatohepatitis in the United States. *Gastroenterology* 2011;141:1249–53.
5. O'Leary JG. Debate — a bridge too far: nonalcoholic fatty liver disease will not exhaust the donor pool. *Liver Transpl* 2014;20(Suppl 2):S38–41.
6. Kopelman PG. Obesity as a medical problem. *Nature* 2000;404:635–43.
7. Choudhury J and Sanyal AJ. Insulin resistance and the pathogenesis of nonalcoholic fatty liver disease. *Clin Liver Dis* 2004;8:575–94, ix.
8. Diehl AM, Clarke J, and Brancati F. Insulin resistance syndrome and nonalcoholic fatty liver disease. *Endocr Pract* 2003;9(Suppl 2):93–6.
9. Schuppan D and Schattenberg JM. Non-alcoholic steatohepatitis: pathogenesis and novel therapeutic approaches. *J Gastroenterol Hepatol* 2013;28(Suppl 1): 68–76.
10. Bellentani S, Tiribelli C, Saccoccio G, *et al.* Prevalence of chronic liver disease in the general population of northern Italy: the Dionysos Study. *Hepatology* 1994;20:1442–9.
11. Marchesini G, Moscatiello S, Di Domizio S, and Forlani G. Obesity-associated liver disease. *J Clin Endocrinol Metab* 2008;93:S74–80.
12. Marchesini G, Brizi M, Morselli-Labate AM, *et al.* Association of nonalcoholic fatty liver disease with insulin resistance. *Am J Med* 1999;107:450–5.
13. Petta S, Miele L, Bugianesi E, *et al.* Glucokinase regulatory protein gene polymorphism affects liver fibrosis in non-alcoholic fatty liver disease. *PLoS ONE* 2014;9:e87523.
14. Bugianesi E, Gastaldelli A, Vanni E, *et al.* Insulin resistance in non-diabetic patients with non-alcoholic fatty liver disease: sites and mechanisms. *Diabetologia* 2005;48:634–42.
15. Petta S, Gastaldelli A, Rebelos E, *et al.* Pathophysiology of non alcoholic fatty liver disease. *Int J Mol Sci* 2016;17:2082.
16. Donnelly KL, Smith CI, Schwarzenberg SJ, Jessurun J, Boldt MD, and Parks EJ. Sources of fatty acids stored in liver and secreted via lipoproteins in patients with nonalcoholic fatty liver disease. *J Clin Invest* 2005;115:1343–51.

17. Bugianesi E, Moscatiello S, Ciaravella MF, and Marchesini G. Insulin resistance in nonalcoholic fatty liver disease. *Curr Pharm Des* 2010;16:1941–51.
18. Bugianesi E, McCullough AJ, and Marchesini G. Insulin resistance: a metabolic pathway to chronic liver disease. *Hepatology* 2005;42:987–1000.
19. Adams LA, Lymp JF, St Sauver J, *et al*. The natural history of nonalcoholic fatty liver disease: a population-based cohort study. *Gastroenterology* 2005;129:113–21.
20. Romeo S, Kozlitina J, Xing C, *et al*. Genetic variation in PNPLA3 confers susceptibility to nonalcoholic fatty liver disease. *Nat Genet* 2008;40:1461–5.
21. Pirola CJ, Gianotti TF, Burgueno AL, *et al*. Epigenetic modification of liver mitochondrial DNA is associated with histological severity of nonalcoholic fatty liver disease. *Gut* 2013;62:1356–63.
22. Argo CK, Northup PG, Al-Osaimi AM, and Caldwell SH. Systematic review of risk factors for fibrosis progression in non-alcoholic steatohepatitis. *J Hepatol* 2009;51:371–9.
23. Lonardo A, Adinolfi LE, Loria P, Carulli N, Ruggiero G, and Day CP. Steatosis and hepatitis C virus: mechanisms and significance for hepatic and extrahepatic disease. *Gastroenterology* 2004;126:586–97.
24. Bressler BL, Guindi M, Tomlinson G, and Heathcote J. High body mass index is an independent risk factor for nonresponse to antiviral treatment in chronic hepatitis C. *Hepatology* 2003;38:639–44.
25. Romero-Gomez M, Del Mar Viloria M, Andrade RJ, *et al*. Insulin resistance impairs sustained response rate to peginterferon plus ribavirin in chronic hepatitis C patients. *Gastroenterology* 2005;128:636–41.
26. Castera L, Pawlotsky JM, and Dhumeaux D. Worsening of steatosis and fibrosis progression in hepatitis C. *Gut* 2003;52:1531.
27. Leandro G, Mangia A, Hui J, *et al*. Relationship between steatosis, inflammation, and fibrosis in chronic hepatitis C: a meta-analysis of individual patient data. *Gastroenterology* 2006;130:1636–42.
28. Jonsson JR, Barrie HD, O'Rourke P, Clouston AD, and Powell EE. Obesity and steatosis influence serum and hepatic inflammatory markers in chronic hepatitis C. *Hepatology* 2008;48:80–7.
29. Bellentani S, Saccoccio G, Masutti F, *et al*. Prevalence of and risk factors for hepatic steatosis in Northern Italy. *Ann Intern Med* 2000;132:112–7.
30. Timoh T, Bloom ME, Siegel RR, Wagman G, Lanier GM, and Vittorio TJ. A perspective on obesity cardiomyopathy. *Obes Res Clin Pract* 2012;6: e175–262.
31. Alpert MA. Obesity cardiomyopathy: pathophysiology and evolution of the clinical syndrome. *Am J Med Sci* 2001;321:225–36.
32. Mottillo S, Filion KB, Genest J, *et al*. The metabolic syndrome and cardiovascular risk a systematic review and meta-analysis. *J Am Coll Cardiol* 2010;56:1113–32.

33. Doggen K, Nobels F, Scheen AJ, Van Crombrugge P, Van Casteren V, and Mathieu C. Cardiovascular risk factors and complications associated with albuminuria and impaired renal function in insulin-treated diabetes. *J Diabetes Complicat* 2013;27:370–5.

34. Huschak G, Busch T, and Kaisers UX. Obesity in anesthesia and intensive care. *Best Pract Res Clin Endocrinol Metab* 2013;27:247–60.

35. Sinha AC and Singh PM. Controversies in perioperative anesthetic management of the morbidly obese: I am a surgeon, why should I care? *Obes Surg* 2015;25:879–87.

36. Therapondos G, Flapan AD, Plevris JN, and Hayes PC. Cardiac morbidity and mortality related to orthotopic liver transplantation. *Liver Transpl* 2004;10:1441–53.

37. Fili D, Vizzini G, Biondo D, *et al.* Clinical burden of screening asymptomatic patients for coronary artery disease prior to liver transplantation. *Am J Transplant* 2009;9:1151–7.

38. Watt KD, Pedersen RA, Kremers WK, Heimbach JK, and Charlton MR. Evolution of causes and risk factors for mortality post-liver transplant: results of the NIDDK long-term follow-up study. *Am J Transplant* 2010;10: 1420–7.

39. Choban PS and Flancbaum L. The impact of obesity on surgical outcomes: a review. *J Am Coll Surg* 1997;185:593–603.

40. Stevens SM, O'Connell BP, and Meyer TA. Obesity related complications in surgery. *Curr Opin Otolaryngol Head Neck Surg* 2015;23:341–7.

41. McKay RE, Malhotra A, Cakmakkaya OS, Hall KT, McKay WR, and Apfel CC. Effect of increased body mass index and anaesthetic duration on recovery of protective airway reflexes after sevoflurane vs desflurane. *Br J Anaesth* 2010;104:175–82.

42. Soens MA, Birnbach DJ, Ranasinghe JS, and van Zundert A. Obstetric anesthesia for the obese and morbidly obese patient: an ounce of prevention is worth more than a pound of treatment. *Acta Anaesthesiol Scand* 2008;52: 6–19.

43. Fontaine GV, Vigil E, Wohlt PD, *et al.* Venous thromboembolism in critically ill medical patients receiving chemoprophylaxis: a focus on obesity and other risk factors. *Clin Appl Thromb Hemost* 2016;22:265–73.

44. Ortiz VE and Kwo J. Obesity: physiologic changes and implications for preoperative management. *BMC Anesthesiol* 2015;15:97.

45. Eichenberger A, Proietti S, Wicky S, *et al.* Morbid obesity and postoperative pulmonary atelectasis: an underestimated problem. *Anesth Analg* 2002;95:1788–92.

46. Fernandez-Bustamante A, Hashimoto S, Serpa Neto A, Moine P, Vidal Melo MF, and Repine JE. Perioperative lung protective ventilation in obese patients. *BMC Anesthesiol* 2015;15:56.

47. Orlic L, Mikolasevic I, Jakopcic I, *et al.* Body mass index: short- and long-term impact on kidney transplantation. *Int J Clin Pract* 2015;69:1357–65.

48. de Heredia FP, Gomez-Martinez S, and Marcos A. Obesity, inflammation and the immune system. *Proc Nutr Soc* 2012;71:332–8.

49. Schaeffer DF, Yoshida EM, Buczkowski AK, *et al.* Surgical morbidity in severely obese liver transplant recipients — a single Canadian Centre Experience. *Ann Hepatol* 2009;8:38–40.

50. Dick AA, Spitzer AL, Seifert CF, *et al.* Liver transplantation at the extremes of the body mass index. *Liver Transpl* 2009;15:968–77.

51. Alizadeh RF, Moghadamyeghaneh Z, Whealon MD, *et al.* Body mass index significantly impacts outcomes of colorectal surgery. *Am Surg* 2016;82:930–5.

52. Lee KT and Mun GH. Effects of obesity on postoperative complications after breast reconstruction using free muscle-sparing transverse rectus abdominis myocutaneous, deep inferior epigastric perforator, and superficial inferior epigastric artery flap: a systematic review and meta-analysis. *Ann Plast Surg* 2016;76:576–84.

53. Govaert JA, Lijftogt N, van Dijk WA, *et al.* Colorectal cancer surgery for obese patients: financial and clinical outcomes of a Dutch population-based registry. *J Surg Oncol* 2016;113:489–95.

54. Adhikary SD, Liu WM, Memtsoudis SG, Davis CM, and Liu J. Body mass index more than 45 kg/m^2 as a cutoff point is associated with dramatically increased postoperative complications in total knee arthroplasty and total hip arthroplasty. *J Arthroplast* 2016;31:749–53.

55. Takeuchi M, Ishii K, Seki H, *et al.* Excessive visceral fat area as a risk factor for early postoperative complications of total gastrectomy for gastric cancer: a retrospective cohort study. *BMC Surg* 2016;16:54.

56. Carrara G, Pecorelli N, De Cobelli F, *et al.* Preoperative sarcopenia determinants in pancreatic cancer patients. *Clin Nutr* 2016. doi: 10.1016/j.clnu.2016.10.014.

57. Pecorelli N, Carrara G, De Cobelli F, *et al.* Effect of sarcopenia and visceral obesity on mortality and pancreatic fistula following pancreatic cancer surgery. *Br J Surg* 2016;103:434–42.

58. Saab S, Lalezari D, Pruthi P, Alper T, and Tong MJ. The impact of obesity on patient survival in liver transplant recipients: a meta-analysis. *Liver Int* 2015;35:164–70.

59. Keeffe EB, Gettys C, and Esquivel CO. Liver transplantation in patients with severe obesity. *Transplantation* 1994;57:309–11.

60. Braunfeld MY, Chan S, Pregler J, *et al.* Liver transplantation in the morbidly obese. *J Clin Anesth* 1996;8:585–90.

61. Nair S, Verma S, and Thuluvath PJ. Obesity and its effect on survival in patients undergoing orthotopic liver transplantation in the United States. *Hepatology* 2002;35:105–9.

62. LaMattina JC, Foley DP, Fernandez LA, *et al.* Complications associated with liver transplantation in the obese recipient. *Clin Transplant* 2012;26:910–8.
63. Hakeem AR, Cockbain AJ, Raza SS, *et al.* Increased morbidity in overweight and obese liver transplant recipients: a single-center experience of 1325 patients from the United Kingdom. *Liver Transpl* 2013;19:551–62.
64. Bambha KM, Dodge JL, Gralla J, Sprague D, and Biggins SW. Low, rather than high, body mass index confers increased risk for post-liver transplant death and graft loss: risk modulated by model for end-stage liver disease. *Liver Transpl* 2015;21:1286–94.
65. Perez-Protto SE, Quintini C, Reynolds LF, *et al.* Comparable graft and patient survival in lean and obese liver transplant recipients. *Liver Transpl* 2013;19:907–15.
66. Ayloo S, Hurton S, Cwinn M, and Molinari M. Impact of body mass index on outcomes of 48281 patients undergoing first time cadaveric liver transplantation. *World J Transplant* 2016;6:356–69.
67. Pannacciulli N, Del Parigi A, Chen K, Le DS, Reiman EM, and Tataranni PA. Brain abnormalities in human obesity: a voxel-based morphometric study. *Neuroimage* 2006;31:1419–25.
68. Terjimanian MN, Harbaugh CM, Hussain A, *et al.* Abdominal adiposity, body composition and survival after liver transplantation. *Clin Transplant* 2016;30:289–94.
69. Carias S, Castellanos AL, Vilchez V, *et al.* Nonalcoholic steatohepatitis is strongly associated with sarcopenic obesity in patients with cirrhosis undergoing liver transplant evaluation. *J Gastroenterol Hepatol* 2016;31:628–33.
70. Sakuma K and Yamaguchi A. Sarcopenic obesity and endocrinal adaptation with age. *Int J Endocrinol* 2013;2013:1–12.
71. Roubenoff R. Sarcopenic obesity: the confluence of two epidemics. *Obes Res* 2004;12:887–8.
72. Batsis JA, Mackenzie TA, Barre LK, Lopez-Jimenez F, and Bartels SJ. Sarcopenia, sarcopenic obesity and mortality in older adults: results from the National Health and Nutrition Examination Survey III. *Eur J Clin Nutr* 2014;68:1001–7.
73. Kim WR, Smith JM, Skeans MA, *et al.* OPTN/SRTR 2012 Annual Data Report: liver. *Am J Transplant* 2014;14(Suppl 1):69–96.
74. Cameron A and Busuttil RW. AASLD/ILTS transplant course: is there an extended donor suitable for everyone? *Liver Transpl* 2005;11:S2–5.
75. Wong TC, Fung JY, Chok KS, *et al.* Excellent outcomes of liver transplantation using severely steatotic grafts from brain-dead donors. *Liver Transpl* 2016;22:226–36.
76. McCormack L, Dutkowski P, El-Badry AM, and Clavien PA. Liver transplantation using fatty livers: always feasible? *J Hepatol* 2011;54:1055–62.

77. Ploeg RJ, D'Alessandro AM, Knechtle SJ, *et al*. Risk factors for primary dysfunction after liver transplantation — a multivariate analysis. *Transplantation* 1993;55:807–13.
78. Kleiner DE, Brunt EM, Van Natta M, *et al*. Design and validation of a histological scoring system for nonalcoholic fatty liver disease. *Hepatology* 2005;41:1313–21.
79. Nativ NI, Maguire TJ, Yarmush G, *et al*. Liver defatting: an alternative approach to enable steatotic liver transplantation. *Am J Transplant* 2012;12:3176–83.
80. Berthiaume F, Barbe L, Mokuno Y, MacDonald AD, Jindal R, and Yarmush ML. Steatosis reversibly increases hepatocyte sensitivity to hypoxia-reoxygenation injury. *J Surg Res* 2009;152:54–60.
81. Serafin A, Rosello-Catafau J, Prats N, Xaus C, Gelpi E, and Peralta C. Ischemic preconditioning increases the tolerance of fatty liver to hepatic ischemia-reperfusion injury in the rat. *Am J Pathol* 2002;161:587–601.
82. Rey JW, Wirges U, Dienes HP, and Fries JW. Hepatic steatosis in organ donors: disparity between surgery and histology? *Transplant Proc* 2009;41:2557–60.
83. Nickkholgh A, Weitz J, Encke J, *et al*. Utilization of extended donor criteria in liver transplantation: a comprehensive review of the literature. *Nephrol Dial Transplant* 2007;22(Suppl 8):viii29–viii36.
84. Silva MA. Putting objectivity into assessment of steatosis. *Transplantation* 2009;88:620–1.
85. El-Badry AM, Breitenstein S, Jochum W, *et al*. Assessment of hepatic steatosis by expert pathologists: the end of a gold standard. *Ann Surg* 2009;250:691–7.
86. Frankel WL, Tranovich JG, Salter L, Bumgardner G, and Baker P. The optimal number of donor biopsy sites to evaluate liver histology for transplantation. *Liver Transpl* 2002;8:1044–50.
87. De Carlis L, Colella G, Sansalone CV, *et al*. Marginal donors in liver transplantation: the role of donor age. *Transplant Proc* 1999;31:397–400.
88. Imber CJ, St Peter SD, Lopez I, Guiver L, and Friend PJ. Current practice regarding the use of fatty livers: a trans-Atlantic survey. *Liver Transpl* 2002;8:545–9.
89. Spitzer AL, Lao OB, Dick AA, *et al*. The biopsied donor liver: incorporating macrosteatosis into high-risk donor assessment. *Liver Transpl* 2010;16:874–84.
90. Chavin KD, Taber DJ, Norcross M, *et al*. Safe use of highly steatotic livers by utilizing a donor/recipient clinical algorithm. *Clin Transplant* 2013;27:732–41.
91. de Graaf EL, Kench J, Dilworth P, *et al*. Grade of deceased donor liver macrovesicular steatosis impacts graft and recipient outcomes more than the Donor Risk Index. *J Gastroenterol Hepatol* 2012;27:540–6.

92. Deroose JP, Kazemier G, Zondervan P, Ijzermans JN, Metselaar HJ, and Alwayn IP. Hepatic steatosis is not always a contraindication for cadaveric liver transplantation. *HPB* 2011;13:417–25.

93. Gao F, Xu X, Ling Q, et al. Efficacy and safety of moderately steatotic donor liver in transplantation. *Hepatobiliary Pancreat Dis Int* 2009;8:29–33.

94. Chu MJ, Dare AJ, Phillips AR, and Bartlett AS. Donor hepatic steatosis and outcome after liver transplantation: a systematic review. *J Gastrointest Surg* 2015;19:1713–24.

95. Thurairajah PH, Syn WK, Neil DA, Stell D, and Haydon G. Orlistat (Xenical)-induced subacute liver failure. *Eur J Gastroenterol Hepatol* 2005;17:1437–8.

96. Yanovski SZ and Yanovski JA. Long-term drug treatment for obesity: a systematic and clinical review. *JAMA* 2014;311:74–86.

97. Halperin F, Ding SA, Simonson DC, et al. Roux-en-Y gastric bypass surgery or lifestyle with intensive medical management in patients with type 2 diabetes: feasibility and 1-year results of a randomized clinical trial. *JAMA Surg* 2014;149:716–26.

98. Picot J, Jones J, Colquitt JL, et al. The clinical effectiveness and cost-effectiveness of bariatric (weight loss) surgery for obesity: a systematic review and economic evaluation. *Health Technol Assess* 2009;13:1–190, 215–357, iii–iv.

99. Colquitt JL, Pickett K, Loveman E, and Frampton GK. Surgery for weight loss in adults. *Cochrane Database Syst Rev* 2014;8:CD003641.

100. Loveman E, Frampton GK, Shepherd J, et al. The clinical effectiveness and cost-effectiveness of long-term weight management schemes for adults: a systematic review. *Health Technol Assess* 2011;15:1–182.

101. Schnetzler B, Kondo-Oestreicher M, Vala D, Khatchatourian G, and Faidutti B. Orlistat decreases the plasma level of cyclosporine and may be responsible for the development of acute rejection episodes. *Transplantation* 2000;70:1540–1.

102. Segev DL, Thompson RE, Locke JE, et al. Prolonged waiting times for liver transplantation in obese patients. *Ann Surg* 2008;248:863–70.

103. O'Leary JG, Landaverde C, Jennings L, Goldstein RM, and Davis GL. Patients with NASH and cryptogenic cirrhosis are less likely than those with hepatitis C to receive liver transplants. *Clin Gastroenterol Hepatol* 2011;9:700–4 e1.

104. Conzen KD, Vachharajani N, Collins KM, et al. Morbid obesity in liver transplant recipients adversely affects longterm graft and patient survival in a single-institution analysis. *HPB* 2015;17:251–7.

105. Keller EJ, Kwo PY, and Helft PR. Ethical considerations surrounding survival benefit-based liver allocation. *Liver Transpl* 2014;20:140–6.

106. Leonard J, Heimbach JK, Malinchoc M, Watt K, and Charlton M. The impact of obesity on long-term outcomes in liver transplant recipients-results of the NIDDK liver transplant database. *Am J Transplant* 2008;8:667–72.

107. Martin P, DiMartini A, Feng S, Brown R, Jr., and Fallon M. Evaluation for liver transplantation in adults: 2013 practice guideline by the American Association for the Study of Liver Diseases and the American Society of Transplantation. *Hepatology* 2014;59:1144–65.
108. Pelletier SJ, Maraschio MA, Schaubel DE, *et al.* Survival benefit of kidney and liver transplantation for obese patients on the waiting list. *Clin Transpl* 2003:77–88.
109. Leyba JL, Llopis SN, and Aulestia SN. Laparoscopic Roux-en-Y astric bypass versus laparoscopic sleeve gastrectomy for the treatment of morbid obesity. A prospective study with 5 years of follow-up. *Obes Surg* 2014;24(12):2094–8.
110. Gumbs AA, Gagner M, Dakin G, and Pomp A. Sleeve gastrectomy for morbid obesity. *Obes Surg* 2007;17:962–9.
111. Zhang Y, Ju W, Sun X, *et al.* Laparoscopic sleeve gastrectomy versus laparoscopic Roux-En-Y gastric bypass for morbid obesity and related comorbidities: a meta-analysis of 21 studies. *Obes Surg* 2015;25(1):19–26.
112. Catheline JM, Fysekidis M, Bachner I, *et al.* Five-year results of sleeve gastrectomy. *J Visc Surg* 2013;150:307–12.
113. Lin MY, Tavakol MM, Sarin A, *et al.* Laparoscopic sleeve gastrectomy is safe and efficacious for pretransplant candidates. *Surg Obes Relat Dis* 2013;9: 653–8.
114. Takata MC, Campos GM, Ciovica R, *et al.* Laparoscopic bariatric surgery improves candidacy in morbidly obese patients awaiting transplantation. *Surg Obes Relat Dis* 2008;4:159–64; discussion 64–5.
115. Taneja S, Gupta S, Wadhawan M, and Goyal N. Single-lobe living donor liver transplant in a morbidly obese cirrhotic patient preceded by laparoscopic sleeve gastrectomy. *Case Rep Transplant* 2013;2013:279651.
116. Al-Nowaylati AR, Al-Haddad BJ, Dorman RB, *et al.* Gastric bypass after liver transplantation. *Liver Transpl* 2013;19:1324–9.
117. Duchini A and Brunson ME. Roux-en-Y gastric bypass for recurrent nonalcoholic steatohepatitis in liver transplant recipients with morbid obesity. *Transplantation* 2001;72:156–9.
118. Lin MY, Tavakol MM, Sarin A, *et al.* Safety and feasibility of sleeve gastrectomy in morbidly obese patients following liver transplantation. *Surg Endosc* 2013;27:81–5.
119. Tichansky DS and Madan AK. Laparoscopic Roux-en-Y gastric bypass is safe and feasible after orthotopic liver transplantation. *Obes Surg* 2005;15:1481–6.
120. Campsen J, Zimmerman M, Shoen J, *et al.* Adjustable gastric banding in a morbidly obese patient during liver transplantation. *Obes Surg* 2008;18: 1625–7.
121. Heimbach JK, Watt KD, Poterucha JJ, *et al.* Combined liver transplantation and gastric sleeve resection for patients with medically complicated obesity and end-stage liver disease. *Am J Transplant* 2013;13:363–8.

122. Selzner N, Selzner M, Jochum W, Amann-Vesti B, Graf R, and Clavien PA. Mouse livers with macrosteatosis are more susceptible to normothermic ischemic injury than those with microsteatosis. *J Hepatol* 2006;44:694–701.
123. Fukumori T, Ohkohchi N, Tsukamoto S, and Satomi S. Why is fatty liver unsuitable for transplantation? Deterioration of mitochondrial ATP synthesis and sinusoidal structure during cold preservation of a liver with steatosis. *Transplant Proc* 1997;29:412–5.
124. Nagrath D, Xu H, Tanimura Y, *et al*. Metabolic preconditioning of donor organs: defatting fatty livers by normothermic perfusion ex vivo. *Metab Eng* 2009;11:274–83.
125. Guarrera JV, Henry SD, Chen SW, *et al*. Hypothermic machine preservation attenuates ischemia/reperfusion markers after liver transplantation: preliminary results. *J Surg Res* 2011;167:e365–73.
126. Perito ER, Rhee S, Glidden D, Roberts JP, and Rosenthal P. Impact of the donor body mass index on the survival of pediatric liver transplant recipients and post-transplant obesity. *Liver Transpl* 2012;18:930–9.
127. Perito ER, Glidden D, Roberts JP, and Rosenthal P. Overweight and obesity in pediatric liver transplant recipients: prevalence and predictors before and after transplant, United Network for Organ Sharing Data, 1987–2010. *Pediatr Transplant* 2012;16:41–9.
128. Yoo HY, Molmenti E, and Thuluvath PJ. The effect of donor body mass index on primary graft nonfunction, retransplantation rate, and early graft and patient survival after liver transplantation. *Liver Transpl* 2003;9:72–8.
129. Beal EW, Tumin D, Conteh LF, *et al*. Impact of recipient and donor obesity match on the outcomes of liver transplantation: all matches are not perfect. *J Transplant* 2016;2016:9709430.
130. Freeman RB, Jamieson N, Schaubel DE, Porte RJ, and Villamil FG. Who should get a liver graft? *J Hepatol* 2009;50:664–73.
131. Sackett DL. Evidence-based medicine. *Spine* 1998;23:1085–6.

14. Liver Transplantation for Metabolic Disease

Patrick McKiernan*,† and Kyle Soltys‡

*Department of Pediatrics, University of Pitttsburgh,
1400 Locust St, Pittsburgh, PA 15219, USA
†Department of Hepatology, Division of Gastroenterology/
Hepatology/Nutrition, Children's Hospital of Pittsburgh of UPMC,
4401 Penn Avenue, Pittsburgh, PA 15224, USA
‡Department of Surgery, University of Pittsburgh, Pittsburgh,
PA 15213, USA

1. Introduction

Liver transplant(ation) (LT) is one of the outstanding successes of high technology medicine. Pediatric LT can now offer a 1 year survival of >90% of whom the vast majority will survive into adulthood with a good quality of life [1]. Inherited metabolic disorders have recently been the indication in approximately 15% of cases with urea cycle disorders, the commonest indication, followed by α-1 antitrypsin deficiency [2].

These indications however are never static. LT is not a "cure" but rather a disorder in itself with a defined acute mortality and a future attrition rate mostly related to the lifelong need for immunosuppression. In an individual child and family, the therapeutic decision has to incorporate the transplant centre's results and experience, the impact of the metabolic defect on the child and the family, the natural history of the defect and whether any new therapies are available or potentially available. As a result, an inherited defect that may be a relative contraindication to transplantation in one era may be a definite indication in another and vice versa.

Assessment for LT is a formal process carried out by the transplant multidisciplinary team. This team should be widely based and incorporate pediatricians, surgeons, anesthetists, nurses, social workers, play therapists, and psychologists. The team should be supported by a metabolic expert where metabolic disease is the indication and should be able to call on other relevant organ-based specialists as required. The process involves a comprehensive evaluation to assess fitness and suitability for transplantation in parallel by providing age-appropriate information to the child and their family [3]. This usually follows an outpatient review and is usually undertaken over 4–5 working days, but the pace should be individually determined.

Prior to formal listing, an individual clinical perioperative protocol should be prepared incorporating instructions for immediate preoperative preparation and investigations, which individuals and teams to contact and outlining intraoperative and early posttransplant management.

In considering the indication and outcome of LT in metabolic disease, two independent factors need to be considered: firstly whether or not the metabolic defect causes significant liver disease and secondly whether or not the defect is confined to the liver. This results in four categories of disorders to consider.

2. Category 1: Intrinsic liver disease with defect confined to the liver

In this group, the indication for transplantation is usually made depending on the severity of the liver disease rather than that of the intrinsic metabolic defect. These indications are well established (Table 1). Where the defect causes a significantly higher risk of developing hepatocellular carcinoma (HCC), e.g., in tyrosinemia, transplantation may be indicated at an earlier stage than if it were based on the severity of liver disease alone.

For this category, the outcome of transplantation will reflect the success of the transplantation programme, the clinical status of the child at transplant and possibly the age at transplant. LT for acute liver failure (ALF) is less successful than elective transplantation [4]. The effect of age at transplantation is more unpredictable. LT in early infancy is less successful, but considering these are very ill children with ALF and that waiting times are usually longer for this age group, this is hardly unexpected [5]. Beyond 6 months of age, age at transplantation has little impact on outcome. Children with established liver disease usually have some degree of portal hypertension and hence tolerate the effect of intraoperative portal vein clamping relatively well.

Table 1. Categories of metabolic disease when considering liver transplantation

	Liver disease (1)	No significant liver disease (2)
Defect confined to liver (a)	α1 antitrypsin deficiency (PiZZ)	Crigler-Najjar
	Tyrosinemia type 1	Primary hyperoxaluria type 1
	Wilson's disease	(preemptive)
	PFIC types 2 ,3 and X	Urea cycle disorders (arginosuccinic
	Urea cycle disorders : ASL	aciduria excepted)
	(arginosuccinic aciduria)	Citrin deficiency
	GSD type I (Adenoma/HCC)	Familial hypercholesterolaemia
	& IIIb	Hemophilia
	Indian childhood cirrhosis	Factor VII deficiency
	Bile acid synthesis disorders	Protein C and S deficiencies
	Hereditary hemochromatosis	Factor H deficiency
		GSD type Ia, (metabolic control)
		Fatty acid oxidation defects
		Acute intermittent porphyria
		Familial Amyloid Polyneuropathy
		Afibrinoginaemia
		S-adenosylhomocysteine hydrolase
		deficiency
Extrahepatic Defect (b)	GSD IIIa and IV	MSUD
	Erythropoietic protoporphyria	Methylmalonic academia
	Lysosomal storage diseases	Propionic acidemia
	Niemann-Pick disease	GSD I non A
	Cystic fibrosis	Primary hyperoxaluria type 1
	Respiratory chain disorders	(with renal failure)
	PFIC 1	
	Cholesterol ester storage disease.	
	Familial amyloid polyneuropathy	

Post transplantation, there is lifelong correction of the metabolic defect, with the possible exception of progressive familial intrahepatic cholestasis type 2 (PFIC2), and the long-term prognosis is similar to that of contemporary LT for other indications [2].

2.1. *Progressive familial intrahepatic cholestasis type 2 (PFIC2)*

PFIC2 is caused by deficiency of the canalicular bile salt transporter (BSEP) due to mutations in *ABCB11*. The commonest clinical presentation of the severe phenotype is with neonatal jaundice and subsequent pruritus. Biochemical tests show normal or low serum GGT activity and liver histology shows severe giant cell hepatitis [6].

Treatment consists of supportive nutritional and medical care with timely partial external biliary diversion. Unfortunately, progression to cirrhosis is common and when this is established, or biliary diversion fails, LT is the only lifesaving option.

LT has overall been very successful and in the majority of cases provides functional correction of the defect. However, as many as 8–10% develop recurrence of cholestasis between 3 months and 10 years post transplant [7]. This has been shown to be due to *de novo* anti-BSEP antibodies which inhibit bile acid transport. This phenomenon is confined to those with severe mutations where there is absent or very low native protein expression. In this setting, BSEP escapes normal immune autotolerance and becomes an immune target when expressed in the allograft.

Treatment options include manipulating immunosuppression, plasmapheresis, and rituximab. Where liver retransplantation has been required, the incidence of recurrent disease is very high.

3. Category 2: Intrinsic liver disease with an extrahepatic defect

The indication for transplantation in this category will usually be as in category 1, i.e., primarily based on the severity of the liver disease. However, in some disorders the timing of transplantation may be impacted by the extrahepatic defect as there may be a relatively short time window in which transplantation is feasible. The metabolic correction of the defect will be immediate and lifelong but long-term survival will reflect not just the outcome of transplantation but the nature and progression of the extrahepatic disease. When counselling families, the fact that LT will not be "curative" should be highlighted. In this group of diseases, pre-emptive transplantation may not be appropriate depending on the nature of the extrahepatic defect. A careful individualized multidisciplinary transplant assessment process should be undertaken and the outcome of transplantation in this group of disorders should be continuously audited.

3.1. Cystic fibrosis

Approximately 5–10% of young people with cystic fibrosis develop cirrhosis and portal hypertension; among them, some develop end-stage liver disease (ESLD). LT has been shown to be very successful in selected cases with excellent medium term survival [8]. Transplantation results in an initial stabilization of lung function and some slowing of the natural rate of deterioration in the first 4 years. In the longer term, respiratory deterioration continues to be the commonest cause of death.

In cystic fibrosis, transplantation needs to be undertaken while there is sufficient pulmonary reserve to support transplantation. Ideally the FEV1 should be greater than 50% predicted and certainly more than 40% predicted. This may prompt consideration of pre-emptive transplantation prior to the development of ESLD if pulmonary function is deteriorating, in order to avoid missing the window of suitability. However, if LT is undertaken too early, ESLD may never have developed prior to the eventual onset of pulmonary insufficiency. In this situation, LT may not result in improved survival. However, the improved quality of life following successful LT also needs to be considered in this complex equation.

3.2. *Mitochondrial liver diseases*

Mitochondrial liver diseases may be due to inherited disorders of respiratory chain proteins or abnormalities of mitochondrial DNA assembly. Unfortunately these disorders are usually multisystemic and when the presentation is with ALF the outlook is very poor. LT for ALF due to a multisystemic defect does not prevent, and may even hasten, neurological deterioration. This is not just an individual tragedy but in an era of organ shortage, it results in the denial or delay of transplantation to someone else. The challenge is to exclude untreatable disorders as quickly and accurately as possible without denying lifesaving LT to those who may benefit.

Rapid and accurate characterization of the underlying defect is increasingly feasible and more is known about the natural history of this group of disorders. LT is contraindicated where liver failure is due to valproate-induced liver failure in children, mutations in polymerase γ, twinkle and deoxyguanine kinase with neurological involvement [9, 10]. On the other hand, children presenting with chronic liver disease due to isolated respiratory chain defect may have an excellent outcome following transplantation. Similarly, occasional children with mitochondrial DNA depletion due to mutations in MPV-17 have good quality long-term survival albeit often complicated by peripheral neuropathy [11]. Where the underlying defect in mitochondrial DNA cannot be defined, a systematic multidisciplinary assessment including evaluation of extrahepatic involvement is important so that individualized advice can be given to affected families. In general, the benefit of any genuine doubt should be given to the child.

3.3. *Progressive familial intrahepatic cholestasis type 1 (PFIC1)*

PFIC1 is caused by a deficiency of a P-type ATPase that is required for ATP-dependent amino phospholipid transport and encoded by the *ATP8B1* gene. FIC1 is also expressed in liver, intestine, and pancreas [12]. Clinical presentation is with jaundice and pruritus in the first year of life which may initially be intermittent but eventually is persistent. Systemic manifestations include diarrhea, pancreatitis, short stature, and sensorineural deafness [13].

The diagnosis is usually suspected when blood tests show normal or low serum GGT activity and normal cholesterol in the setting of cholestasis. Liver histology shows a rather bland intrahepatic cholestasis with little necrotic or inflammatory activity.

Treatment options are similar to PFIC2 but many progress to ESLD, usually in the second decade of life. For these children, LT is the only option.

Despite excellent survival, the extrahepatic manifestations of the disease limit the benefit of transplantation. Diarrhea is usually worsened, catch-up growth is rare, and pancreatitis persists [13]. A unique complication is the development of microvesicular steatohepatitis in approximately two-thirds of cases within months of transplant [13, 14]. This is usually accompanied by progressive fibrosis and may lead to ESLD requiring retransplantation. Steatosis is also highly associated with those who develop posttransplant diarrhea.

The mechanism of this complication is unclear but is presumably related to the interaction of normal bile from the allograft in an affected intestine with abnormal bile acid absorption. Interestingly, recurrence of steatosis appears to be associated with the severity of the underlying mutation [14]. Using bile acid sequestrants is logical but of uncertain benefit. Post transplant biliary diversion appears to have the potential to reverse steatosis and prevent fibrosis progression [15, 16].

As a result, in PFIC1, alternatives to transplantation such as biliary diversion should be maximized and transplantation reserved for ESLD. Post transplant biliary diversion should be considered at an early stage if steatohepatitis develops.

4. Category 3: No intrinsic liver disease with defect confined to liver

This category utilizes transplantation as a highly effective and realistic form of gene therapy. In individual disorders, the decision on transplantation should be assessed by a multidisciplinary team taking into account the success of transplantation, the prognosis of the underlying metabolic defect, the quality of life associated with treatment of the disease for the child and the family and the risk of irreversible disease in other organs including kidney, brain and heart.

In children without liver disease, the technical aspects of transplantation, especially removal of the native liver, are usually straightforward. However these children have not had pre-existing portal hypertension and are sensitive to the haemodynamic effect of portal vein clamping and as a result more susceptible to early liver dysfunction. It follows that surgical expertise and selection of suitable high-quality donor organs are particularly crucial to success. For this group of diseases, transplantation results in a lifelong correction of the metabolic defect and the long-term prognosis is similar to that of contemporary LT for other indications unless irreversible disease-related complications have occurred.

4.1. Urea cycle disorders

Urea cycle defects (UCDs) are due to defects in any one of six enzymes involved in the detoxification and elimination of ammonia. The clinical manifestations of UCD are with encephalopathy due to hyperammonemia, although acute liver dysfunction is increasingly recognized. The most severe defects present in the newborn period and have a poor prognosis with a high risk of severe neurological injury even with prospective treatment. Those who present later have milder defects but are still at risk of suffering neurological sequelae [17].

LT for UCD results in a complete functional correction of the metabolic defect, allowing a normal diet, abolishing the risk of hyperammonemia, and transforming the quality of life for affected children and their families [18]. Due to the persistent intestinal defect, citrulline levels remain low in carbamoyl phosphate synthetase and ornithine transcarbamylase deficiencies (OTCDs) and high in argininosuccinate synthase deficiency (citrullinemia). The former is of uncertain significance and responds to supplementation, while the latter appears of no consequence.

There is protection against further neurological damage and there may even be some recovery of pre-existing impairment where transplantation is undertaken early and in particular if carried out before 1 year of age [19].

Transplantation should be considered early where there is severe disease and ideally before any neurological insult. The "honeymoon period" before further acute decompensation is usually shorter than previously thought [20]. As a result, transplantation should be planned after 3 months which allows maximization of medical therapy, aggressive vaccination and avoids the higher technical risks of neonatal transplantation [18, 20]. For milder, later onset cases, the indication will be recurrent metabolic instability. Each case should be reviewed on its merits, taking account of familial preferences [19].

Decision making in argininosuccinic aciduria (ASA) is more nuanced. Clinically, the metabolic defect is milder but children frequently develop progressive liver disease. It is however rare for transplantation to be indicated solely because of the severity of liver disease during childhood. Another concern is that the enzyme is expressed in the brain and hence the impact of transplantation on neurologic outcome is less predictable. However, the limited clinical experience with transplantation has been encouraging with excellent outcome to date [21, 22].

4.2. *Primary hyperoxaluria type 1*

This is due to deficiency of hepatic alanine glycoxalate transaminases and shows considerable phenotypic variability. The defect causes overproduction of oxalate which results in nephrocalcinosis and urolithiasis which may in turn cause renal insufficiency. As renal insufficiency progresses, and in particular as glomerular filtration rate (GFR) falls below 40 mL/min/1.74 m^2, oxalate starts to accumulate setting the seeds of systemic oxalosis [23]. Conventional dialysis is relatively inefficient in removing oxalate and renal impairment marks the transition from a disease curable by LT into a multisystemic disease with long-term cardiovascular, ocular, renal, urological, and orthopedic manifestations. In the most severe phenotype, renal failure develops in infancy and for the remainder, approximately 50% will develop end-stage renal disease during childhood [23].

LT completely corrects the primary biochemical defect, and ideally should be undertaken when there is evidence of progressive renal disease despite maximal medical treatment, but before GFR falls below 40–50 mL/min/1.74 m^2. For this pre-emptive group, the medium term outlook is excellent with long-term preservation of native renal function, although some will eventually require renal transplantation [24]. Even if they do require future renal transplantation, they avoid the morbidity associated with systemic oxalosis.

For those with established renal failure, combined liver kidney transplant is required for survival. The presence of systemic oxalosis increases the immediate perioperative risks, and subsequent to transplantation, the huge accumulated oxalate load must be excreted via the grafted kidney. This is associated with a significant risk of recurrent renal oxalosis [25]. In severely affected infants with renal failure, combined transplantation may be unrealistic. A staged procedure, with early LT to arrest oxalate production followed by renal transplantation when feasible (approximately 10 kg), may be the only option [26]. However, cardiovascular complications of systemic oxalosis may still develop following LT while on dialysis which may preclude future renal transplantation and hence prove ultimately fatal.

4.3. *Atypical hemolytic uremic syndrome*

This may result from genetic defects in a number of complement factors, most commonly factor H and rarely factor I. These disorders have a high risk of progression to end-stage renal disease but unfortunately commonly recur following isolated renal transplant. The majority of complement factors are synthesized within the liver and combined liver and kidney, or isolated liver, transplant results in complete correction of the defect. The success of transplantation is dependent on using preoperative and perioperative plasma exchange to prevent fatal, uncontrolled complement activation in the perioperative period. The indications for combined liver and kidney transplantation are to treat renal failure and to reduce the risk of renal recurrence. Isolated LT may be occasionally indicated when plasma exchange is not feasible or tolerated [27].

The availability and extraordinary efficacy of Eculizumab, a monoclonal antibody blocking C5 activation and the formation of the pathogenic membrane attack complex, has meant that transplantation will probably be reserved for occasional cases [28]. Eculizumab appears to prevent renal recurrence and to replace the need for plasma exchange therapy, but it is very expensive and it is not yet clear whether treatment needs to be continued lifelong [29].

5. Category 4: No liver disease and extrahepatic defect

These disorders largely consist of the organic acidemias and type 1 non-A glycogen storage disease. The indications for LT will be similar to those of category 3. Long-term outcome will be related not just to the success of transplantation but to the severity of the extrahepatic defect.

5.1. *Organic acidemias*

The organic acidemias are a severe group of disorders where children are at risk from recurrent metabolic instability and face a significant cumulative risk of developing systemic complications, particularly neurological damage but also including renal and cardiac disease despite intrusive medical and nutritional support. These defects are expressed within the liver but also in muscle and other organs.

LT results in a clinically important partial correction of the metabolic defect in propionic acidemia (PA) [30]. Dietary restriction can be minimized and there is complete protection against metabolic crises with reversal of cardiomyopathy. Early experience of transplantation was however associated with a high morbidity and mortality in young children which may well have been at least partly an era effect [31]. Recent experience has been much more positive with long-term survival rates of greater than 80% with excellent quality of life [32]. In this era, it is preferable that where children with PA are being considered for transplant that this is done relatively early as the risk of systemic complications is progressive. Despite the partial correction of the defect, living-related transplantation from heterozygote donors has been as effective as cadaveric transplantation [33].

Methylmalonic acidemia has a very similar presentation and clinical course to PA but has the additional significant risk of developing renal failure from the second decade of life. LT may be considered either early because of the severity of the metabolic defect or later in combination with kidney transplantation where renal failure develops. The metabolic effect of transplantation is similar to that of PA but the risk of neurological deterioration persists [34].

In maple syrup urine disease (MSUD), LT only replaces approximately 10% of enzyme activity, yet the functional correction is much more complete with excellent control of amino acids whether from dietary sources and muscle turnover. Management is transformed by transplantation allowing a normal diet, almost complete protection from metabolic decompensation, prevention of new neurological damage, and improvement in neuroimaging appearances [35, 36]. Because of the limited enzymatic correction, living-related transplant from a heterozygote donor while effective, is associated with residual risk of metabolic decompensation and should be avoided where possible [37, 38].

5.2. Glycogen storage disease type 1 non-A

In this disorder, LT corrects the metabolic defect and reduces frequency of hospitalization. Neutropenia persists, albeit often milder and GCSF requirements decrease. In addition, the manifestations of inflammatory bowel disease usually decrease post transplantation [39].

5.3. *S-adenosylhomocysteine hydrolase deficiency (SAHHD)*

Methyl-group donation is crucial to a wide range of cellular processes which are concentrated in the liver but are present in all tissues. S-adenosylmethionine (SAM) is the universal methyl donor, forming S-adenosylhomocysteine (SAH). This is in turn metabolised to homocysteine by SAHH. SAHHD results in an abnormal SAM/SAH ratio which inhibits transmethylation throughout the body. Clinically this presents in infancy with a multisystemic disorder including microcephaly, developmental delay, growth failure, and coagulopathy.

In a single case report, LT resulted in resolution of the coagulopathy, a significant increase in hepatic methylation products, and improvement of the SAM/SAH ratio [40]. This was accompanied by accelerated developmental progress, increased head growth, and an improvement in brain MRI appearance. This provided strong indirect evidence that not only was the hepatic defect corrected but also that normalization of the SAM/SAH ratio stimulated cerebral methyltransferase activity. This represents a novel way to cross the blood–brain barrier by using LT to impact on cerebral intracellular processes.

5.4. *Domino transplant*

Where the recipient does not have intrinsic liver disease, the possibility of using the explant liver for a domino transplant exists. Here the explanted liver is used to transplant another recipient with the expectation that the disease would either not be clinically expressed, or if it is expressed that it could be managed easily and would not cause short-term clinical sequelae. A significant advantage of the domino procedure is that the donor is hemodynamically stable, short graft ischemia times can be achieved and there is no impact on the overall donor organ pool. However, the need to use the domino organ immediately after the original transplant produces logistical difficulties. As a result, this is better undertaken in high volume, well-resourced centres where parallel operating is feasible. Organs from patients with MSUD have been used very successfully, even in pediatric recipients, without any untoward clinical or biochemical consequence [41]. The commonest use of domino transplant has been from donors with familial amyloid polyneuropathy. Although recipients express the disease, it takes many years to become clinically relevant and this does not impact on overall survival when used for older recipients [42]. Domino organs from patients with familial hypercholesterolemia and methylmalonic acidemia have also been used successfully [43]. However, organs from patients with acute porphyria and oxalosis result in rapid onset of severe disease in the recipient and should not be utilized [42].

Cadaveric donation has been the dominant organ source in most programmes with most donors being adults. As a result, donor organs for children are surgically modified. These are either reduced size or split LTs. In the latter, the organ is used to benefit two recipients, usually an adult and a child. In all cases, the native liver is removed and the graft placed in the same (orthotopic) position.

5.4.1. *Living-related liver transplantation (LRLT)*

Access to cadaveric liver donation varies widely throughout the world and its availability is the main driver for LRLT. LRLT has largely utilized left-lobe donation from a parent to child, although adult-to-adult donation is very successful in experienced hands. The long-term outcome of LRLT is slightly superior to cadaveric transplantation, but the major advantage in unstable metabolic disease is that the procedure can be scheduled, ensuring the donor is in ideal condition.

Most inherited metabolic diseases are autosomal recessive; hence parents are obligate heterozygotes and typically have 50% of normal enzyme activity. This does not seem to affect either the risk to the donor parent or the efficacy of metabolic control in the recipient for most disorders [44, 45].

In α-1 antitrypsin deficiency (A1ATD), the great majority of heterozygous parents will be clinically normal but the heterozygous MZ state is a known cofactor for other liver diseases. Where cadaveric MZ donors have been used inadvertently, α-1 antitrypsin granules can be found on follow-up biopsies [46]. So in theory, these parents might be at greater future risk from hepatic resection and their recipient children may be receiving a less than ideal graft. However, these are only theoretical concerns and several living-related transplants have been undertaken in A1ATD without reported adverse outcome for either donor or recipient [47].

In MSUD, because cadaveric transplantation only corrects approximately 10% of the defect, the use of an obligate heterozygous donor might result in an incomplete correction. However, where LRLT has been used, it has significantly ameliorated the disease, albeit with some residual risk of decompensation [37]. Another example is the X-linked inherited disorder OTCD. While there is rarely a metabolic risk associated with a paternal donor, a maternal donor is very likely to be a carrier and possibly partially affected. While this would normally preclude maternal donation if there were alternatives, the use of a partially affected donor results in significantly improved metabolic control as the recipient develops the phenotype of the donor [48].

5.5. *Auxiliary liver transplantation (LT)*

In auxiliary LT, not all of the recipient liver is removed and a partial donor graft is placed orthotopically. This may be considered where there is no primary liver disease and where a partial correction is likely to be effective. The major advantage of auxiliary LT is that the native liver is retained as a "safety net" if the graft fails or if gene therapy becomes available, where-upon immunosuppression could be withdrawn. The major disadvantage of the procedure is that the surgery is more complex with the need to preferentially divert portal venous blood flow to the graft by native portal vein banding. In experienced hands, this can be very effective and long-term stable graft function can be achieved [49].

In practice, the use of auxiliary LT has largely been confined to Crigler–Najjar syndrome and in occasional cases of UCDs or PA [50].The recent description of the successful use of a domino graft from a patient with PA as an auxiliary implant into a patient with Crigler–Najjar syndrome may extend the role of the technique [51]. The recipient had effective clearance of bilirubin without manifestations of PA. This raises the possibility of patients with differing metabolic diseases undertaking partial liver exchanges without any impact on the donor pool.

5.6. *Hepatocyte transplantation*

Hepatocytes can be efficiently isolated from donor livers and transplanted either immediately as fresh cells or thawed following cryopreservation when needed. Transplantation is minimally invasive requiring only infusion into to the portal vein using either a percutaneous or surgically placed catheter and can be repeated. Although HLA matching is not required, levels of immunosuppression compared to whole organ transplantation are necessary.

More than 30 subjects have received hepatocyte transplants for metabolic disease. In general, the procedure and immunosuppression have been well tolerated, but the metabolic effect has been modest and usually short lived. The major role for the first generation of this procedure appears to be in newborn infants with severe forms of urea cycle disorders where it appears to provide some stability and acts as a bridge to subsequent LT [52].

Methods to improve the efficacy of hepatocyte transplantation are needed and these need to be multifaceted [53]. Options include increasing the number of cells transplanted, improving the hepatocyte repopulation rate, or using different cell types. Increasing cell numbers will be problematic as the number of organs where cells can be harvested and which are not used for immediate organ transplantation are increasingly rare. In addition, larger cell volumes may not be tolerated due to the risk of acute portal hypertension during the infusion. Efforts to increase hepatocyte repopulation may require a noxious stimulus to the native liver to provide a survival advantage to transplanted cells, hence changing the risk–benefit balance.

An alternative is to use stem cells, which may retain proliferative potential to repopulate the liver. Donor derived stem cells will still require immunosuppression [53] but can be reliably produced in sufficient amounts in clinically approved conditions [54]. Pilot studies have been undertaken demonstrating proof of therapeutic potential and safety of the technique [55]. The ability to develop patient specific induced pleuripotent stem cells from which functional hepatocyte-like cells can be produced is a major advance [56]. These could in theory be genetically corrected and then transplanted, without the need for immunosuppression.

6. Conclusion

Liver transplant(ation) (LT) is now very successful with >85% long term survival into adult life. When considering the impact of LT for metabolic disease, two independent factors need to be considered: whether or not the defect causes significant liver disease and whether or not it is confined to the liver. When considering transplantation, many factors need to be considered including the local success of transplantation, the impact of the metabolic disease on the patient and family, and the potential for future therapeutic developments.

Where transplantation is undertaken for a liver-based defect there is a lifelong complete correction of the defect. Where there is a residual extrahepatic defect, this will have an impact on the outcome of LT and the severity of this defect must be considered as part of the transplant assessment process. Access to a multidisciplinary team with expertise in metabolic disease, liver disease, and other relevant organ-based specialists is crucial.

Most children will receive transplantation from cadaveric donor but living-related transplantation from a heterozygote parent is usually safe and effective. Auxiliary LT has a small but useful role where partial correction of the defect is helpful and there is a future prospect of gene therapy.

The first generation of hepatocyte transplants have shown proof of principle but to date have had a rather modest and temporary metabolic effect. Stem cells may have the potential to produce a more sustained and significant metabolic correction, but must be shown to be effective in controlled trials.

References

1. McKiernan PJ. Long-term care following paediatric liver transplantation. ArchDisChild EducPractEd. 2010.
2. Arnon R, Kerkar N, Davis MK, Anand R, Yin W, and Gonzalez-Peralta RP. Liver transplantation in children with metabolic diseases: the studies of pediatric liver transplantation experience. *PediatrTransplant* 2010;14(6):796–805.
3. Squires RH, Ng V, Romero R, Ekong U, Hardikar W, Emre S, *et al*. Evaluation of the pediatric patient for liver transplantation: 2014 practice guideline by the american association for the study of liver diseases, american society of transplantation and the north american society for pediatric gastroenterology, hepatology and nutrition. *Hepatology* 2014;60(1):362–98.
4. Sze YK, Dhawan A, Taylor RM, Bansal S, Mieli-Vergani G, Rela M, *et al*. Pediatric liver transplantation for metabolic liver disease: experience at King's College Hospital. *Transplantation* 2009;87(1):87–93.
5. Gelas T, McKiernan PJ, Kelly DA, Mayer DA, Mirza DF, and Sharif K. ABO-incompatible pediatric liver transplantation in very small recipients: Birmingham's experience. *Pediatr Transplant* 2011;15(7):706–11.
6. Davit-Spraul A, Gonzales E, Baussan C, and Jacquemin E. Progressive familial intrahepatic cholestasis. *Orphanet J Rare Dis* 2009;4:1.
7. Kubitz R, Droge C, Kluge S, Stross C, Walter N, Keitel V, *et al*. Autoimmune BSEP disease: disease recurrence after liver transplantation for progressive familial intrahepatic cholestasis. *Clin Rev Allergy Immunol* 2015;48(2–3):273–84.
8. Dowman JK, Watson D, Loganathan S, Gunson BK, Hodson J, Mirza DF, *et al*. Long-term impact of liver transplantation on respiratory function and nutritional status in children and adults with cystic fibrosis. *Am J Transplant* 2012;12(4):954–64.
9. Mindikoglu AL, King D, Magder LS, Ozolek JA, Mazariegos GV, and Shneider BL. Valproic acid-associated acute liver failure in children: case report and analysis of liver transplantation outcomes in the United States. *J Pediatr* 2011;158(5):802–7.
10. Sokal EM, Sokol R, Cormier V, Lacaille F, McKiernan P, Van Spronsen FJ, *et al*. Liver transplantation in mitochondrial respiratory chain disorders. *Eur J Pediatr* 1999;158(Suppl 2):S81–S4.

11. Rahman S. Gastrointestinal and hepatic manifestations of mitochondrial disorders. *J Inherit Metab Dis* 2013;36(4):659–73.

12. Paulusma CC, Elferink RP, and Jansen PL. Progressive familial intrahepatic cholestasis type 1. *Semin Liver Dis* 2010;30(2):117–24.

13. Lykavieris P, van Mil S, Cresteil D, Fabre M, Hadchouel M, Klomp L, et al. Progressive familial intrahepatic cholestasis type 1 and extrahepatic features: no catch-up of stature growth, exacerbation of diarrhea, and appearance of liver steatosis after liver transplantation. *J Hepatol* 2003;39(3):447–52.

14. Miyagawa-Hayashino A, Egawa H, Yorifuji T, Hasegawa M, Haga H, Tsuruyama T, et al. Allograft steatohepatitis in progressive familial intrahepatic cholestasis type 1 after living donor liver transplantation. *Liver Transpl* 2009;15(6):610–8.

15. Nicastro E, Stephenne X, Smets F, Fusaro F, de Magnee C, Reding R, et al. Recovery of graft steatosis and protein-losing enteropathy after biliary diversion in a PFIC 1 liver transplanted child. *Pediatr Transplant* 2012;16(5):E177–82.

16. Usui M, Isaji S, Das BC, Kobayashi M, Osawa I, Iida T, et al. Liver retransplantation with external biliary diversion for progressive familial intrahepatic cholestasis type 1: a case report. *Pediatr Transplant* 2009;13(5):611–4.

17. Haberle J, Boddaert N, Burlina A, Chakrapani A, Dixon M, Huemer M, et al. Suggested guidelines for the diagnosis and management of urea cycle disorders. *Orphanet J Rare Dis* 2012;7:32.

18. Leonard JV and McKiernan PJ. The role of liver transplantation in urea cycle disorders. *Mol Genet Metab* 2004;81(Suppl 1):S74–8.

19. Campeau PM, Pivalizza PJ, Miller G, McBride K, Karpen S, Goss J, et al. Early orthotopic liver transplantation in urea cycle defects: follow up of a developmental outcome study. *Mol Genet Metab* 2010;100(Suppl 1):S84–7.

20. Ah Mew N, Krivitzky L, McCarter R, Batshaw M, and Tuchman M. Urea Cycle Disorders Consortium of the Rare Diseases Clinical Research N. Clinical outcomes of neonatal onset proximal versus distal urea cycle disorders do not differ. *J Pediatr* 2013;162(2):324–9 e1.

21. Marble M, McGoey RR, Mannick E, Keats B, Ng SS, Deputy S, et al. Living related liver transplant in a patient with argininosuccinic aciduria and cirrhosis: metabolic follow-up. *J Pediatr Gastroenterol Nutr* 2008;46(4):453–6.

22. Newnham T, Hardikar W, Allen K, Wellard RM, Hamilton C, Angus P, et al. Liver transplantation for argininosuccinic aciduria: clinical, biochemical, and metabolic outcome. *Liver Transplant* 2008;14(1):41–5.

23. Cochat P and Rumsby G. Primary hyperoxaluria. *N Engl J Med* 2013;369(7):649–58.

24. Perera MT, Sharif K, Lloyd C, Foster K, Hulton SA, Mirza DF, et al. Preemptive liver transplantation for primary hyperoxaluria (PH-I) arrests long-term renal function deterioration. *Nephrol Dial Transplant* 2010;26(1):354–9.

25. Perera MT, McKiernan PJ, Sharif K, Milford DV, Lloyd C, Mayer DA, *et al.* Renal function recovery in children undergoing combined liver kidney transplants. *Transplantation* 2009;87(10):1584–9.
26. Sasaki K, Sakamoto S, Uchida H, Shigeta T, Matsunami M, Kanazawa H, *et al.* Two-step transplantation for primary hyperoxaluria: a winning strategy to prevent progression of systemic oxalosis in early onset renal insufficiency cases. *Pediatr Transplant* 2015;19(1):E1–6.
27. Saland JM, Ruggenenti P, and Remuzzi G. Liver-kidney transplantation to cure atypical hemolytic uremic syndrome. *J Am Soc Nephrol* 2009;20(5):940–9.
28. Greenbaum LA, Fila M, Ardissino G, Al-Akash SI, Evans J, Henning P, *et al.* Eculizumab is a safe and effective treatment in pediatric patients with atypical hemolytic uremic syndrome. *Kidney Int* 2016;89(3):701–11.
29. Zuber J, Quintrec ML, Krid S, Bertoye C, Gueutin V, Lahoche A, *et al.* Eculizumab for atypical hemolytic uremic syndrome recurrence in renal transplantation. *Am J Transplant* 2012;12(12):3337–54.
30. Leonard JV, Walter JH, and McKiernan PJ. The management of organic acidaemias: the role of transplantation. *J Inherit Metab Dis* 2001;24(2):309–11.
31. Charbit-Henrion F, Lacaille F, McKiernan P, Girard M, de LP, Valayannopoulos V, *et al.* Early and late complications after liver transplantation for propionic acidemia in children: a two centers study. *Am J Transplant* 2015;15(3):786–91.
32. Celik N SK, Bond G, Sun Q, Vockley G, Sindhi R, and Mazariegos G. Liver transplantation for propionic acidemia: a review of the United States Scientific Registry for Transplant Recipients (SRTR) and Non-US Case Series. *Am J Transplant* 2016;16:766.
33. Kasahara M, Sakamoto S, Horikawa R, Koji U, Mizuta K, Shinkai M, *et al.* Living donor liver transplantation for pediatric patients with metabolic disorders: the Japanese multicenter registry. *Pediatr Transplant* 2014; 18(1):6–15.
34. Chakrapani A, Sivakumar P, McKiernan PJ, and Leonard JV. Metabolic stroke in methylmalonic acidemia five years after liver transplantation. *J Pediatr* 2002;140(2):261–3.
35. Mazariegos GV, Morton DH, Sindhi R, Soltys K, Nayyar N, Bond G, *et al.* Liver transplantation for classical maple syrup urine disease: long-term follow-up in 37 patients and comparative United Network for Organ Sharing experience. *J Pediatr* 2012;160(1):116–21 e1.
36. Diaz VM, Camarena C, de la Vega A, Martinez-Pardo M, Diaz C, Lopez M, *et al.* Liver transplantation for classical maple syrup urine disease: long-term follow-up. *J Pediatr Gastroenterol Nutr* 2014;59(5):636–9.
37. Al-Shamsi A, Baker A, Dhawan A, and Hertecant J. Acute metabolic crises in maple syrup urine disease after liver transplantation from a related heterozygous living donor. *JIMD Reports* 2016, Vol. 30, Heidelberg: Springer.

38. Feier F, Schwartz IV, Benkert AR, Seda Neto J, Miura I, Chapchap P, *et al.* Living related versus deceased donor liver transplantation for maple syrup urine disease. *Mol Genet Metab* 2016;117(3):336–43.

39. Boers SJ, Visser G, Smit PG, and Fuchs SA. Liver transplantation in glycogen storage disease type I. *Orphanet J Rare Dis* 2014;9:47.

40. Strauss KA, Ferreira C, Bottiglieri T, Zhao X, Arning E, Zhang S, *et al.* Liver transplantation for treatment of severe S-adenosylhomocysteine hydrolase deficiency. *Mol GenetMetab* 2015;116(1-2):44–52.

41. Celik N, Squires RH, Vockley J, Sindhi R, and Mazariegos G. Liver transplantation for maple syrup urine disease: a global domino effect. *Pediatr Transplant* 2016;20(3):350–1.

42. Popescu I and Dima SO. Domino liver transplantation: how far can we push the paradigm? *Liver Transpl* 2012;18(1):22–8.

43. Khanna A, Gish R, Winter SC, Nyhan WL, and Barshop BA. Successful domino liver transplantation from a patient with methylmalonic acidemia. *JIMD Reports* 2015, Heidelberg: Springer.

44. Morioka D, Takada Y, Kasahara M, Ito T, Uryuhara K, Ogawa K, *et al.* Living donor liver transplantation for noncirrhotic inheritable metabolic liver diseases: impact of the use of heterozygous donors. *Transplantation* 2005;80(5):623–8.

45. Pham TA, Enns GM, and Esquivel CO. Living donor liver transplantation for inborn errors of metabolism — an underutilized resource in the United States. *Pediatr Transplant* 2016;20(6):770–3.

46. Roelandt P, Dobbels P, Komuta M, Corveleyn A, Emonds MP, Roskams T, *et al.* Heterozygous alpha1-antitrypsin Z allele mutation in presumed healthy donor livers used for transplantation. *Eur J Gastroenterol Hepatol* 2013;25(11):1335–9.

47. Tannuri AC, Gibelli NE, Ricardi LR, Santos MM, Maksoud-Filho JG, Pinho-Apezzato ML, *et al.* Living related donor liver transplantation in children. *Transplant Proc* 2011;43(1):161–4.

48. Nagasaka H, Yorifuji T, Egawa H, Kikuta H, Tanaka K, and Kobayashi K. Successful living-donor liver transplantation from an asymptomatic carrier mother in ornithine transcarbamylase deficiency. *J Pediatr* 2001;138(3):432–4.

49. Rela M, Bharathan A, Palaniappan K, Cherian PT, and Reddy MS. Portal flow modulation in auxiliary partial orthotopic liver transplantation. *Pediatr Transplant* 2015;19(3):255–60.

50. Rela M, Muiesan P, Vilca-Melendez H, Dhawan A, Baker A, Mieli-Vergani G, *et al.* Auxiliary partial orthotopic liver transplantation for Crigler-Najjar syndrome type I. *Ann Surg* 1999;229(4):565–9.

51. Govil S, Shanmugam NP, Reddy MS, Narasimhan G, and Rela M. A metabolic chimera: two defective genotypes make a normal phenotype. *Liver Transpl* 2015;21(11):1453–4.

52. Hughes RD, Mitry RR, and Dhawan A. Current status of hepatocyte transplantation. *Transplantation* 2012;93(4):342–7.

53. Puppi J, Strom SC, Hughes RD, Bansal S, Castell JV, Dagher I, *et al.* Improving the techniques for human hepatocyte transplantation: report from a consensus meeting in London. *Cell Transplant* 2012;21(1):1–10.

54. Najimi M, Defresne F, and Sokal EM. Concise review: updated advances and current challenges in cell therapy for inborn liver metabolic defects. *Stem Cell Transl Med* 2016;5(8):1117–25.

55. Dobbelaere D, Semts F, McKiernan, *et al.* Phase I/II multicenter trial of liver derived mesenchymal stem cells (HepastemR) for the treatment of urea cycle disorder and Crigler Najjar syndrome. Interim analysis at 6 months post infusion. *J Inherit Metab Dis* 2014;37:S27.

56. Yusa K, Rashid ST, Strick-Marchand H, Varela I, Liu PQ, Paschon DE, *et al.* Targeted gene correction of α1-antitrypsin deficiency in induced pluripotent stem cells. *Nature* 2011;478(7369):391.

15. Fulminant Hepatic Failure: Integrating Devices with Liver Transplantation

Nigel Heaton and Shirin Elizabeth Khorsandi

*King's Health Partners at Denmark Hill Campus,
Institute of Liver Studies, Kings College Hospital NHSFT, London,
SE59RS, UK*

1. Introduction

Acute liver failure (ALF), which is synonymous with fulminant hepatic failure, is a rare life-threatening condition that typically occurs in the context of no pre-existing liver disease. Clinically, the conscious level declines as brain edema, hypoglycemia, and extrahepatic organ failure evolve [1]. ALF produces cardiovascular instability, renal failure, brain edema, and death due to irreversible shock, cerebral herniation, or development of multiorgan failure.

Originally, fulminant hepatic failure was defined as a severe liver injury, potentially reversible in nature, with the onset of encephalopathy occurring within 8 weeks of the first symptoms in the absence of pre-existing liver disease [2]. However, it is increasingly recognized that there are ALF clinical phenotype subtypes that are defined by the time it takes for encephalopathy to develop from first symptoms [3]. In hyperacute liver failure, this is usually less than a week and the etiology is typically acetaminophen toxicity or viral, while the slower evolving subacute liver failure is second to a drug-induced liver injury or etiology remains indeterminate [2, 3]. Subacute liver failure has a poorer outcome compared to hyperacute in the absence of liver transplant(ation) (LT) [2, 3]. Establishing the correct etiology in ALF is important as diagnosis impacts on treatment choices as well as helping with the prognostic assessment, e.g., acetaminophen toxicity is increasingly managed medically.

Over the past four decades the outcomes for ALF have significantly improved from a survival rate of 16.7% in 1973 to 62.2% in 2008 [3]. A patient presenting in 1984 had an 80% likelihood of dying from severe cerebral edema and intracranial hypertension; this has now been reduced to 20%, reflecting improvement in liver intensive care and the application of criteria to select patients for LT [4–6]. The decline in the incidence of cerebral edema and intracranial hypertension over time also highlights the importance of earlier disease recognition, better initial treatment such as body temperature control, plasma tonicity, systemic hemodynamics, and the early use of renal replacement therapy, with the greatest benefit resulting from early institution of intensive care.

Recommendations in the management of adult ALF have been made [7, 8] but selection criteria are less well defined in pediatric ALF [9, 10]. In children, the classical (adult) ALF definition of encephalopathy onset within 8 weeks of liver injury is difficult to apply as children may either present with ALF revealing an underlying metabolic disease with liver involvement or have encephalopathy unrelated to ALF. In pediatric ALF, liver-related encephalopathy is a late complication, associated with a poor prognosis. As a result, the definition of ALF in children has been modified to a multisystem disorder with severe impairment of liver function, with or without encephalopathy, with no underlying chronic liver disease [11, 12].

Intensive care management of ALF in both children and adults are to prevent or treat its major complications which include encephalopathy, brain edema, intracranial hypertension, bleeding, hepatorenal syndrome, infection, and ultimately, multiorgan failure. The aim of supportive care is to provide an environment and time for the liver to recover function and if not, to support the patient until a suitable liver graft becomes available for transplant to proceed. The rarity of ALF combined with its variable etiology, rapidity, and severity of presentation means that the evidence basis for best supportive care is limited [2, 3, 8]. The following sections of this chapter highlight some of the devices that have been developed and applied to the assessment, support, and monitoring of patients with ALF. This is followed by a summary of some of the concepts and current developments in the evolving field of artificial and bioartificial liver support.

2. Devices for assessment/prognostication in acute liver failure (ALF)

Early identification of which ALF patient will not recover with medical therapy alone will help to expedite the decision regarding LT and widens the window of opportunity for a donor liver to become available. As a result, a variety of prognostic systems and markers have been utilized. The most widely used and established is the King's College Criteria [4]. However, its accuracy in identifying patients needing transplant declines in nonacetaminophen ALF [13, 14]. Additionally, King's College Criteria is a poor negative predictor in children, mainly because in adults, severity of organ dysfunction is associated with hepatic encephalopathy and outcome. As a consequence, it has been proposed that the Pediatric Risk of Mortality (PRISM) score more accurately assesses the severity of ALF in children [15–17] and infants <90 days presenting additional dilemmas, with better spontaneous survival (>60%) than expected being found [18].

A number of different prognostic predictors in ALF of varying applicability in adults and children have been described including Clichy's criteria, liver histology, Model for End-stage Liver Disease (MELD), Pediatric End-stage Liver Disease (PELD), Acute Physiology and Chronic Health Evaluation II (APACHE2), and PRISM score. However, many of these fail to provide consistent and reproducible results [14, 16]. Other tests that have also been evaluated involve the administration of a variety of drugs to assess the functional liver reserve with a measuring device at the bedside.

Indocyanine green (ICG), a water soluble, inert anionic compound is the most well known. Administered as an intravenous injection, it binds to albumin and β lipoproteins in plasma. ICG is mainly excreted in the bile without being metabolized and undergoes no enterohepatic recirculation. ICG has been used to assess liver function before hepatectomy, in LT donor and recipients, in chronic liver disease and in the critically ill [19]. Typically, the rate of disappearance of ICG from the plasma (ICG-PDR) is used as a marker of liver function and normally should be >18%/minute [20]. However, ICG clearance is decreased by reduced hepatic blood flow, either as a result of local (hepatosplanchnic) or systemic hypoperfusion, or if there is reduced ICG extraction because of hepatocyte dysfunction or hyperbilirubinemia.

The measurement of ICG clearance can either be performed using an intravascular fiberoptic (invasive) or transcutaneous noninvasive pulse dye densitometry (PDD) sensor placed on a digit [21]. The principle used to measure arterial ICG concentration is based on the difference in wavelength absorbance between oxyhemoglobin (905 nm) and ICG (805 nm). There are two systems available for ICG PDD measurement; both calculate the rate constant (k) of the ICG indicator dilution curve by backward dynamic extrapolation of the elimination phase. The ICG-PDR is then calculated by multiplying k by 100. ICG-PDR and the ICG retention ratio after 15 minutes (ICGR15) are the main ICG variables used in assessing liver function; normal values are >18%/minute and <10%, respectively [20].

There is some data to support the use of ICG clearance as a tool for ALF prognostic assessment. In a small study on adult patients ($n = 25$), ICG-PDR >6.3% was associated with spontaneous liver recovery (sensitivity 86% and specificity of 89%) but most of the patients studied did not fulfill ALF criteria for transplant. However, a similar cutoff value was found in ALF occurring after major hepatectomy in adults, where MARS® (Molecular Adsorbent Recirculating System) was used as bridging treatment. For children, <5.9%/minute was predictive of the need for transplantation [22, 23].

Another bedside test that has been used in ALF to identify the need for transplant is a noninvasive breath test based on cytochrome P450 1A2 capacity. A ^{13}C labeled methacetin solution is injected intravenously, and metabolized by the hepatocyte cytochrome P450 1A2 into paracetamol and $^{13}CO_2$. After 60 minutes, 40 breaths are analyzed for $^{13}CO_2/^{12}CO_2$ ratio using a modified nondispersive isotope selective infrared spectroscopy based device [24]. In one small retrospective pilot study of nonacetaminophen induced ALF ($n = 12$), a cutoff value of 38 μg/kg/hour was found to be predictive for a negative outcome, suggesting that this system could be useful in predicting individual ALF prognosis [25]. However, the King's College Criteria remains the standard in ALF prognostic guidance, with alternative clinical scoring systems and bedside functional tests for liver recovery, requiring further prospective study for their validation to support widespread adoption.

3. Monitoring

3.1. *General*

In the context of ALF, grade 3–4 encephalopathy leads to semielective intubation and ventilation or in patients with grade 1 or 2 that are undergoing sedation or an intervention, rather than respiratory failure. Additionally, in ALF with its associated coagulopathy ± renal dysfunction, invasive cardiovascular monitoring and bedside ECHO is often needed to allow for optimal fluid and vasoactive drug management.

3.2. Cardiovascular

Monitoring the cardiac index (CI) either in liver intensive care or theatre enables goal-directed optimization of the stroke volume and CI. Measurement of CI with the pulmonary artery catheter is regarded as the gold standard but less invasive techniques are gaining popularity and these are based on transpulmonary thermodilution or arterial waveform analysis.

The pulse contour cardiac output (PiCCO) system (Pulsion Medical System; Munich, Germany) is a continuous cardiac output (CO) monitor, which uses a femoral arterial catheter with a thermistor to analyze pulse contour. The device uses an algorithm to analyze the arterial pressure waveform calculating the pulsatile systolic area in order to give data on preload (intrathoracic blood volume), afterload, myocardial contractility, CO and extravascular lung water index [26]. It is initially calibrated by using thermodilution to estimate cardiac output. CO measured by PiCCO and thermodilution are comparable [27, 28]. Other devices that make use of proprietary pulse power algorithms to calculate the CO are the Lithium Dilution Cardiac Output (LiDCO) (LiDCO Ltd; Cambridge, UK) and FloTrac/Vigileo (Edwards Life-Sciences LLC, Irvine, CA) [29]. The ideal hemodynamic monitoring device is to be determined and presently, transplant institutional practice determines which system is used [30].

3.3. Neuromonitoring

ALF produces cerebral edema and raised intracranial pressure (ICP) in 15–20% of patients [31, 32]. The development of grade 3 or 4 encephalopathy is a poor prognostic marker dependent on etiology in adults, as this is associated with intracranial hypertension and brain herniation [33]. Worsening of encephalopathy and the Cushing reflex (systemic hypertension and bradycardia) with altered pupillary reflexes and decerebrate rigidity occur late in ALF. At this point, therapeutic interventions such as transplant or aggressive intensive care management start to become futile. As a consequence, ICP monitoring is helpful to allow for pre-emptive management such as initiating continuous hemofiltration to lower plasma ammonia [32–34]. Targets in managing cerebral edema are to maintain ICP

<20 mmHg and cerebral perfusion pressure >60 mmHg either by reducing brain volume or cerebral blood flow.

3.3.1. Invasive

The use of invasive neuromonitoring in ALF, i.e., subdural devices based on saline-filled transducers and electrical impedance is becoming less common, through a combination of associated complications and the lack of randomized trial data showing a benefit from their use. Additionally, the occurrence of intracranial hypertension in ALF appears to be declining [3, 5]. Bleeding complications occurs in 8–10% and fatal bleeds more rarely. However, it permits continuous monitoring to be performed, allowing for more responsive treatment of raised ICP in ALF, especially in the optimization for transplant to be undertaken [35, 36].

3.3.2. Noninvasive

Noninvasive neuromonitoring techniques including Transcranial Doppler (TCD), Optic Nerve Sheath Diameter (ONSD) and jugular bulb oxygen saturations are increasingly utilized as they avoid the complications of invasive neuromonitoring. TCD estimates the ICP from blood flow waveform characteristics in the middle cerebral artery, by calculating the pulsatility index (PI), which is systolic minus diastolic flow velocity divided by mean flow velocity [37]. The utility of TCD in ICP measurement in ALF has not been prospectively validated but it does correlate with invasively measured ICP [38].

The ONSD measures the diameter of the optic nerve sheath using transocular ultrasound, the expansion of the nerve sheath diameter correlates with invasively measured ICP. Many of the noninvasive neuromonitoring techniques require training, have variation between observers, are not continuous, and are regarded by as not being as accurate as invasive ICP monitoring, but they can distinguish between normal and raised ICP (>20 mmHg).

Jugular bulb oximetry ($SjvO_2$), measures the unused oxygen by the brain that is determined by cerebral blood flow and cerebral metabolic activity, therefore providing an indirect continuous assessment of cerebral blood flow. The technique involves insertion of fiberoptic oximeter into the jugular bulb. Normal $SjvO_2$ is 55–70%. Cerebral blood flow is inversely related to the arterial–jugular venous oxygen content difference, so <55% represents compromise [39]. With all the aforementioned noninvasive ICP monitoring devices, and other systems such as transcranial near infrared reflective spectroscopy (NIRS) [40] and pupillometry [41], validation in ALF needs to be done, in order to establish the ideal monitoring that can guide treatment.

4. Support

4.1. *General*

Respiratory dysfunction is uncommon in the early phases of ALF and the goals of respiratory care are similar to that of other critical illnesses. However, in fulminant ALF that escalates into multiorgan failure, in selected candidates, extracorporeal membrane oxygenation (ECMO) has been undertaken, either venovenous (VV) for respiratory failure or venoarterial (VA) for combined cardiac and respiratory failure. Indications for ECMO in ALF are respiratory and/or cardiac failure that is refractory to standard intensive care support and is anticipated to be reversible on LT. ALF is normally regarded as a relative contraindication because of the perceived risk of intracranial hemorrhage from coagulopathy combined with a raised ICP. There has been one case report of successful management of a child with fulminant Wilsons requiring ECMO support for pulmonary hemorrhage and subsequent LT [42]. And institutionally, five out of nine ALF patients have survived after being supported and/or bridged to LT with VA or VV ECMO. The overall reported experience is limited, but VV ECMO in the postoperative setting has met with a greater likelihood of survival. Pretransplant ECMO has been associated with a higher mortality and morbidity (including fungal sepsis as a late complication) and further understanding of patient selection is required [43].

A low arterial blood pressure with systemic vasodilation, with or without sepsis is common in ALF [44] and cardiovascular support in ALF is not significantly different to that used in other critical illnesses, with targets in care being maintenance of circulating volume, systemic perfusion, and oxygen delivery. Renal dysfunction occurs in more than 50% of patients with ALF and continuous rather than intermittent renal replacement therapy is preferred in order to achieve better metabolic and hemodynamic stability, as well as control of hyperammonia and acid–base disturbances [45]. Plasma ammonia >150–200 mmol/L is a risk factor for intracranial hypertension and early institution of continuous hemofiltration (adults and children) before the onset of significant renal dysfunction should be adopted to clear ammonia [32, 46–48].

4.2. Liver support systems

4.2.1. Overview

A key aspects in ALF management is to replace or preserve organ function in order to avoid the multiorgan failure, while waiting for either liver regeneration or transplantation [3, 4]. However, the main determinants of the clinical presentation in ALF have not been fully defined but the accumulation of inflammatory mediators, toxins, and metabolites that are produced and/or not cleared by the failing liver are thought to be central. Based on these ideas, liver support systems have been designed that remove both water-soluble toxins (e.g., ammonia) and lipophilic albumin-bound toxins (e.g., bilirubin, bile acids, aromatic amino acid metabolites, medium chain fatty acids, cytokines).

Initial liver support strategies were therefore based on hemodialysis, hemofiltration, or hemoperfusion, evolving with the addition of charcoal/albumin adsorption (hemodiabsorption). But it was recognized that liver synthetic and metabolic functions were not being supported, leading to the introduction of a cellular component in circuit design. Present liver support systems can broadly be divided into the artificial and bioartificial. In the artificial liver support system, the focus is on detoxification using a combination of filtration and/or adsorption while in the bioartificial, the use of hepatocytes (human/zoonotic) for synthetic and detoxification is emphasized [49].

4.2.2. Artificial

Most liver support systems are composed of a number of therapeutic modules/units that are joined together. These modules can range from conventional hemodialysis or hemofiltration units to custom-designed adsorptive modules. The artificial liver support systems with the most clinical data are Molecular Adsorbent Recirculating System (MARS®; Gambro, Stockholm, Sweden) and the fractionated plasma separation and adsorption system (Prometheus®, Fresenius Medical Care, Bad Homburg, Germany); both systems combine filtration with adsorption. MARS® is a high-flux hollow-fiber hemodiafilter that uses albumin as the acceptor molecule for lipophilic toxins. The recirculated albumin is regenerated, by passing it through an anion exchanger and charcoal adsorber [50]. While in Prometheus®, the fractionated plasma separation and adsorption system uses an albumin-permeable polysulfone membrane, combined with conventional, high-flux dialysis [51].

Similar in concept to MARS®, single-pass albumin dialysis (SPAD®) uses a standard renal replacement therapy machine and is based on a high-flux hollow-fiber hemodiafilter with an albumin solution in counter directional flow. But the albumin solution is discarded after passing through the filter rather than recirculated as in MARS® [52]. While in the Hepa Wash® system (Hepa Wash GmbH, Munich, Germany) albumin is regenerated with adsorbers, by using changes in pH and temperature [53]. In another design, selective plasma exchange therapy (SEPET™, Arbios Systems, Allendale, NJ, USA) fractionated plasma separation is combined with single-pass albumin dialysis; the albumin fraction is then discarded and replaced with electrolytes, albumin, and fresh frozen plasma [54]. Despite increasingly sophisticated device design and sorbents, the clinical evidence for the survival benefit in ALF is not substantive (see Section 4.2.4) [55, 56].

4.2.3. *Bioartificial*

The basic concept in the design of a bioartificial liver support system is to combine detoxification with the added benefit of hepatocyte synthetic and regulatory function. The biological component being fulfilled by the use of an extracorporeal bioreactor either a whole liver or 3D liver cell culture that allow for perfusion. The first liver support system used was an extracorporeal whole liver perfusion system in dogs via an Eck (portocaval) fistula [57, 58]. This was then repeated in pigs and humans [59, 60]. But this system was not the most practical or the best use of a donor liver, requiring the organ to be connected to the patient's blood stream with a modified heart–lung machine.

In bioartificial design, hepatocytes are cultured in a cell-housing bioreactor that processes circulated plasma or blood from the patient. Alternative bioreactor designs for cell housing are hollow fiber, packed bed, flat bed, and perfused bed [61]. But there are a number of limitations in these designs such as restricted convectional movement, poor cellular nutritional gradients, and poor hepatocyte growth [62].

In the HepatAssist™ system (Alliqua Inc., Langhorne, PA, USA), plasma ultrafiltrate from the patient is passed through an activated charcoal adsorber and oxygenator prior to the modified dialysis cartridge that houses cryopreserved porcine hepatocytes [63, 64]. The Extracorporeal Liver Assist Device (ELAD®; Vital Therapies Inc., San Diego, CA, USA) has a similar arrangement with a charcoal adsorber and membrane oxygenator, but uses a hepatoblastoma cell line [65] separated from plasma with a hollow-fiber membrane, while in the Modular Extracorporeal Liver Support (MELS) system, the bioreactor houses either porcine [66] or human hepatocytes [67] and consists of two columns of hydrophilic polyethersulfone membrane combined with hollow hydrophobic fibers for oxygenation. In the Academisch Medisch Centrum Bioartificial Liver (AMC-BAL), there is no separating membrane, so the plasma is in direct contact with the bioreactor cells to enable better mass exchange [68].

A key aspect limiting bioartificial liver device development is finding the ideal cell to populate the bioreactors. The ideal bioreactor hepatocyte should be human, safe, metabolically active, and easily expandable. But human hepatocytes are impractical in terms of both quantity and availability. Primary hepatocytes are able to divide *in vivo* but once in culture, outside their normal cell niche, start to dedifferentiate and stop dividing. Cryopreservation then leads to further loss in viability and functionality. Ideally, primary hepatocytes should be isolated a few days before use, which adds to logistics and cost, limiting the applicability of these systems.

In contrast, bioreactors that use established cultured hepatocyte cell lines are easier to handle, can be prepared and integrated into the bioreactors in advance. However, established hepatocyte cell lines in culture are heavily passaged, leading to genetic drift and loss of hepatocyte phenotype [69]. C3A, a human hepatoblastoma cell line, used in the ELAD® system, can hypothetically metastasize if there is a break in the fiber circuits [65], while porcine hepatocytes that are used in the AMC-BAL and HepatAssistTM systems have problems with metabolic biocompatibility, immunogenicity, and risk of xenozoonoses [66]. Additionally, poorer survival is experienced when xenogenic systems are used for liver support in humans [63, 70]. For now, there is a moratorium on xenotransplantation in Europe but in other countries there are less restrictions.

Other technical issues are related to the membranes that limit mass exchange and the column arrangement of the hollow fibers that result in low flow rates (100–200 mL/minute) in the bioreactors [71]. As a consequence, new bioreactor designs, e.g., spheroids, are being explored in order to create a more physiological relationship between the hepatocyte and patient blood to improve mass exchange and cell health [72].

4.2.4. Trials

Well-designed trials in ALF are difficult to undertake; the condition is rare and heterogeneous in etiology and presentation. Therefore, most of the clinical studies on liver support systems are nonblinded, uncontrolled, and insufficiently powered. There is increasing evidence that just the use of hemofiltration or plasma exchange can help with ammonia clearance and immune system dysfunction to reduce the risk of brain edema and multiorgan failure in ALF [32, 46–48, 55]. Plasmapheresis, synonymous with plasma replacement or exchange therapy with fresh frozen plasma, in ALF has been shown to be safe, reduce encephalopathy and vasopressor need, as well as improve hepatic based nitrogen homeostasis [73–78]. In a recent prospective, randomized, controlled multicenter trial (n = 182 ALF, n = 90 standard medical therapy vs. n = 92 plasmapheresis), plasmapheresis was found to improve transplant-free survival, with the main benefit on survival being seen in patients who did not have transplant [79]. Enthusiasm for the addition of sorbents such as charcoal to the liver support circuits in the 1970s declined, after a randomized control trial in the 1980s failed to show benefit (see Table 1). The perceived benefit reflected more an improvement

Table 1. Summary of published randomized trials on liver support systems (artificial and bioartificial) used in ALF that compare liver support to standard medical therapy (SMT). BioLogic-DT system (HemoCleanse Inc, West Lafayette, IN, USA) is based on hemodiabsorption with activated charcoal. Molecular Adsorbent Recirculation System (MARS®; Gambro, Stockholm, Sweden) uses a hollow-fiber hemodiafilter that regenerates albumin with an anion exchanger and charcoal adsorber. The Extracorporeal Liver Assist Device (ELAD®; Vital Therapies Inc., San Diego, CA, USA) uses a charcoal adsorber and membrane oxygenator, with hepatoblastoma cell line. HepatAssist™ system (Alliqua Inc., Langhorne, PA, USA) uses an activated charcoal adsorber and oxygenator with cryopreserved porcine hepatocytes

	Reference	Liver support system	Multicenter	Sample size Liver support	SMT
Artificial	Redeker 1973[93]	Whole blood exchange	No	15	13
	O'Grady 1988[94]	Charcoal hemoperfusion	No	29	33
	#Hughes 1994[95]	Biologic-DT	No	5	5
	#Mazariegos 1997[96]	Biologic-DT	No	5	5
	El Banayosy 2004[97]	MARS	No	14	13
	*Larsen 2016[79]	Plasmapheresis	Yes	92	90
Bioartificial	Ellis 1996[65]	ELAD	No	12	12
	#Stevens 2001[98]	HepatAssist	Yes	73	74
	#Demetriou 2004[64]	HepatAssist	Yes	85	86

Note: *Not included in the meta-analyses of liver support.

#Duplicate institutional data [89–91].

in liver intensive care management, rather than from the liver support system per se [4–6]. This has implications for the introduction and use of artificial liver support and the value of clinical trials in assessing possible benefit.

There have been five large prospective randomized controlled trials using MARS® [56, 80–83] not all necessarily applicable in the scenario of ALF. The conclusions are that MARS® is safe and results in better biochemistry and improvement in encephalopathy but no benefit on survival is found. Similarly, with two studies that have compared MARS® and Prometheus®, the RELIEF trial (n = 189) [56], and HELIOS study (n = 145) [84], no survival benefit was found. Otherwise, clinical data on SPAD is in the form of case reports and series [85, 86]. Bioartificial liver support has mainly be assessed in small studies [66–68, 87, 88], apart from the HepatAssist™ system where a randomized study has been undertaken in ALF or primary nonfunction after LT. In that study, no improvement in 30-day survival was found (n = 171, HepatAssist™ vs. standard care), but on subgroup analysis, survival in ALF was found to be better [64].

The clinical effectiveness of liver support systems, both artificial and bioartificial, have been summarized in three major systematic reviews and meta-analysis (see Table 1) [89–91]. Two studies summarized data from trials for liver support systems (n = 5) in ALF from 1973 to 2001 and concluded that there was no survival benefit from their use [89, 90]. However, a more recent meta-analysis based on randomized control trials (n = 3) from 1996 to 2004 concluded that there was a survival benefit from the use of liver support in ALF [91]. However, no individual randomized control trial has showed a survival benefit from liver support in ALF. But one trial, after subgroup analysis, taking into account the confounding factors then, demonstrated a survival benefit in ALF [64].

The explanation for no clear survival benefit, being demonstrated in artificial and bioartificial liver support systems, may be related to a number of factors in addition to trial design, such as insufficient detoxification or insufficient hepatocyte mass to fulfill metabolic needs. But fundamentally, all the functions of the liver have not been fully characterized. Similarly, the environment and pathways involved in liver regeneration have not been fully determined and our ability to optimize these remains limited. Therefore, unselective adsorption may be removing elements that are important for liver regeneration. In addition, the benefit of liver support may be more evident in certain ALF subgroups (e.g., hyperacute liver failure secondary to acetaminophen toxicity) that have a higher rate of liver regeneration and recovery.

5. Conclusion

The actual pathophysiology in ALF that determines multiorgan failure or whether a liver will recover is still not fully understood. But over the past few decades, advances in patient care have significantly improved survival from what was regarded as a fatal illness. ALF is a potentially reversible disease caused by a critical loss of functioning hepatocyte mass [92] and being able to use devices to assess liver functional reserve, monitor and support during the illness of ALF will improve care. The use of liver support systems (artificial or bioartificial) in ALF, while awaiting transplant or liver regeneration, has been explored over the past few decades, with limited survival benefit. Continuing developments in nanomaterials, tissue bioengineering, and induced pluripotent stem cells will change the design of liver support systems for application in the near future.

References

1. O'Grady JG, Schalm SW, and Williams R. Acute liver failure: redefining the syndromes. *Lancet* 1993;342:273–5.
2. Bernal W and Wendon J. Acute liver failure. *N Engl J Med* 2013;369:2525–34.
3. Bernal W, Hyyrylainen A, Gera A, *et al.* Lessons from look back in acute liver failure? A single centre experience of 3300 patients. *J Hepatol* 2013;59:74–80.
4. O'Grady JG, Alexander GJ, Hayllar KM, and Williams R. Early indicators of prognosis in fulminant hepatic failure. *Gastroenterology* 1989;97:439–45.
5. Bernal W, Lee WM, Wendon J, *et al.* Acute liver failure: a curable disease by 2024? *J Hepatol* 2015;62:S112–20.
6. Bernal W, Auzinger G, Sizer E, *et al.* Intensive care management of acute liver failure. *Semin Liver Dis* 2008;28:188–200.
7. Stravitz RT, Kramer AH, Davern T, *et al.* Intensive care of patients with acute liver failure: recommendations of the U. S. Acute Liver Failure Study Group. *Crit Care Med* 2007;35:2498–508.
8. Lee WM, Stravitz RT, and Larson AM. Introduction to the revised American Association for the Study of Liver Diseases Position Paper on acute liver failure 2011. *Hepatology* 2012;55:965–7.
9. Bhaduri BR and Mieli-Vergani G. Fulminant hepatic failure: pediatric aspects. *Semin Liver Dis* 1996;16:349–55.
10. Squires RH, Jr., Shneider BL, Bucuvalas J, *et al.* Acute liver failure in children: the first 348 patients in the pediatric acute liver failure study group. *J Pediatr* 2006;148:652–8.
11. Dhawan A. Etiology and prognosis of acute liver failure in children. *Liver Transpl* 2008;14:S80–4.

12. Shanmugam NP, Bansal S, Greenough A, *et al.* Neonatal liver failure: aetiologies and management-state of the art. *Eur J Pediatr* 2011;170:573–81.
13. Bailey B, Amre DK, and Gaudreault P. Fulminant hepatic failure secondary to acetaminophen poisoning: a systematic review and meta-analysis of prognostic criteria determining the need for liver transplantation. *Crit Care Med* 2003;31:299–305.
14. McPhail MJ, Wendon JA, and Bernal W. Meta-analysis of performance of Kings's College Hospital Criteria in prediction of outcome in non-paracetamol-induced acute liver failure. *J Hepatol* 2010; 53:492–9.
15. Tissières P, Prontera W, Chevret L, and Devictor D. The pediatric risk of mortality score in infants and children with fulminant liver failure. *Pediatr Transplant* 2003;7:64–8.
16. Jain V and Dhawan A. Prognostic modelling in paediatric acute liver failure. *Liver Transpl* 2016. doi: 10.1002/lt.24501.
17. Ciocca M, Ramonet M, Cuarterolo M, *et al.* Prognosis factors in pediatric acute liver failure. *Arch Dis Child* 2008;3:48–51.
18. Sundaram SS, Alonso EM, Narkewicz MR, *et al.* Characterization and outcomes of young infants with acute liver failure. *J Pediatr* 2011;159:813–8.
19. Vos J, Wietasch KG, Absalom AR, *et al.* Green light for liver function monitoring using indocyanine green? An overview of current clinical applications. *Anaesthesia* 2014;69:1364–76.
20. Fox IJ, Brooker LG, Heseltine DW, *et al.* A tricarbocyanine dye for continuous recording of dilution curves in whole blood independent of variations in blood oxygen saturation. *Proc Staff Meet Mayo Clinic* 1957;32:478–84.
21. Sakka SG, Reinhart K, and Meier-Hellmann A. Comparison of invasive and noninvasive measurements of indocyanine green plasma disappearance rate in critically ill patients with mechanical ventilation and stable hemodynamics. *Intensive Care Med* 2000;26:1553–6.
22. Merle U, Sieg O, Stremmel W, *et al.* Sensitivity and specificity of plasma disappearance rate of indocyanine green as a prognostic indicator in acute liver failure. *BMC Gastroenterol* 2009;9:91.
23. Inderbitzin D, Muggli B, Ringger A, *et al.* Molecular absorbent recirculating system for the treatment of acute liver failure in surgical patients. *J Gastrointest Surg* 2005;9:1155–61.
24. Stockmann M, Lock JF, Riecke B, *et al.* Prediction of postoperative outcome after hepatectomy with a new bedside test for maximal liver function capacity. *Ann Surg* 2009;250:119–25.
25. Lock JF, Kotobi AN, Malinowski M, *et al.* Predicting the prognosis in acute liver failure: results from a retrospective pilot study using the LiMAx test. *Ann Hepatol* 2013;12:556–62.
26. Diaz S, Perez-Pena J, Sanz J, *et al.* Haemodynamic monitoring and liver function evaluation by pulsion cold system Z-201 (PCS) during orthotopic liver transplantation. *Clin Transplant* 2003;17:47–55.

27. Della Rocca G, Costa MG, Coccia C, *et al.* Preload and haemodynamic assessment during liver transplantation: a comparison between the pulmonary artery catheter and transpulmonary indicator dilution techniques. *Eur J Anaesthesiol* 2002;19:868–87.

28. Della Rocca G, Costa MG, Pompei L, *et al.* Continuous and intermittent cardiac output measurement: pulmonary artery catheter versus aortic transpulmonary technique. *Br J Anaesth* 2002;88:350–6.

29. Button D, Weibel L, Reuthebuch O, *et al.* Clinical evaluation of the FloTrac/Vigileo™ system and two established continuous cardiac output monitoring devices in patients undergoing cardiac surgery. *Br J Anaesth* 2007;99:329–36.

30. Krenn C-G, De Wolf AM. Current approach to intra-operative monitoring in liver transplantation. *Curr Opin Organ Transpl* 2008;13:285–90.

31. Murphy N, Auzinger G, Bernal W, *et al.* The effect of hypertonic sodium chloride on intracranial pressure in patients with acute liver failure. *Hepatology* 2004;39:464–70.

32. Bernal W, Hall C, Karvellas CJ, *et al.* Arterial ammonia and clinical risk factors for encephalopathy and intracranial hypertension in acute liver failure. *Hepatology* 2007;46:1844–52.

33. Clemmesen JO, Larsen FS, Kondrup J, *et al.* Cerebral herniation in patients with acute liver failure is correlated with arterial ammonia concentration. *Hepatology* 1999;29: 648–53.

34. Hoofnagle JH, Carithers RL Jr, *et al.* Fulminant hepatic failure: summary of a workshop. *Hepatology* 1995;21:240–52.

35. Vaquero J, Fontana RJ, Larson AM, *et al.* Complications and use of intracranial pressure monitoring in patients with acute liver failure and severe encephalopathy. *Liver Transpl* 2005;11:1581–9.

36. Karvellas CJ, Fix OK, Battenhouse H, *et al.* Outcomes and complications of intracranial pressure monitoring in acute liver failure: a retrospective cohort study. *Crit Care Med* 2014;42:1157–67.

37. Aggarwal S, Brooks DM, Kang Y, *et al.* Noninvasive monitoring of cerebral perfusion pressure in patients with acute liver failure using transcranial Doppler ultrasonography. *Liver Transpl* 2008;14:1048–57.

38. Abdo A, Lopez O, Fernandez A, *et al.* Transcranial Doppler sonography in fulminant hepatic failure. *Transplant Proc* 2003;35:1859–60.

39. Aggarwal S, Kramer D, Yonas H, *et al.* Cerebral hemodynamic and metabolic changes in fulminant hepatic failure: a retrospective study. *Hepatology* 1994;19:80–87.

40. Nielsen HB, Tofteng F, Wang LP, and Larsen FS. Cerebral oxygenation determined by near infrared spectrophotometry in patients with fulminant hepatic failure. *J Hepatol* 2003;38:188–92.

41. Larson MD and Singh V. Portable infrared pupillometry in critical care. *Crit Care* 2016;20:161.

42. Son SK, Oh SH, Kim KM, *et al.* Successful liver transplantation following veno-arterial extracorporeal membrane oxygenation in a child with fulminant Wilson

disease and severe pulmonary hemorrhage: a case report. *Pediatr Transplant* 2012;16:E281–5.

43. Auzinger G, Willars C, Loveridge R, *et al*. Extracorporeal membrane oxygenation before and after adult liver transplantation: worth the effort? *Crit Care* 2014; 18:203.

44. Karvellas CJ, Pink F, McPhail M, *et al*. Predictors of bacteraemia and mortality in patients with acute liver failure. *Intensive Care Med* 2009;35:1390–6.

45. Davenport A. Continuous renal replacement therapies in patients with liver disease. *Semin Dial* 2009;22:169–72.

46. Slack AJ, Auzinger G, Willars C, *et al*. Ammonia clearance with haemofiltration in adults with liver disease. *Liver Int* 2014;34:42–48.

47. Merouani A and Jouvet P. High-volume hemofiltration for critically ill children with acute liver failure: a standard treatment? *Pediatr Crit Care Med* 2014;15:681–3.

48. Deep A, Stewart CE, Dhawan A, and Douiri A. Effect of continuous renal replacement therapy on outcome in pediatric acute liver failure. *Crit Care Med* 2016;44(10):1910–9.

49. Struecker B, Raschzok N, and Sauer IM. Liver support strategies: cutting-edge technologies. *Nat Rev Gastroenterol Hepatol* 2014;11:166–76.

50. Mitzner SR. Extracorporeal liver support — albumin dialysis with the Molecular Adsorbent Recirculating System (MARS). *Ann Hepatol* 2011;10: S21–28.

51. Rifai K. Fractionated plasma separation and adsorption: current practice and future options. *Liver Int* 2011;31:13–15.

52. Sauer IM, Goetz M, Steffen I, *et al*. In vitro comparison of the molecular adsorbent recirculation system (MARS) and single-pass albumin dialysis (SPAD). *Hepatology* 2004;39:1408–14.

53. Al-Chalabi A, Matevossian E, Thaden AK, *et al*. Evaluation of the Hepa Wash®treatment in pigs with acute liver failure. *BMC Gastroenterol* 2013;13:83.

54. Rozga J, Umehara Y, Trofimenko A, *et al*. A novel plasma filtration therapy for hepatic failure: preclinical studies. *Ther Apher Dial* 2006;10:138–44.

55. Saliba F, Camus C, Durand F, *et al*. Albumin dialysis with a non cell artificial liver support device in patients with acute liver failure: a randomized, controlled trial. *Ann Intern Med* 2013;159:522–31.

56. Banares R, Nevens F, Larsen FS, *et al*. Extracorporeal albumin dialysis with the molecular adsorbent recirculating system in acute-on-chronic liver failure: the RELIEF trial. *Hepatology* 2013;57:1153–62.

57. Starzl TE, Porter KA, and Francavilla A. The Eck fistula in animals and humans. *Curr Probl Surg* 1983;20:687–752.

58. Otto JJ, Pender JC, Cleary JH, *et al*. The use of a donor liver in experimental animals with elevated blood ammonia. *Surgery* 1958;43:301–9.

59. Sen PK, Bhalerao RA, Parulkar GP, *et al*. Use of isolated perfused cadaveric liver in the management of hepatic failure. *Surgery* 1966;59:774–81.

60. Eiseman B, Liem DS, and Raffucci F. Heterologous liver perfusion in treatment of hepatic failure. *Ann Surg* 1965;162:329–45.
61. Park JK and Lee DH. Bioartificial liver systems: current status and future perspective. *J Biosci Bioeng* 2005;99:311–9.
62. Jain E, Damaniaa A, Shakyaa AK, *et al.* Fabrication of macroporous cryogels as potential hepatocyte carriers for bioartificial liver support. *Colloids Surf B: Biointerfaces* 2015;136:761–71.
63. Pascher A, Sauer IM, Hammer C, *et al.* Extracorporeal liver perfusion as hepatic assist in acute liver failure: a review of world experience. *Xenotransplantation* 2002;9:309–24.
64. Demetriou AA, Brown RS, Busuttil RW, *et al.* Prospective, randomized, multicenter, controlled trial of a bioartificial liver in treating acute liver failure. *Ann Surg* 2004;239:660–7.
65. Ellis AJ, Hughes RD, Wendon JA, *et al.* Pilot-controlled trial of the extracorporeal liver assist device in acute liver failure. *Hepatology* 1996;24:1446–51.
66. Sauer IM, Kardassis D, Zeillinger K, *et al.* Clinical extracorporeal hybrid liver support — phase I study with primary porcine liver cells. *Xenotransplantation* 2003;10:460–9.
67. Sauer IM, Zeilinger K, Pless G, *et al.* Extracorporeal liver support based on primary human liver cells and albumin dialysis — treatment of a patient with primary graft non-function. *J Hepatol* 2003;39:649–53.
68. van de Kerkhove MP, Di Florio E, Scuderi V, *et al.* Phase I clinical trial with the AMC-bioartificial liver. *Int J Artif Organs* 2002;25:950–9.
69. Sussman NL and Kelly JH. Artificial Liver. *Clin Gastroenterol Hepatol* 2014;12:1439–42.
70. Pascher A, Sauer IM, and Neuhaus P. Analysis of allogeneic versus xenogeneic auxiliary organ perfusion in liver failure reveals superior efficacy of human livers. *Int J Artif Organs* 2002;25:1006–12.
71. Iwata H and Ueda Y. Pharmacokinetic considerations in development of a bioartificial liver. *Clin Pharmacokinet* 2004;43:211–25.
72. Hoekstra R, van Wenum M, and Chamuleau RA. Pivotal preclinical trial of the spheroid reservoir bioartificial liver. *J Hepatol* 2015;63:1051–2.
73. Kondrup J, Almdal T, Vilstrup H, and Tygstrup N. High volume plasma exchange in fulminant hepatic failure. *Int J Artif Organs* 1992;15:669–76.
74. Nakamura T, Ushiyama C, Suzuki S, *et al.* Effect of plasma exchange on serum tissue inhibitor of metalloproteinase 1 and cytokine concentrations in patients with fulminant hepatitis. *Blood Purif* 2000;18:50–54.
75. Larsen FS, Hansen BA, Ejlersen E, *et al.* Systemic vascular resistance during high volume plasmapheresis in patients with fulminant hepatic failure: relationship with oxygen consumption. *Eur J Gastroenterol Hepatol* 1995;7:887–92.
76. Larsen FS, Hansen BA, Ejlersen E, *et al.* Cerebral blood flow, oxygen metabolism and transcranial Doppler sonography during high volume plasmapheresis in fulminant hepatic failure. *Eur J Gastroenterol Hepatol* 1996;8:261–5.

77. Clemmesen JO, Kondrup J, Nielsen LB, *et al.* Effects of high-volume plasmapheresis on ammonia, urea, and amino acids in patients with acute liver failure. *Am J Gastroenterol* 2001;96:1217–23.

78. Clemmesen JO, Gerbes AL, Gülberg V, *et al.* Hepatic blood flow and splanchnic oxygen consumption in patients with liver failure. Effect of high-volume plasmapheresis. *Hepatology* 1999;29:347–55.

79. Larsen FS, Schmidt LE, Bernsmeier C, *et al.* High-volume plasma exchange in patients with acute liver failure: an open randomised controlled trial. *J Hepatol* 2016;64:69–78.

80. Mitzner SR, Stange J, Klammt S, *et al.* Improvement of hepatorenal syndrome with extracorporeal albumin dialysis MARS: results of a prospective, randomized, controlled clinical trial. *Liver Transpl* 2000;6:277–86.

81. Heemann U, Treichel U, Loock J, *et al.* Albumin dialysis in cirrhosis with superimposed acute liver injury: a prospective, controlled study. *Hepatology* 2002;36:949–58.

82. Sen S, Davies NA, Mookerjee RP, *et al.* Pathophysiological effects of albumin dialysis in acute-on-chronic liver failure: a randomized controlled study. *Liver Transpl* 2004;10;1109–19.

83. Hassanein TI, Tofteng F, Brown RS Jr, *et al.* Randomized controlled study of extracorporeal albumin dialysis for hepatic encephalopathy in advanced cirrhosis. *Hepatology* 2007;46:1853–62.

84. Kortgen A, Rauchfuss F, Götz M, *et al.* Albumin dialysis in liver failure: comparison of molecular adsorbent recirculating system and single pass albumin dialysis — a retrospective analysis. *Ther Apher Dial* 2009;13:419–25.

85. Ringe H, Varnholt V, Zimmering M, *et al.* Continuous veno-venous single pass albumin hemodiafiltration in children with acute liver failure. *Pediatr Crit Care Med* 2011;12;257–64.

86. Karvellas CJ, Bagshaw SM, McDermid RC, *et al.* A case-control study of single-pass albumin dialysis for acetaminophen- induced acute liver failure. *Blood Purif* 2009;28:151–8.

87. Ellis AJ, Hughes RD, Wendon JA, *et al.* Pilot-controlled trial of the extracorporeal liver assist device in acute liver failure. *Hepatology* 1996;24:1446–51.

88. van de Kerkhove MP, Di Florio E, Scuderi V, *et al.* Bridging a patient with acute liver failure to liver transplantation by the AMC-bioartificial liver. *Cell Transplant* 2003;12(6):563–8.

89. Kjaergard LL, Liu J, Als-Nielsen B, and Gluud C. Artificial and bioartificial support systems for acute and acute-on-chronic liver failure. *JAMA* 2003;289:217–22.

90. Liu JP, Gluud LL, Als-Nielsen B, and Gluud C. Artificial and bioartificial support systems for liver failure. *Cochrane Database Syst Rev* 2004;1:CD003628. doi: 10.1002/14651858.CD003628.pub2.

91. Stutchfield BM, Simpson K, and Wigmore SJ. Systematic review and meta-analysis of survival following extracorporeal liver support. *Br J Surg* 2011;98:623–31.
92. Remien CH, Adler FR, Waddoups L, *et al.* Mathematical modeling of liver injury and dysfunction after acetaminophen overdose: early discrimination between survival and death. *Hepatology* 2012;56:727–34.
93. Redeker AG and Yamahiro HS. Controlled trial of exchange-transfusion therapy in fulminant hepatitis. *Lancet* 1973;1:3–6.
94. O'Grady JG, Gimson AE, O'Brien CJ, *et al.* Controlled trials of charcoal hemoperfusion and prognostic factors in fulminant hepatic failure. *Gastroenterology* 1988;94:1186–92.
95. Hughes RD, Pucknell A, Routley D, *et al.* Evaluation of the BioLogic-DT sorbent-suspension dialyser in patients with fulminant hepatic failure. *Int J Artif Organs* 1994;17:657–62.
96. Mazariegos GV, Ash SR, and Patzer JF. Preliminary results: randomized clinical trial of the BioLogic-DT in treatment of acute hepatic failure (AHF) with coma. *Artif Organs* 1997;21:529.
97. El Banayosy A, Kizner L, Schueler V, *et al.* First use of the Molecular Adsorbent Recirculating System technique on patients with hypoxic liver failure after cardiogenic shock. *ASAIO J* 2004;50:332–7.
98. Stevens C, Busuttil RW, Han S, *et al.* An interim analysis of a phase II/III prospective randomized multicenter controlled trial of the HepatAssist Bioartificial Liver Support System for the treatment of fulminant hepatic failure. *Hepatology* 2001;34:299A.

16. Future Directions in Liver Replacement Therapy: Liver Xenotransplantation

Burcin Ekser* and David K. C. Cooper[†]

*Transplant Division, Department of Surgery, Indiana University
School of Medicine, Indianapolis, IN, USA
[†]Xenotransplantation Program, Department of Surgery,
University of Alabama at Birmingham (UAB), 703 19th Street South,
ZRB 701, Birmingham, AL 35233, USA

1. Introduction

Liver transplant(ation) (LT) is an established curative therapy for end-stage liver disease either in its chronic or acute/fulminant form. One-year, 3-year, and 5-year patient survival rates post LT are 90%, >80%, and >70%, respectively [1]. Although patient survival is good compared to patients on the waiting list, LT is limited by the shortage of deceased human donor organs. For example, in patients with acute liver failure (ALF), usually induced by chemical or viral hepatitis, the onset of disease is sudden and identification of a suitable donor organ is frequently not possible before permanent neurologic injury and/or death occurs.

In the USA, in July 2016, the United Network for Organ Sharing (UNOS) waiting list for LT was close to 15,000 [1]. In 2015, almost 3,000 patients were removed from the waiting list because they died before a suitable donor liver became available. (They either died on the waiting list or became too sick for a transplant and died after removal from the waiting list.) Because of these deaths, the number of patients on the waiting list for LT has not changed much during the last decade, in contrast to the number waiting for kidney grafts which has increased annually.

For patients with end-stage failure of kidneys, hearts, or even lungs, mechanical support is available, e.g., dialysis, ventricular assist devices, or extracorporeal membrane oxygenation, and is largely successful. There is no similar device for patients in hepatic failure. The molecular adsorbent recirculating system (MARS) does not provide a level of support comparable to those for other organs. There is, therefore, a need for a form of biologic support for patients with severe liver failure.

Liver xenotransplantation, using pig organs, could resolve the shortage of suitable donor organs (Table 1) [2–6]. The prompt availability of a pig liver would be particularly important in a patient with ALF in whom spontaneous recovery does not occur or in whom all therapeutic measures fail. Alternative potential solutions (that will not be discussed here) include (i) an artificial liver device, (ii) the transplantation of hepatocytes or (iii) hepatocyte-like expanded human stem cells, and (iv) *ex vivo* pig or nonhuman primate (NHP) liver perfusion (although clinical experience will be summarized). Regenerative medicine techniques whereby a human or pig liver is decellularized and recelluarized with cells from the potential recipient would not be applicable to patients with ALF.

Based on experience in the pig-to-NHP (preclinical) LT model, this chapter will discuss the potential therapeutic impact of liver xenotransplantation — particularly with regard to the management of patients with ALF. The remaining barriers — that currently do not yet justify clinical trials — will be summarized. Experiences of *in vitro* studies or in small animal models will not be discussed unless they were cornerstones of research in this field.

2. Clinical experience with liver xenotransplantation

The history of clinical xenotransplantation has recently been reviewed [7], and goes back to the 17th century when blood transfusion from animals to humans was practiced. In the early 19th century, skin and corneal xenotransplants were attempted, and in the early 20th century kidney and other organ transplants were carried out clinically without success. A small breakthrough was achieved by Reemtsma and his colleagues who transplanted chimpanzee kidneys into patients with renal failure in the mid-1960s, with one patient surviving for 9 months.

Table 1. The advantages and disadvantages of the pig as a potential source of organs and cells for humans, in contrast with those of the baboon in this role. (Reproduced with permission from Ref. [127]. Copyright © 2015 Taylor & Francis.)

	Pig	Baboon
Availability	Unlimited	Limited
Breeding potential	Good	Poor
Period to reproductive maturity	4–8 months	3–5 years
Length of pregnancy	114 ± 2 days	173–193 days
Number of offspring	5–12	1–2
Growth	Rapid (adult human size within 6 months)**	Slow (9 years to reach maximum size)
Size of adult organs	Adequate	Inadequate*
Cost of maintenance	Significantly lower	High
Anatomical similarity to humans	Moderately close	Close
Physiological similarity to humans	Moderately close	Close
Relationship of immune system to humans	Distant	Close
Knowledge of tissue typing	Considerable (in selected herds)	Limited
Necessity for blood type compatibility with humans	Probably unimportant	Important
Experience with genetic engineering	Considerable	None
Risk of transfer of infection (xenozoonosis)	Low	High
Availability of specific pathogen-free animals	Yes	No
Public opinion	More in favor	Mixed

Note: *The size of certain organs, e.g., the heart, would be inadequate for transplantation into adult humans.

**Breeds of miniature swine are approximately 50% of the weight of domestic pigs at birth and sexual maturity, and reach a maximum weight of approximately 30% of standard breeds.

The first clinical attempts at liver xenotransplantation were by Starzl *et al.*, who carried out transplants between NHPs and young patients in Colorado in the 1960s, but without great success [8].

Only one clinical attempt of pig liver xenotransplantation has been reported. In 1995, Makowka and his colleagues performed a heterotopic wild-type (i.e., genetically-unmodified) pig liver xenotransplant with the aim of carrying out orthotopic liver allotransplantation when a human donor became available, at which time the auxiliary pig liver would have been removed [9, 10]. The patient was a 26-year-old woman with fulminant liver failure secondary to acute-on-chronic liver failure due to a 14-year history of autoimmune hepatitis and hepatitis C. She was admitted to hospital with grade III encephalopathy and listed under UNOS's highest priority, status 1. Despite aggressive medical therapy, the patient continued to deteriorate, with increasing encephalopathy and coagulopathy.

Before transplantation, circulating natural antipig antibodies were removed by plasmapheresis and *ex vivo* perfusion of the donor pig kidneys (to which antipig antibodies would bind). After transplantation, the liver xenograft clearly functioned, as documented by bile production, stabilization of prothrombin levels, and reduction in the levels of lactic acid and the enzymes aspartate aminotransferase and alanine aminotransferase. Unfortunately, this did not result in any improvement in the neurologic status of the patient, who died after 34 hours from irreversible brain damage. A liver allograft had not become available. No mention was made as to whether thrombocytopenia was documented, as seen in pig-to-NHP models (see the following).

Despite the removal of >90% of the recipient's natural xenoantibodies prior to transplantation, antipig antibody rapidly returned and was associated with complement-mediated injury of the graft. A liver biopsy obtained 3 hours post transplantation showed deposition of antibody and complement components, and endothelial swelling, suggesting early graft rejection [10]. At autopsy, the pig liver showed thrombosis and ischemic necrosis.

Nevertheless, this experience demonstrated the ability of a pig liver to function, at least temporarily, in a human recipient and to provide some metabolic support during ALF.

3. Clinical experience with *ex vivo* pig liver perfusion

Early experience has been reviewed previously [2, 11]. Initial experience using human livers was documented in the 1960s and 1970s. In the late 1960s and early 1970s, at least 141 *ex vivo* pig liver perfusions were performed to treat 87 patients with liver failure, but then this therapeutic approach was largely superseded for several years by orthotopic liver allotransplantation. Neurologic improvement to at least hepatic coma grade 3 or 2 was documented in many patients. In 1994, Chari and Collins and their colleagues reported their clinical experience using wild-type pig liver perfusion in four patients, but only one patient survived [12, 13]. In 2000, Horslen *et al.* at the University of Nebraska used human or pig livers to bridge 14 patients to allotransplantation [14]. Patient selection criteria were that the patient (1) was an acceptable candidate for LT, (2) had encephalopathy with progression to grade 4 coma despite medical management, (3) had undergone endotracheal intubation, and (4) had a marginal cerebral perfusion pressure. If no human liver became available, *ex vivo* liver perfusion would be initiated. This therapy maintained low ammonia levels for 48 hours, but did not lower bilirubin levels.

With the development of the techniques of genetic engineering, and the availability of genetically engineered pigs (discussed in the following), Levy *et al.* attempted a small clinical trial using livers from pigs transgenic for the human complement-regulatory proteins, CD55 (human decay-accelerating factor (hDAF)) and CD59 [15]. They extracorporeally perfused these genetically engineered pig livers in two patients with acute hepatic failure for 6.5 hours and 10 hours, respectively, as bridging to successful allotransplantation.

4. Experience with experimental pig liver xenotransplantation

For a number of reasons, it is very unlikely that NHPs will be used as sources of livers for clinical xenotransplantation (Table 1). Therefore, the pig-to-NHP model is increasingly being investigated to assess strategies aimed at advancing toward clinical liver xenotransplantation (Figure 1).

There has been significantly more experimental experience in the transplantation of pig hearts and kidneys than livers. A wild-type pig organ transplanted into a NHP is rapidly bound by primate antipig antibodies that activate the complement cascade, resulting in destruction of the graft (hyperacute rejection) (reviewed in Ref. [16]). Innate immune cells, e.g., neutrophils, macrophages, may also be involved in injury to the graft. If antibody binding is delayed, e.g., by pretransplant plasmapheresis or perfusion of the recipient blood through a pig organ, graft injury is delayed, but only for hours or a few days. Efforts to overcome the humoral response have largely been directed to genetic manipulation of the pig to protect the organ graft from antibody-mediated complement injury. However, transplantation of pig livers and lungs is associated with additional pathobiologic problems not seen in pig heart or kidney transplantation [6].

Experimental pig liver xenotransplantation in NHPs was initiated using wild-type pig livers in 1968 by Calne *et al.* [17–19]. They reported seven pig-to-baboon orthotopic liver xenografts using either no immunosuppressive therapy or a combination of azathioprine and methylprednisolone

	1968	1970	1994	1998	2000	2005	2010	2012	2014	2015		2016
Pig Type	WT	WT	WT	WT	hCD55	hCD55 hCD59.HT	GTKO hCD46	GTKO	GTKO	GTKO	GTKO	GTKO
Immuno-suppression	Aza Cs	ALG	Gal abs. WBI ATG pig BM	CsA Cs	CyP CsA Cs	CyP CsA Cs	ATG FK MMF Cs	ATG CVF a-CD154 LoCD2b Aza+Cs	ATG CVF FK Cs	ATG CVF a-CD154 FK MMF Cs	ATG CVF FK Cs	ATG CVF Bela FK Cs
Max. Survival (days)	<4	<1	<3	<1	8	1	7	9	15	14	7	25
Type of Transplant	OLT	OLT	OLT	OLT	OLT	OLT	OLT	OLT	HLT	HLT	OLT	OLT

Figure 1. Timeline in experimental pig liver xenotransplantation in NHPs. (Adapted with permission from Ref. [5]. Copyright © 2016 Wolters Kluwer Health, Inc.)

Note: a-CD154 = anti-CD154 monoclonal antibodies; ALG, antilymphocyte globulin; ATG, antithymocyte globulin; Aza, azathioprine; Bela, belatacept; BM, bone marrow; Cs, corticosteroids; CsA, cyclosporine; CVF, cobra venom factor; CyP, cyclophosphamide; FK, tacrolimus; Gal abs, extracorporeal anti-Gal antibody adsorption; GTKO, α1,3-galactosyltransferase gene-knockout; hCD46, expression of the human regulator of complement, hCD46; hCD55, expression of the human regulator of complement, CD55; HLT, heterotopic LT; HT, H-transferase; LoCD2b, anti-CD2 monoclonal antibody; MMF, mycophenolate mofetil; OLT, orthotopic LT; WBI, whole body irradiation; WT, wild type.

(the standard therapy available at that time) (Table 2). Survival of the baboons was limited to hours. Four baboons died from uncontrollable hemorrhage within 6–30 hours, although the remaining three baboons, which were given human fibrinogen, did not bleed. The longest survival was recorded as 84 hours (3½ days). This group also transplanted a pig liver into a chimpanzee, but survival remained only 8 hours (Table 2).

Despite (1) the use of different NHP species as recipients, (2) the administration of more potent immunosuppressive agents (and sometimes aggressive immunomodulation), and (3) pretransplant depletion of antipig antibodies by plasmapheresis or perfusion of another pig organ, the survival of liver xenografts remained largely limited to hours until the year 2000 (Table 2). For example, Powelson *et al.* attempted to adsorb antipig antibodies by perfusing the recipient's blood through a pig kidney or liver, but this did not result in significant prolongation of liver graft function [20].

A step forward was taken when the major carbohydrate antigen on pig vascular endothelial cells, against which humans have preformed antipig antibodies, was identified as galactose-α1,3-galactose (Gal) ([21]; reviewed

Table 2. Experimental pig liver xenotransplantation in NHPs (1968–1999).

Recipient	Type of transplant	No.	Immunosuppressive therapy	Survival (hours)	First author [reference]
Baboon	Orthotopic	7	none (*n* = 3), Cs (*n* = 2), AZA + Cs (*n* = 2)	6, 6, 9, 19, 30, 36, 84	Calne [17]
Rhesus	Orthotopic	3	ALG	12, 12, 12	Calne [19]
Chimpanzee	Orthotopic	1	None	8	Calne [19]
Cynomolgous	Orthotopic	4	EIA (organ) + WBI + TI + ATG + pig bone marrow	2, 4, 5, 13, 72, 75	Powelson [20]
Baboon	Orthotopic	2	EIA (organ) + WBI + TI + ATG + pig bone marrow		Powelson [20]
Rhesus	Orthotopic	6	None (*n* = 3), CsA + Cs + Dashen (*n* = 3)	2–5.5	Luo [68]
Baboon	Heterotopic	2	CyP + CsA + Cs	2, 2	Luo [68]

Note: ALG, antilymphocyte globulin; ATG, antithymocyte globulin; AZA, azathioprine; Cs, corticosteroids; CsA, cyclosporine; CyP, cyclophosphamide; EIA, extracorporeal immunoadsorption (through an immunoaffinity column of αGal oligosaccharide or by perfusion of a pig kidney or liver; TI, thymic irradiation; WBI, whole body irradiation.

in Ref. [22]). With the discovery that Gal was a major target, efforts were made to remove specifically anti-Gal antibodies from the potential recipient, using immunoabsorption with immunoaffinity columns of synthetic Gal oligosaccharides [23, 24]. Despite immense efforts in this respect, pig kidney or heart graft function remained limited.

5. Genetic engineering of organ-source pigs

When genetic engineering techniques were achieved in pigs, this opened the way to a different approach to overcome the barriers of xenotransplantation by modifying the *donor,* and not just immunosuppressing the recipient. It should be stressed that xenotransplantation, for the first time, offers the possibility of this major advantage.

It was known that *pig* complement-regulatory proteins were not very effective at protecting transplanted pig organs from *primate* complement-mediated injury [6, 16]. To regulate injury of the pig graft from the host's complement cascade, at least two independent groups made the suggestion

Table 3. Timeline for application of evolving techniques for genetic engineering of pigs employed in xenotransplantation. (Adapted with permission from Ref. [6]. Copyright © 2015 John Wiley & Sons.)

Year	Genetic engineering technique
1992	Microinjection of randomly integrating transgenes
2000	Somatic cell nuclear transfer (SCNT)
2002	Homologous recombination
2011	Zinc finger nucleases (ZFNs)
2013	Transcription activator-like effector nucleases (TALENs)
2014	CRISPR/cas9*

Note: *CRISPR/cas9, cluster randomly interspaced short palindromic repeats and the associated protein 9.

of genetically engineering pigs that expressed a *human* complement-regulatory protein, e.g., CD55 (decay-accelerating factor) [25, 26]. In the early 1990s, the production of pigs expressing human CD55 was achieved by microinjection of DNA directly into the pronucleus of a fertilized egg (Table 3) [27, 28]. Numerous studies in pig-to-NHP models demonstrated that the expression of human CD55 prolonged pig heart, kidney, and liver graft survival (the latter is discussed in the following) (reviewed in Refs. [23] and [24]).

A second major step forward in genetic engineering of pigs was taken when the gene for the α1,3-galactosyltransferase enzyme (that is responsible for the addition of Gal to the surface of the pig cells) was deleted (providing GTKO pigs) [29–31]. Nuclear transfer was combined with homologous recombination technology, resulting in GTKO pigs that were used as sources of organs for experimental transplantation in NHPs. GTKO pig organs (heart, kidney, liver, lungs) showed prolonged survival in preclinical studies, especially when baboon recipients were preselected for low levels of the remaining antipig antibodies (so-called anti-non-Gal antibodies) [32].

More efficient genetic engineering techniques, such as zinc finger nucleases, and transcription activator-like effector nucleases (TALENS), have subsequently been introduced (Table 3) (reviewed in Ref. [33]). The most recent technology, CRISPR/cas9 (cluster randomly interspaced short palindromic repeats and the associated protein 9), has already increased the speed and reduced the cost by which genetic modifications can be made.

Several groups have reported the production of genetically modified pigs using CRISPR technology (reviewed in Ref. [34]). The most important of these pigs to date has been the "triple knock-out" pigs (that do not express Gal or the other two definitively identified antigenic targets for antipig antibodies, namely N-glycolylneuraminic acid (Neu5Gc) [35], or SD(a) (through KO of the gene for the enzyme beta-1,4-N-acetyl-galactosaminyltransferase-2 (B4GalNT2)) [36].

GTKO has been combined with expression of one or more human complement-regulatory proteins, and also by one or more human coagulation-regulatory proteins (e.g., thrombomodulin, endothelial protein C receptor, CD39), which inhibit the coagulation dysregulation that has been documented after pig heart or kidney transplantation in NHPs [16, 37].

Kidneys, hearts, and islets from pigs with up to six genetic modifications have been transplanted into NHPs, with survival in some cases for months or even years [32, 38–44]. Although currently livers from pigs with only four to five different genetic modifications have been transplanted into NHPs (see the following), there are >25 different genetically engineered pigs available worldwide (Table 4), some of which have been sources of organs for kidney, heart, or lung xenotransplantation experiments.

6. Genetically engineered pig liver xenotransplantation in NHPs

The first liver xenotransplantation experiments using genetically engineered pigs were reported by Ramirez *et al.* in 2000 [45, 46]. They transplanted two livers from pigs expressing CD55 (hDAF) into baboons, with three wild-type pig livers being transplanted as controls. Baboons with wild-type pig livers survived for only hours, whereas those with livers transgenic for CD55 survived for 4 days and 8 days, respectively (Table 5). Neither liver graft demonstrated histopathologic features of hyperacute rejection.

This study indicated that, when hyperacute rejection is abrogated by the expression of hCD55, the porcine liver can maintain reasonable levels of coagulation factors and proteins in the baboon for up to 8 days, although factors 2, 7, and 10 decreased significantly. (Rodent studies confirmed that that the recipient of a liver xenograft progressively acquires the protein profile of the donor species [47–49].) However, in a subsequent brief report by Ramirez *et al.*, livers transplanted from pigs transgenic for two human complement-regulatory proteins (CD55, CD59) and H-transferase into baboons were associated with disappointing results, with survival for only 13–24 hours [46] (Table 5).

In our own studies in Pittsburgh, we reported our experience of orthotopic pig liver xenotransplantation in baboons with grafts from GTKO pigs

Table 4. Selected genetically modified pigs currently available for xenotransplantation research. (Adapted with permission from Ref. [6]. Copyright © 2015 John Wiley & Sons.)

Complement regulation by human complement-regulatory gene expression

CD46 (membrane cofactor protein)

CD55 (decay-accelerating factor)

CD59 (protectin or membrane inhibitor of reactive lysis)

Gal or non-Gal antigen "masking" or deletion

Human H-transferase gene expression (expression of blood type O antigen)

Endo-β-galactosidase C (reduction of Gal antigen expression)

α1,3-galactosyltransferase gene-knockout (GTKO)

Cytidine monophosphate-*N*-acetylneuraminic acid hydroxylase (CMAH) gene-knockout (NeuGcKO)

β4GalNT2 (β1,4 *N*-acetylgalactosaminyltransferase) gene-knockout (β4GalNT2KO)

Suppression of cellular immune response by gene expression or downregulation

CIITA-DN (MHC class II transactivator knockdown, resulting in swine leukocyte antigen class II knockdown)

Class I MHC-knockout (MHC-IKO)

HLA-E/human β2-microglobulin (inhibits human natural killer cell cytotoxicity)

Human FAS ligand (CD95L)

Human GnT-III (*N*-acetylglucosaminyltransferase III) gene

Porcine CTLA4-Ig (cytotoxic T-lymphocyte antigen 4 or CD152)

Human TRAIL (tumor necrosis factor-α-related apoptosis-inducing ligand)

Anticoagulation and anti-inflammatory gene expression or deletion

von Willebrand factor (vWF)-deficient (natural mutant)

Human tissue factor pathway inhibitor (TFPI)

Human thrombomodulin

Human endothelial protein C receptor (EPCR)

Human CD39 (ectonucleoside triphosphate diphosphohydrolase-1)

Anticoagulation, anti-inflammatory, and antiapoptotic gene expression

Human A20 (tumor necrosis factor-α-induced protein 3)

Human heme oxygenase-1 (HO-1)

Human CD47 (species-specific interaction with SIRP-α inhibits phagocytosis)

Porcine asialoglycoprotein receptor 1 gene-knockout (ASGR1-KO) (decreases platelet phagocytosis)

Human signal regulatory protein α (SIRPα) (decreases platelet phagocytosis by "self" recognition)

Prevention of porcine endogenous retrovirus (PERV) activation

PERV siRNA

Table 5.   Experimental pig liver xenotransplantation in NHPs (2000–2016).

Pig type	Recipient	Type of transplant	No.	Immunosuppressive therapy	Survival (days)	Author [reference]
WT	Baboon	Orthotopic	3	CyP + CsA + Cs	<1, <1, <1	Ramirez [45]
hCD55	Baboon	Orthotopic	2	CyP + CsA + Cs	4, 8	Ramirez [45]
hCD55. CD59. HT	Baboon	Orthotopic	5	CyP + Dac + RTX + CsA + MMF + Cs	<1, <1, <1, <1, 1	Ramirez [46]
WT	Baboon	Orthotopic	1	None	<1	Ekser [51]
GTKO	Baboon	Orthotopic	2	ATG + FK + MMF + Cs	<1, 6	Ekser [51]
GTKO hCD46	Baboon	Orthotopic	8	ATG + FK + MMF + Cs ($n = 5$), CyP + FK + MMF + Cs ($n = 3$)	<1, <1, 1, 4, 5, 6, 6, 7	Ekser [51]
GTKO	Baboon	Orthotopic	3	ATG + LoCD2b + CVF + anti-CD154 + Aza + Cs	6, 8, 9	Kim [53]
GTKO	Baboon	Heterotopic	3	ATG + CVF + FK + Cs	6, 9, 15	Yeh [54]
GTKO	Tibetan Monkey	Heterotopic	3	ATG + CVF + FK + anti-CD154 + Cs	2, 5, 14	Ji [57]
GTKO	Baboon	Orthotopic	6	ATG + CVF + FK + Cs	1, 3, 5, 5, 6, 7	Navarro-Alvarez [55]
GTKO	Baboon	Orthotopic	1	ATG + CVF + Bela + FK + Cs	25	Shah [56]

Note: ATG, antithymocyte globulin; CD46, membrane cofactor protein, CD55, decay-accelerating factor; CD59, homologous restriction factor (protectin); Cs, corticosteroids; CsA, cyclosporine; CyP, cyclophosphamide; Dac, daclizumab; FK, tacrolimus; GTKO, α1,3-galactosyltransferase gene-knockout; h, human; HT, H-transferase (α1,2-fucosyltransferase); MMF, mycophenolate mofetil; RTX, rituximab; TI, thymic irradiation; WBI, whole body irradiation; WT, wild type.

or GTKO pigs transgenic for the human complement-regulatory protein, CD46 (GTKO/hCD46 pigs), using a clinically applicable immunosuppressive regimen (Table 5) [4, 50–52]. Profound thrombocytopenia developed within 1 hour post transplantation (Figure 2), which persisted throughout the period of follow-up, eventually resulting in spontaneous hemorrhages in various native organs and in the graft, limiting recipient survival to a maximum of 7 days. However, throughout much of this time, hepatic function was documented near-normal to normal (as assessed by liver enzymes, coagulation factors, coagulation assays, and production of porcine-specific proteins) [50].

Kim *et al.* reported GTKO miniature swine orthotopic liver xenotransplantation in baboons with an intensive immunosuppressive regimen (Table 5) [53]. Their initial three cases survived 6 days, 8 days, and 9 days, respectively. The 6-day survivor died of spontaneous hemorrhage associated

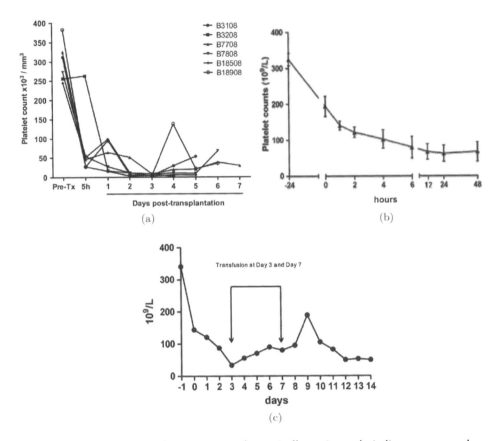

Figure 2. Platelet counts after experimental genetically engineered pig liver xenotransplantation. Platelet counts after (a) GTKO/hCD46 orthotopic pig LT in baboons ($n = 6$) that survived from 4 to 7 days, (b) GTKO Wu Zhishan miniature swine heterotopic left liver lobe transplantation in Tibetan monkeys ($n = 3$; mean ± SD) within the first 48 hours, and (c) in a Tibetan monkey that survived for 14 days. (Reproduced with permission from Ref. [5]. Copyright © 2016 Wolters Kluwer Health, Inc.)

with profound thrombocytopenia, as observed by our group previously [51]. In the 8- and 9-day survivors, loss of platelets was ameliorated to some extent by blocking fibrinolysis by the administration of aminocaproic acid. Although thrombocytopenia was marginal (platelet counts remained between 40,000/mm^3 and 50,000/mm^3), the baboons suffered severe blood loss and sepsis.

In the same model, Yeh *et al.* went on to assess the effect of maintaining the recipient liver *in situ* and transplanting the pig liver heterotopically [54]. Although thrombocytopenia developed as before, the presence of baboon coagulation factors prevented severe spontaneous hemorrhage from occurring. However, features of thrombotic microangiopathy and ischemia developed in the graft (as seen in pig hearts and kidneys), resulting in graft failure in two cases. Survival in three experiments was limited to 6 days, 9 days, and 15 days, respectively, with sepsis being a major cause of death.

Navarro-Alvarez *et al.* reported seven further cases (six new, one historical) of orthotopic GTKO pig-to-baboon liver xenotransplantation [55] in which they sought to determine the effects of the administration of human coagulation factors (Table 5). Graft and recipient survival was 1 day and 3 days (with bolus administration) and 5–7 days (with continuous administration), which was not different from survival of a historical control baboon (6 days). Platelet counts were maintained, but the baboons quickly developed large vessel thrombosis and thrombotic microangiopathy. Several deaths were from infection.

The most recent report by Shah *et al.* [56] documented 25-day survival of a GTKO pig liver graft in a baboon treated with a human prothrombinase concentrate complex (Table 5). Immunosuppressive therapy included induction with anti-thymocyte globulin and cobra venom factor, with maintenance with belatacept, tacrolimus, and methylprednisolone. Abnormalities of liver function developed by day 7, but were thought to be associated with rejection, and were reversed by a course of steroid pulses. Early thrombocytopenia began to recover by day 11 (without the need for platelet transfusions), and the platelet count was maximal on day 21 ($614,000/mm^3$). Euthanasia was necessary on day 25 from the development of plantar ulcerations (associated with peripheral edema), progressive cholestasis, hemolysis, and a rising direct bilirubin. The liver showed no macroscopic features of necrosis with all vessels free of thrombus.

This and previous reports provided encouragement that a pig liver graft might maintain life in a patient with fulminant hepatic failure for sufficient time until either recovery of the native liver occurs (if the pig liver had been transplanted heterotopically) or until an allograft becomes available.

Another recent experience in heterotopic pig liver xenotransplantation was reported by Ji *et al.* [57]. They inserted left liver lobes from GTKO miniature swine as auxiliary grafts into Tibetan monkeys (Table 5). Their innovative surgical technique is illustrated in Figure 3. Although it requires native splenectomy, their technique has the advantage that none of the native liver needs to be excised as the graft fits comfortably into the splenic fossa. However, in acute/fulminant liver failure it may be detrimental to leave the necrotic native liver *in situ*. Furthermore, the transplantation of a

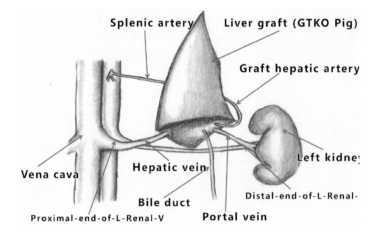

Figure 3. Surgical technique of pig left liver lobe transplantation in Tibetan monkeys (reported in Ref. [57]). After native splenectomy, the pig liver graft was placed in the splenic recess. The recipient's left renal vein was divided, the distal end being anastomosed to the graft portal vein, and the proximal end to the graft hepatic vein. The graft hepatic artery was anastomosed end-to-end to the recipient splenic artery (using a microvascular technique with an operating microscope). After reperfusion, the bile duct was drained through the abdominal wall to allow measurement of bile drainage. (Using the same technique in clinical cases of allotransplantation, the bile duct was drained into a Roux-en-Y jejunal loop). (Adapted with permission from Ref. [5]. Copyright © 2016 Wolters Kluwer Health, Inc.)

small left liver lobe may be insufficient to support the patient, and this remains to be investigated.

In the above studies, various immunosuppressive regimens have been administered, ranging from conventional therapy to novel agents that induce T cell costimulation blockade (Table 5). In pig heart, kidney, or islet xenotransplantation, T cell costimulation blockade (first introduced into xenotransplantation by Buhler *et al.* [58]) has proved effective in preventing the adaptive immune response, allowing graft and recipient survival for months or even years [32, 38–40, 42–44, 59].

7. Surgical considerations

Our own studies indicated that donor (pig) selection is important in order to avoid liver size mismatch [51]. In a series of 10 pig-to-baboon LTs, the native liver proved to be 2.31% of a baboon's total body weight, whereas this ratio is greater in pigs (3.61% of total body weight). We concluded that the liver graft/body weight ratio in the pig is 64% greater than in the baboon. When the pig liver is too large, abdominal closure may prove impossible. We concluded that the donor pig weight should be 40–50% smaller than the recipient baboon weight. Whether this will apply when clinical pig xenotransplantation is introduced will require investigation.

There are differences in the anatomy of pig and human livers that have to be considered. The pig liver has three main lobes — right lateral, median, and left lateral. The median lobe is further subdivided by a deep umbilical fissure, which extends almost to the hilum. Unlike the human liver, the left lateral lobe of the pig liver is consistently the largest of the three lobes. The inferior vena cava is intraparenchymal and runs within the caudate lobe (as a part of the median lobe). Filipponi *et al.* suggested that, due to the prominent fissures in the pig liver, it is much easier to divide the pig liver anatomically into right and left hemilivers than the human liver [60, 61].

The anatomy of the portal and hepatic veins of the pig liver is similar to that of the human liver, but the hepatic vein sometimes divides into four branches before draining into the inferior vena cava. Owing to the intra-parenchymal and thin-walled nature of the inferior vena cava in the pig, and the fact that the right hepatic artery may branch immediately after entering the liver, resection of the right lateral lobe is extremely difficult and cannot be performed without the risk of devascularization of the left and median lobes [61, 62].

In the experimental laboratory, the donor pig and recipient baboon may be small (e.g., 4 kg and 8 kg, respectively), and therefore both recipient and donor bile ducts are of small diameter. Pig bile is significantly more viscous than human and baboon bile (see the following) [63] and so, when the bile ducts are small, the viscous bile may obstruct the duct, particularly if there is any narrowing at the site of duct anastomosis. A Roux-en-Y choledocho-jejunostomy is therefore preferred for bile duct drainage, unless external biliary drainage (through a pediatric tube or T-tube) is employed [54] (which is difficult to manage in an NHP, and is a risk for infection).

Finally, all of the surgical groups involved in this field have performed splenectomy in order to reduce thrombocytopenia. Whether splenectomy is immunologically beneficial to the outcome is uncertain (discussed in the following).

8. Immunological considerations

8.1. *The impact of pig complement on the liver graft*

Despite some negative aspects of pig liver xenotransplantation, there may be some advantages in comparison with xenotransplantation of the pig heart or kidney. As the liver is the major site of synthesis of complement proteins, except for C1q, factor D, properdin, and C7, impaired hepatic synthetic function contributes to complement deficiency in patients with hepatic disease [64–66]. The level of complement membrane attack complex activity may be much lower than that seen in healthy subjects, reducing the possibility of early graft injury.

Furthermore, after pig LT in humans (or NHPs), the graft will produce *pig* complement. *In vitro* studies by Hara and his colleagues indicated that (1) in the presence of *human* antibodies, *pig* complement is associated with less lysis of pig cells than *human* complement (and thus may be associated with less graft injury), (2) lysis by pig complement of GTKO pig cells is significantly less than of wild-type pig cells, and (3) the expression of a *human* complement-regulatory protein (such as CD55 or CD46) on the pig cell can reduce *pig* complement-induced lysis of the cells [67]. In *ex vivo* liver perfusion with human blood, survival of hCD55 pig livers for up to 72 hours indicated that a pig liver expressing both pig and human complement-regulatory proteins may provide some protection from injury by pig complement [68, 69].

Independent of the low complement levels seen in patients with hepatic failure, numerous studies have shown that the liver is more resistant than other solid organs to injury from preformed antigraft antibodies [70–73]. In some studies, human serum caused significantly less cytotoxicity when incubated with porcine hepatic sinusoidal endothelial cells than with porcine aortic endothelial cells (25% vs. 72%) [71]. This relative resistance to injury could possibly be related to the liver's ability to clear soluble immune complexes [71] or to less binding of human IgM and IgG to porcine hepatic sinusoidal endothelial cells when compared to aortic endothelial cells, suggesting lower expression of antigens [74].

8.2. *Investigation of the mechanisms of platelet loss*

The studies summarized above have identified certain barriers specific to the liver that need to be overcome. The major outstanding problem preventing successful long-term pig liver graft survival is the rapid loss of platelets from the recipient within minutes or hours of the transplant [75]. Evidence has been presented to indicate that (1) primate platelets are phagocytosed by pig liver macrophages (Kupffer cells) and sinusoidal endothelial cells [76–80] or (2) may be lost in platelet–leukocyte aggregates in the graft and in certain recipient organs [76, 81].

Potential factors that may contribute towards the phagocytosis are complex and are being investigated in several laboratories. They include (1) the activity of the asialoglycoprotein receptor-1 (ASGR1) present on sinusoidal endothelial cells, and of the macrophage antigen complex-1 (CD11b/CD18; Mac-1), a surface integrin receptor on Kupffer cells, (2) interspecies incompatibility and phagocytic dysregulation in the porcine signal regulatory protein-alpha (SIRPα)/human CD47 pathway, and (3) upregulation of tissue factor expression on donor sinusoidal endothelial cells activated by the immune response, as well as on recipient platelets and mononuclear cells [82–86].

In addition to the reported loss of platelets in NHPs, the *ex vivo* perfusion of a pig liver with human blood demonstrated that pig macrophages continuously phagocytosed human erythrocytes [69, 87, 88]. This was unrelated to antibody binding and complement activation, but was associated with direct recognition of erythrocytes by pig Kupffer cells. A pig liver removed approximately one unit of human erythrocytes from the circulation every 24 hours. Phagocytosis of recipient erythrocytes has *not* been documented in most studies in NHPs, suggesting that the expression of N-glycolylneuraminic acid (NeuGc) on pig erythrocytes and the production of anti-NeuGc antibodies in humans (but *not* in NHPs which, like pigs, express NeuGc) may be playing a role (reviewed in Ref. [89]).

Pigs in which the gene for the enzyme that adds NeuGc to underlying carbohydrate chains has been deleted have recently become available [35], and Butler *et al.* have demonstrated that the transplantation of a liver from a GTKO/NeuGcKO pig significantly reduced xenogeneic consumption of human platelets in an *ex vivo* perfusion study [34].

An alternative approach is to administer human coagulation factors [56], but modification of the pig organ would be much preferable.

8.3. *The potential of sensitization to pig antigens*

If a pig liver is employed to bridge the patient to allotransplantation, will exposure to pig tissues result in the production of anti-pig antibodies that might cross-react with alloantigens, thus preventing or being detrimental to subsequent allotransplantation? Studies of cross-reactivity between antispecies antibodies and/or sensitized T cells are few (reviewed in Ref. [90]), but there has been little evidence for the development of cross-reactive cytotoxic antibodies or activated T cells that might mediate humoral or accelerated cellular rejection of a subsequent allograft [91–93].

In the two cases (mentioned above) where patients underwent successful liver allotransplantation following relatively transient bridging by *ex vivo* hemoperfusion of porcine livers, the patients did not develop antibodies cross-reactive with human leukocyte antigens (HLA) [15]. Bridging with a bioartificial liver, which incorporated porcine hepatocytes, has also been followed by successful liver allotransplantation [94]. On the basis of this very limited experience, and that in experimental studies [91], a liver allograft transplanted after a bridging pig xenograft would not appear to be at increased risk of either humoral or cellular rejection.

Furthermore, current evidence suggests that a patient who is highly sensitized to HLA might be at no greater risk of rejecting a pig xenograft [90, 95, 96] though there are data that question this conclusion ([97, 98]; Tector AJ, personal communication).

9. Histopathology of pig liver xenotransplantation

In untreated NHPs, wild-type pig livers have generally undergone early antibody-mediated rejection (intravascular thrombosis, hemorrhagic necrosis, endothelial cell injury, deposition of IgM, IgG, C3), though no intravascular fibrin aggregation is seen (Figure 4(a)) [45, 99]. Subsequently, our own group provided sequential data on the development of hyperacute rejection in this model [52, 100].

Early after transplantation of a liver from a genetically engineered pig, microscopic and immunohistochemical examination of a liver biopsy has been almost normal, with minimal (patchy) or no deposition of IgM, IgG, C3, C4d, and C5b-9. At necropsy some days later, some livers showed macroscopic changes consistent with cholestasis, except for some patchy dark areas which microscopically showed hemorrhagic necrosis, platelet–fibrin thrombi, monocyte/macrophage margination, and vascular endothelial cell hypertrophy (Figure 4(c)) [52, 68]. No cell infiltration was seen. Confocal microscopy confirmed tissue factor expression on platelets and platelet and platelet/leukocyte aggregates in liver sinusoids. The minimal or absent deposition of immunoglobulin or complement fractions and absence of a cellular infiltrate suggest that neither antibody- nor cell-mediated rejection was playing a major role in injury (Figure 4(b)).

Nevertheless, platelet loss and platelet–leukocyte aggregation would appear to be a major problem [81, 101]. If the native liver remains *in situ*, the production of primate coagulation factors leads to the development of thrombotic microangiopathy in the graft, resulting in ischemic injury and graft destruction [54], just as in pig heart and kidney xenografts.

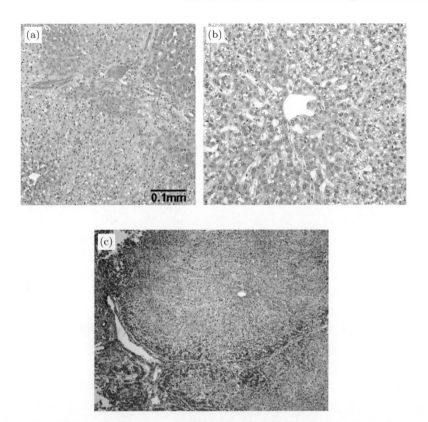

Figure 4. Histopathology after pig-to-NHP LT. Histopathology of (a) hyperacute rejection (<24 hours) in a wild-type pig liver transplanted orthotopically into a baboon, (b) a GTKO/hCD46 orthotopic pig liver graft in a baboon that survived for 6 days, and (c) a pig left liver lobe graft in a Tibetan monkey that survived for 14 days. (a) WT pig-to-baboon liver xenotransplantation at 1 hour (×200). Severe hepatocellular vacuolar change, focal hepatocyte necrosis, and few thrombi. (b) Vacuolar hepatocellular cytoplasmic change with minimal hepatocellular necrosis on postoperative day 6 (×200). (c) The graft shows some lymphocyte infiltration in the portal area, but no major features of antibody-mediated or cellular rejection (×100).

10. Physiological considerations

Most aspects of physiologic compatibility between pig and human have been sparsely investigated or not investigated at all, in part because it is difficult to accurately assess true hepatic function in the presence of an ongoing immune or inflammatory response [102–105]. However, there appear to be few major differences in hepatic function between pigs and humans (and NHPs) even when the pig has been genetically modified [50]. The increased viscosity of pig bile was mentioned above [63].

Nevertheless, incompatibilities between pig and human hepatic function are almost certain to be present, though some of these may be relative rather than absolute hurdles. If a function, e.g., the synthesis of a key protein, is found to be essential, and that function cannot be achieved by the pig liver, genetic modification of the source pig can be carried out to produce its human protein counterpart.

11. Potential infectious risks

The potential risks of the transfer of microorganisms with the pig organ to the human recipient and, more importantly, of the potential transfer of a porcine infectious agent into the community are now considered to be small [106–112]. Indeed, the use of animal organs might have some advantages with regard to recurrence of disease, such as viral hepatitis, as some viruses are species specific. For example, following pig-to-baboon organ transplantation, porcine cytomegalovirus has not been documented to infect the host baboon, and baboon cytomegalovirus has not been seen to infect the transplanted pig organ [113, 114].

Nevertheless, porcine endogenous retroviruses (PERVs) are present in the genome of every pig cell, and will therefore be transplanted with the organ, although the risk of PERVs causing any disease process in the recipient or in the community is considered low [110–112]. Donor pigs that lack functional PERV-C with low copy numbers of PERV-A/B have been identified, and could be selected as the infection risk is considered particularly low. Nonimmunosuppressed patients exposed to microencapsulated porcine islets from a colony of "PERV-low" pigs in a New Zealand clinical trial have shown no evidence of PERV infection [110]. Similarly, burn patients treated with wild-type pig skin transplants did not develop evidence of infection [115].

There are techniques to minimize this potential risk further, if this is believed to be essential. Activation of PERV can be inhibited using siRNA technology [116–118] and, using the new CRISPR/Cas9 technology, it is possible to render pig cells PERV-negative [119], and so it is likely that PERV-negative pigs could become available in the future. Furthermore, there are increasing data that PERV may be susceptible to certain antiretroviral agents [120, 121].

12. Selection of patients for clinical pig liver xenotransplantation

The considerable progress in pig organ xenotransplantation into NHPs that has been made in the past few years has largely been confined to heart and kidney xenotransplantation, as the barriers associated with pig liver or lung xenotransplantation are more complex [86, 122]. Although prolonged function (i.e., weeks or months) of a transplanted pig liver in a primate cannot yet be guaranteed, in rapidly deteriorating patients with ALF, the use of a pig liver in the clinic might be justified if the patient is likely to die without some form of intervention [11, 123]. Support during the critical period when the patient is in ALF may be aimed at (1) "bridging" the patient to liver allotransplantation in order to prevent irreversible cerebral injury, or (2) gaining time for regeneration of a damaged native liver, if this is considered likely.

Patients with ALF, e.g., from acetaminophen toxicity, may benefit from pig liver support in the form of daily *ex vivo* blood perfusion through an isolated genetically engineered pig liver while the native liver recovers. This would not commit the surgical team or patient to an LT, nor would it require significant immunosuppressive therapy. In patients with prolonged, but potentially reversible, liver dysfunction, an alternative would be temporary auxiliary (heterotopic) liver xenotransplantation, which would provide support until the native liver had recovered, at which time the pig liver could be excised [124, 125].

Orthotopic pig liver xenotransplantation would be preferable if the state of the native liver was increasing the risk of death, or if no recovery of the native liver is anticipated [11, 125]. However, this might still be carried out with the aim of replacing the pig graft with an allograft when one becomes available. Destination therapy by pig liver xenotransplantation would probably only be considered if initial trials of *ex vivo* pig liver support or bridging with a pig liver graft are associated with results that suggest moderately long-term graft survival can be anticipated.

13. Regulation of clinical trials of xenotransplantation

The US FDA suggests that xenotransplantation should be limited to "patients with serious or life-threatening diseases for whom adequately safe and effective alternative therapies are not available," while limiting patients to those "who have potential for a clinically significant improvement with increased quality of life following the procedure" (http://www.fda.gov/cber/guidelines.htm).

These patients should be disadvantaged or excluded from obtaining a human organ. Nevertheless, they should fulfill the general criteria for an organ, i.e., they must pass (1) medical (e.g., current negative cancer screening, negative infectious disease workup, adequate function of other organs), (2) surgical (e.g., adequate vascular targets for anastomosis), and (3) psychosocial (e.g., no active uncontrolled psychiatric disease, adequate history of compliance, adequate caregiver and social support) evaluations [125]. Patients who do not fulfill these criteria are unlikely to do well after xenotransplantation.

One subject that requires careful consideration is that of obtaining informed consent for what will be a novel form of therapy. How will consent be obtained when a patient has a hepatic encephalopathy? Consent from all patients at the time they are added to the waiting list has been suggested. However, consent obtained in an emergency from legal representatives would not be very different from that obtained for patients in clinical trials of trauma and resuscitation.

14. Comment

Progress in the transplantation of pig organs into NHPs is currently advancing rapidly [126, 127]. With further genetic manipulation of the organ-source pig, combined with novel immunosuppressive therapy, it is likely that bridging to liver allotransplantation by either *ex vivo* pig liver perfusion or transplantation will be successful within the near future. With the experience gained, destination therapy with pig liver xenotransplantation will become a reality, thus resolving the critical problem of donor liver availability.

Acknowledgments

Work on xenotransplantation in the Thomas E. Starzl Transplantation Institute of the University of Pittsburgh is, or has been, supported in part by NIH grants #U19 AI090959, #U01 AI068642, and # R21 A1074844, and by Sponsored Research Agreements between the University of Pittsburgh and Revivicor, Inc., Blacksburg, VA.

Disclosure

No author has a conflict of interest.

References

1. United Network for Organ Sharing. http://www.unos.org. (Accessed October 20, 2015).
2. Hara H, Gridelli B, Lin YJ, Marcos A, and Cooper DK. Liver xenografts for the treatment of acute liver failure: clinical and experimental experience and remaining immunologic barriers. *Liver Transpl* 2008;14:425–34.

3. Ekser B, Gridelli B, Veroux M, and Cooper DK. Clinical pig liver xenotransplantation: how far do we have to go? *Xenotransplantation* 2011;18:158–67.
4. Ekser B, Ezzelarab M, Hara H, *et al*. Clinical xenotransplantation: the next medical revolution? *Lancet* 2012;379:672–83.
5. Cooper DK, Dou KF, Tao KS, Yang ZX, Tector AJ, and Ekser B. Pig liver xenotransplantation: a review of progress toward the clinic. *Transplantation* 2016;100:2039–47.
6. Cooper DK, Ekser B, Ramsoondar J, Phelps C, and Ayares D. The role of genetically-engineered pigs in xenotransplantation research. *J Pathol* 2016;238:288–99.
7. Cooper DK, Ekser B, and Tector AJ. A brief history of clinical xenotransplantation. *Int J Surg* 2015;23:205–10.
8. Starzl TE. Orthotopic heterotransplantation. In: Starzl TE, Ed. *Experience in Hepatic Transplantation*. Philadelphia: WB Saunders, 1969, p. 408.
9. Makowa L, Cramer DV, Hoffman A, *et al*. The use of a pig liver xenograft for temporary support of a patient with fulminant hepatic failure. *Transplantation* 1995;59:1654–9.
10. Makowka L, Wu GD, Hoffman A, *et al*. Immunohistopathologic lesions associated with the rejection of a pig-to-human liver xenograft. *Transplant Proc* 1994;26:1074–5.
11. Ekser B, Gridelli B, Tector AJ, and Cooper DK. Pig liver xenotransplantation as a bridge to allotransplantation: which patients might benefit? *Transplantation* 2009;88:1041–9.
12. Chari RS, Collins BH, Magee JC, *et al*. Brief report: treatment of hepatic failure with ex vivo pig-liver perfusion followed by liver transplantation. *N Engl J Med* 1994;331:234–7.
13. Collins BH, Chari RS, Magee JC, *et al*. Mechanisms of injury in porcine livers perfused with blood of patients with fulminant hepatic failure. *Transplantation* 1994;58:1162–71.
14. Horslen SP, Hammel JM, Fristoe LW, *et al*. Extracorporeal liver perfusion using human and pig livers for acute liver failure. *Transplantation* 2000;70:1472–8.
15. Levy MF, Crippin J, Sutton S, *et al*. Liver allotransplantation after extracorporeal hepatic support with transgenic (hCD55/hCD59) porcine livers: clinical results and lack of pig-to-human transmission of the porcine endogenous retrovirus. *Transplantation* 2000;69:272–80.
16. Cooper DK, Ezzelarab MB, Hara H, *et al*. The pathobiology of pig-to-primate xenotransplantation: a historical review. *Xenotransplantation* 2016;23:83–105.
17. Calne RY, White HJ, Herbertson BM, *et al*. Pig to baboon liver xenografts. *Lancet* 1968;7553:1176–8.
18. Calne RY. Organ transplantation between widely disparate species. *Transplant Proc* 1970;2:550–6.

19. Calne RY, Davis DR, Pena JR, *et al.* Hepatic allografts and xenografts in primates. *Lancet* 1970;7638:103–6.

20. Powelson J, Cosimi AB, Austen W, Jr, *et al.* Porcine-to-primate orthotopic liver transplantation. *Transplant Proc* 1994;26:1353–4.

21. Good AH, Cooper DK, Malcolm AJ, *et al.* Identification of carbohydrate structures that bind human antiporcine antibodies: implications for discordant xenografting in humans. *Transplant Proc* 1992;24:559–62.

22. Kobayashi T and Cooper DK. Anti-Gal, alpha-Gal epitopes, and xenotransplantation. *Subcell Biochem* 1999;32:229–57.

23. Lambrigts D, Sachs DH, and Cooper DK. Discordant organ xenotransplantation in primates: world experience and current status. *Transplantation* 1998;66:547–61.

24. Cooper DK, Satyananda V, Ekser B, *et al.* Progress in pig-to-nonhuman primate transplantation models (1998–2013): a comprehensive review of the literature. *Xenotransplantation* 2014;21:397–419.

25. Dalmasso AP, Vercellotti GM, Platt JL, and Bach FH. Inhibition of complement-mediated endothelial cell cytotoxicity by decay-accelerating factor. Potential for prevention of xenograft hyperacute rejection. *Transplantation* 1991;52:530–3.

26. White DJ, Oglesby T, Liszewski MK, *et al.* Expression of human decay accelerating factor or membrane cofactor protein genes on mouse cells inhibits lysis by human complement. *Transpl Int* 1992;5(Suppl 1):S648–50.

27. White DJG, Langford GA, Cozzi E, and Young VK. Production of pigs transgenic for human DAF: a strategy for xenotransplantation. *Xenotransplantation* 1995;2:213–7.

28. Cozzi E and White DJ. The generation of transgenic pigs as potential organ donors for humans. *Nat Med* 1995;1:964–6.

29. Cooper DK, Koren E, and Oriol R. Genetically engineered pigs. *Lancet* 1993;342:682–3.

30. Phelps CJ, Koike C, Vaught TD, *et al.* Production of alpha 1,3-galactosyltransferase-deficient pigs. *Science* 2003;299:411–4.

31. Kolber-Simonds D, Lai L, Watt SR, *et al.* Production of alpha-1,3-galactosyltransferase null pigs by means of nuclear transfer with fibroblasts bearing loss of heterozygosity mutations. *Proc Natl Acad Sci USA* 2004;101:7335–40.

32. Higginbotham L, Mathews D, Breeden CA, *et al.* Pre-transplant antibody screening and anti-CD154 costimulation blockade promote long-term xenograft survival in a pig-to-primate kidney transplant model. *Xenotransplantation* 2015;22:221–30.

33. Butler JR, Ladowski JM, Martens GR, Tector M, and Tector AJ. Recent advances in genome editing and creation of genetically modified pigs. *Int J Surg* 2015;23:217–22.

34. Butler JR, Paris LL, Blankenship RL, *et al*. Silencing porcine CMAH and GGTA1 genes significantly reduces xenogeneic consumption of human platelets by porcine livers. *Transplantation* 2016;100:571–6.
35. Lutz AJ, Li P, Estrada JL, *et al*. Double knockout pigs deficient in N-glycolylneuraminic acid and galactose alpha-1,3-galactose reduce the humoral barrier to xenotransplantation. *Xenotransplantation* 2013;20: 27–35.
36. Li P, Estrada JL, Burlak C, *et al*. Efficient generation of genetically distinct pigs in a single pregnancy using multiplexed single-guide RNA and carbohydrate selection. *Xenotransplantation* 2015;22:20–31.
37. Cowan PJ, Robson SC, and d'Apice AJ. Controlling coagulation dysregulation in xenotransplantation. *Curr Opin Organ Transplant* 2011;16:214–21.
38. Mohiuddin MM, Singh AK, Corcoran PC, *et al*. One-year heterotopic cardiac xenograft survival in a pig to baboon model. *Am J Transplant* 2014;14: 488–9.
39. Mohiuddin MM, Reichart B, Byrne GW, and McGregor CG. Current status of pig heart xenotransplantation. *Int J Surg* 2015;23:234–9.
40. Mohuddin MM, Singh AK, Corcoran PC, *et al*. Chimeric 2C10R4 anti-CD40 antibody therapy is critical for long-term survival of GTKO.hCD46.hTBM pig-to-primate cardiac xenograft. *Nat Commun* 2016;7:11138.
41. Iwase H and Kobayashi T. Current status of pig kidney xenotransplantation. *Int J Surg* 2015;23:229–33.
42. van der Windt DJ, Bottino R, Casu A, *et al*. Long-term controlled normoglycemia in diabetic non-human primates after transplantation with hCD46 transgenic porcine islets. *Am J Transplant* 2009;9:2716–26.
43. Bottino R, Wijkstrom M, van der Windt DJ, *et al*. Pig-to-monkey islet xenotransplantation using multi-transgenic pigs. *Am J Transplant* 2014;14:2275–87.
44. Park CG, Bottino R, and Hawthorne WJ. Current status of islet xenotransplantation. *Int J Surg* 2015;23:261–6.
45. Ramirez P, Chavez R, Majado M, *et al*. Life-supporting human complement regulator decay accelerating factor transgenic pig liver xenograft maintains the metabolic function and coagulation in the nonhuman primate for up to 8 days. *Transplantation* 2000;70:989–98.
46. Ramirez P, Montoya MJ, Rios A, *et al*. Prevention of hyperacute rejection in a model of orthotopic liver xenotransplantation from pig to baboon using polytransgenic pig livers (CD55, CD59, and H-transferase). *Transplant Proc* 2005;37:4103–6.
47. Valdivia LA, Fung JJ, Demetris AJ, *et al*. Donor species complement after liver xenotransplantation. The mechanism of protection from hyperacute rejection. *Transplantation* 1994;57:918–22.
48. Valdivia LA, Lewis JH, Celli S, *et al*. Hamster coagulation and serum proteins in rat recipients of hamster xenografts. *Transplantation* 1993;56:489–90.

49. Celli S, Valdivia LA, Fung JJ, and Kelly RH. Early recipient-donor switch of the complement type after liver xenotransplantation. *Immunol Invest* 1997;26:589–600.
50. Ekser B, Echeverri GJ, Hassett AC, et al. Hepatic function after genetically engineered pig liver transplantation in baboons. *Transplantation* 2010;90: 483–93.
51. Ekser B, Long C, Echeverri GJ, et al. Impact of thrombocytopenia on survival of baboons with genetically modified pig liver transplants: clinical relevance. *Am J Transplant* 2010;10:273–85.
52. Ekser B, Klein E, He J, et al. Genetically-engineered pig-to-baboon liver xeno-transplantation: histopathology of xenografts and native organs. PLoS ONE 2012;7:e29720.
53. Kim K, Schuetz C, Elias N, et al. Up to 9-day survival and control of throm-bocytopenia following alpha1,3-galactosyl transferase knockout swine liver xenotransplantation in baboons. *Xenotransplantation* 2012;19:256–64.
54. Yeh H, Machaidze Z, Wamala I, et al. Increased transfusion-free survival following auxiliary pig liver xenotransplantation. *Xenotransplantation* 2014;21:454–64.
55. Navarro-Alvarez N, Shah JA, Zhu A, et al. The effects of exogenous admin-istration of human coagulation factors following pig-to-baboon liver xenotransplantation. *Am J Transplant* 2016;16:1715–25.
56. Shah JA, Navarro-Alvarez N, DeFazio M, et al. A bridge to somewhere: 25-day survival after pig-to-baboon liver xenotransplantation. *Ann Surg* 2016;263:1069–71.
57. Ji H, Li X, Yue S, et al. Pig BMSCs transfected with human TFPI combat species incompatibility and regulate the human TF pathway in vitro and in a rodent model. *Cell Physiol Biochem* 2015;36:233–49.
58. Buhler L, Awwad M, Basker M, et al. High-dose porcine hematopoietic cell transplantation combined with CD40 ligand blockade in baboons prevents an induced anti-pig humoral response. *Transplantation* 2000;69:2296–304.
59. Iwase H, Liu H, Wijkstrom M, et al. Pig kidney graft survival in a baboon for 136 days: longest life-supporting organ graft survival to date. *Xenotransplantation* 2015;22:302–9.
60. Filipponi F, Leoncini G, Campatelli A, et al. Segmental organization of the pig liver: anatomical basis of controlled partition for experimental grafting. *Eur Surg Res* 1995;27:151–7.
61. Court FG, Wemyss-Holden SA, Morrison CP, et al. Segmental nature of the porcine liver and its potential as a model for experimental partial hepatec-tomy. *Br J Surg* 2003;90:440–4.
62. Camprodon R, Solsona J, Guerrero JA, Mendoza CG, Segura J, and Fabregat JM. Intrahepatic vascular division in the pig: basis for partial hepatectomies. *Arch Surg* 1977;112:38–40.

63. Kobayashi T, Taniguchi S, Ye Y, Niekrasz M, Nour B, and Cooper DK. Comparison of bile chemistry between humans, baboons, and pigs: implications for clinical and experimental liver xenotransplantation. *Lab Anim Sci* 1998;48:197–200.

64. Colten HR. Biosynthesis of complement. *Adv Immunol* 1976;22:67–118.

65. Ellison RT, 3rd, Horsburgh CR, Jr, and Curd J. Complement levels in patients with hepatic dysfunction. *Dig Dis Sci* 1990;35:231–5.

66. Tector AJ, Fridell JA, Ruiz P, *et al.* Experimental discordant hepatic xenotransplantation in the recipient with liver failure: implications for clinical bridging trials. *J Am Coll Surg* 2000;191:54–64.

67. Hara H, Campanile N, Tai HC, *et al.* An in vitro model of pig liver xenotransplantation — pig complement is associated with reduced lysis of wild-type and genetically modified pig cells. *Xenotransplantation* 2010;17:370–8.

68. Luo Y, Kosanke S, Mieles L, *et al.* Comparative histopathology of hepatic allografts and xenografts in the nonhuman primate. *Xenotransplantation* 1998;5:197–206.

69. Rees MA, Butler AJ, Chavez-Cartaya G, *et al.* Prolonged function of extracorporeal hDAF transgenic pig livers perfused with human blood. *Transplantation* 2002;73:1194–202.

70. Nakamura K, Murase N, Becich MJ, *et al.* Liver allograft rejection in sensitized recipients. Observations in a clinically relevant small animal model. *Am J Pathol* 1993;142:1383–91.

71. Tector AJ, Elias N, Rosenberg L, *et al.* Mechanisms of resistance to injury in pig livers perfused with blood from patients in liver failure. *Transplant Proc* 1997;29:966–9.

72. Tector AJ, Chen X, Soderland C, and Tchervenkov JI. Complement activation in discordant hepatic xenotransplantation. *Xenotransplantation* 1998;5:257–61.

73. Platt JL. Xenotransplantation of the liver: is more complement control needed? *Liver Transpl* 2001;7:933–4.

74. Cattan P, Zhang B, Braet F, *et al.* Comparison between aortic and sinusoidal liver endothelial cells as targets of hyperacute xenogeneic rejection in the pig to human combination. *Transplantation* 1996;62:803–10.

75. Ekser B, Lin CC, Long C, *et al.* Potential factors influencing the development of thrombocytopenia and consumptive coagulopathy after genetically modified pig liver xenotransplantation. *Transpl Int* 2012;25:882–96.

76. Peng Q, Yeh H, Wei L, *et al.* Mechanisms of xenogeneic baboon platelet aggregation and phagocytosis by porcine liver sinusoidal endothelial cells. *PLoS ONE* 2012;7:e47273.

77. Paris LL, Chihara RK, Reyes LM, *et al.* ASGR1 expressed by porcine enriched liver sinusoidal endothelial cells mediates human platelet phagocytosis in vitro. *Xenotransplantation* 2011;18:245–51.

78. Paris LL, Chihara RK, Sidner RA, Tector AJ, and Burlak C. Differences in human and porcine platelet oligosaccharides may influence phagocytosis by liver sinusoidal cells in vitro. *Xenotransplantation* 2012;19:31–9.

79. Paris LL, Estrada JL, Li P, *et al.* Reduced human platelet uptake by pig livers deficient in the asialoglycoprotein receptor 1 protein. *Xenotransplantation* 2015;22:203–10.

80. Chihara RK, Paris LL, Reyes LM, *et al.* Primary porcine Kupffer cell phagocytosis of human platelets involves the CD18 receptor. *Transplantation* 2011;92:739–44.

81. Ezzelarab M, Ekser B, Gridelli B, Iwase H, Ayares D, and Cooper DK. Thrombocytopenia after pig-to-baboon liver xenotransplantation: where do platelets go? *Xenotransplantation* 2011;18:320–7.

82. Ide K, Ohdan H, Kobayashi T, Hara H, Ishiyama K, and Asahara T. Antibody- and complement-independent phagocytotic and cytolytic activities of human macrophages toward porcine cells. *Xenotransplantation* 2005;12:181–8.

83. Ide K, Wang H, Tahara H, *et al.* Role for CD47-SIRPalpha signaling in xenograft rejection by macrophages. *Proc Natl Acad Sci USA* 2007;104:5062–6.

84. Navarro-Alvarez N and Yang YG. CD47: a new player in phagocytosis and xenograft rejection. *Cell Mol Immunol* 2011;8:285–8.

85. Bongoni AK, Kiermeir D, Denoyelle J, *et al.* Porcine extrahepatic vascular endothelial asialoglycoprotein receptor 1 mediates xenogeneic platelet phagocytosis in vitro and in human-to-pig ex vivo xenoperfusion. *Transplantation* 2015;99:693–701.

86. Yang YG. CD47 in xenograft rejection and tolerance induction. *Xenotransplantation* 2010;17:267–73.

87. Luo Y, Levy G, Ding J, *et al.* HDAF transgenic pig livers are protected from hyperacute rejection during ex vivo perfusion with human blood. *Xenotransplantation* 2002;9:36–44.

88. Rees MA, Butler AJ, Negus MC, Davies HF, and Friend PJ. Classical pathway complement destruction is not responsible for the loss of human erythrocytes during porcine liver perfusion. *Transplantation* 2004;77:1416–23.

89. Padler-Karavani V, and Varki A. Potential impact of the non-human sialic acid N-glycolylneuraminic acid on transplant rejection risk. *Xenotransplantation* 2011;18:1–5.

90. Cooper DK, Tseng YL, and Saidman SL. Alloantibody and xenoantibody cross-reactivity in transplantation. *Transplantation* 2004;77:1–5.

91. Ye Y, Luo Y, Kobayashi T, *et al.* Secondary organ allografting after a primary "bridging" xenotransplant. *Transplantation* 1995;60:19–22.

92. Baertschiger RM, Dor FJ, Prabharasuth D, Kuwaki K, and Cooper DK. Absence of humoral and cellular alloreactivity in baboons sensitized to pig antigens. *Xenotransplantation* 2004;11:27–32.

93. Key T, Schuurman HJ, and Taylor CJ. Does exposure to swine leukocyte antigens after pig-to-nonhuman primate xenotransplantation provoke antibodies that cross-react with human leukocyte antigens? *Xenotransplantation* 2004;11:452–6.

94. Baquerizo A, Mhoyan A, Kearns-Jonker M, *et al*. Characterization of human xenoreactive antibodies in liver failure patients exposed to pig hepatocytes after bioartificial liver treatment: an ex vivo model of pig to human xenotransplantation. *Transplantation* 1999;67:5–18.

95. Hara H, Ezzelarab M, Rood PP, *et al*. Allosensitized humans are at no greater risk of humoral rejection of GT-KO pig organs than other humans. *Xenotransplantation* 2006;13:357–65.

96. Wong BS, Yamada K, Okumi M, *et al*. Allosensitization does not increase the risk of xenoreactivity to alpha1,3-galactosyltransferase gene-knockout miniature swine in patients on transplantation waiting lists. *Transplantation* 2006;82:314–9.

97. Oostingh GJ, Davies HF, Bradley JA, and Taylor CJ. Comparison of allogeneic and xenogeneic in vitro T-cell proliferative responses in sensitized patients awaiting kidney transplantation. *Xenotransplantation* 2003;10:545–51.

98. Oostingh GJ, Davies HF, Tang KC, Bradley JA, and Taylor CJ. Sensitisation to swine leukocyte antigens in patients with broadly reactive HLA specific antibodies. *Am J Transplant* 2002;2:267–73.

99. Ramirez P, Yelamos J, Parrilla P, and Chavez R. Hepatic xenotransplantation will benefit from strategies aimed to reduce complement activation. *Liver Transpl* 2001;7:562–3.

100. Ekser B, Burlak C, Waldman JP, *et al*. Immunobiology of liver xenotransplantation. *Expert Rev Clin Immunol* 2012;8:621–34.

101. Burlak C, Paris LL, Chihara RK, *et al*. The fate of human platelets perfused through the pig liver: implications for xenotransplantation. *Xenotransplantation* 2010;17:350–61.

102. Hammer C. Evolutionary obstacles to xenotransplantation. In: Cooper DKC, Kemp E, Platt J, and White DJG, Eds. *Xenotransplantation*, 2nd ed. Heidelberg: Springer, 1997, pp. 716–35.

103. Hammer C. Physiological obstacles after xenotransplantation. *Ann N Y Acad Sci* 1998;862:19–27.

104. Kanazawa A and Platt JL. Prospects for xenotransplantation of the liver. *Semin Liver Dis* 2000;20:511–22.

105. Ibrahim Z, Busch J, Awwad M, Wagner R, Wells K, and Cooper DK. Selected physiologic compatibilities and incompatibilities between human and porcine organ systems. *Xenotransplantation* 2006;13:488–99.

106. Paradis K, Langford G, Long Z, *et al*. Search for cross-species transmission of porcine endogenous retrovirus in patients treated with living pig tissue. The XEN 111 Study Group. *Science* 1999;285:1236–41.

107. Onions D, Cooper DK, Alexander TJ, *et al.* An approach to the control of disease transmission in pig-to-human xenotransplantation. *Xenotransplantation* 2000;7:143–55.

108. Fishman JA. Screening of source animals and clinical monitoring for xeno-transplantation. *Xenotransplantation* 2007;14:349–52.

109. Fishman JA and Patience C. Xenotransplantation: infectious risk revisited. *Am J Transplant* 2004;4:1383–90.

110. Wynyard S, Nathu D, Garkavenko O, Denner J, and Elliott R. Microbiological safety of the first clinical pig islet xenotransplantation trial in New Zealand. *Xenotransplantation* 2014;21:309–23.

111. Denner J and Mueller NJ. Preventing transfer of infectious agents. *Int J Surg* 2015;23:306–11.

112. Denner J and Tonjes RR. Infection barriers to successful xenotransplantation focusing on porcine endogenous retroviruses. *Clin Microbiol Rev* 2012;25:318–43.

113. Mueller NJ, Kuwaki K, Dor FJ, *et al.* Reduction of consumptive coagulopathy using porcine cytomegalovirus-free cardiac porcine grafts in pig-to-primate xenotransplantation. *Transplantation* 2004;78:1449–53.

114. Mueller NJ, Livingston C, Knosalla C, *et al.* Activation of porcine cytomega-lovirus, but not porcine lymphotropic herpesvirus, in pig-to-baboon xenotransplantation. *J Infect Dis* 2004;189:1628–33.

115. Scobie L, Padler-Karavani V, Le Bas-Bernardet S, *et al.* Long-term IgG response to porcine Neu5Gc antigens without transmission of PERV in burn patients treated with porcine skin xenografts. *J Immunol* 2013;191:2907–15.

116. Dieckhoff B, Karlas A, Hofmann A, *et al.* Inhibition of porcine endogenous retroviruses (PERVs) in primary porcine cells by RNA interference using len-tiviral vectors. *Arch Virol* 2007;152:629–34.

117. Dieckhoff B, Petersen B, Kues WA, Kurth R, Niemann H, and Denner J. Knockdown of porcine endogenous retrovirus (PERV) expression by PERV-specific shRNA in transgenic pigs. *Xenotransplantation* 2008;15:36–45.

118. Ramsoondar J, Vaught T, Ball S, *et al.* Production of transgenic pigs that express porcine endogenous retrovirus small interfering RNAs. *Xenotrans-plantation* 2009;16:164–80.

119. Yang L, Guell M, Niu D, *et al.* Genome-wide inactivation of porcine endog-enous retroviruses (PERVs). *Science* 2015;350:1101–4.

120. Wilhelm M, Fishman JA, Pontikis R, Aubertin AM, and Wilhelm FX. Susceptibility of recombinant porcine endogenous retrovirus reverse tran-scriptase to nucleoside and non-nucleoside inhibitors. *Cell Mol Life Sci* 2002;59:2184–90.

121. Argaw T, Colon-Moran W, and Wilson C. Susceptibility of porcine endoge-nous retrovirus to anti-retroviral inhibitors. *Xenotransplantation* 2016;23:151–8.

122. Cooper DK, Ekser B, Burlak C, *et al.* Clinical lung xenotransplantation — what donor genetic modifications may be necessary? *Xenotransplantation* 2012;19: 144–58.

123. Horton PJ, Chaudhury P, Rochon C, Metrakos P, and Tchervenkov J. Should trials of liver xenotransplantation proceed in toxic fulminant hepatic failure? *Xenotransplantation* 2006;13:483.

124. Mieles L, Ye Y, Luo Y, *et al.* Auxiliary liver allografting and xenografting in the nonhuman primate. *Transplantation* 1995;59:1670–6.

125. Cooper DK, Wijkstrom M, Hariharan S, *et al.* Selection of patients for initial clinical trials of solid organ xenotransplantation. *Transplantation* 2017; 101(7):1551–8.

126. Tector J. New hope for liver xenotransplantation. *Ann Surg* 2016;263:1072.

127. Cooper DK and Bottino R. Recent advances in understanding xenotransplantation: implications for the clinic. *Expert Rev Clin Immunol* 2015;11:1379–90.

Index